# From the book...

### Marin Headlands

The hills surrounding Gerbode Valley, part of the Marin Headlands, are vibrant in the spring with wildflowers, and alive with birdsong and avian acrobatics most of the year, but especially during the fall raptor migration.

### Ring Mountain Open Space Preserve

Its slopes are home to a wonderful array of trees, shrubs, and wildflowers, some quite rare, and one, the Tiburon Mariposa lily, is found nowhere else in the world. As a vantage point with great views, Ring Mountain's summit rivals better-known Bay Area peaks.

### Annadel State Park

This park is one of the best places in the North Bay to see wild turkeys—look in damp ravines or along the edges of clearings for large flocks of these dark, iridescent birds, which are slightly smaller than their domestic cousins.

### Sonoma Coast State Beach: Bodega Head Loop

Daubs of color are added to the scene by the yellow-and-red flowers of seaside paintbrush, and the magenta blooms of iceplant, a succulent that carpets California's coastal dunes and sandy roadside embankments. Just offshore, lines of brown pelicans or cormorants may be cruising low over the waves.

### Napa River Ecological Reserve

Be sure to stop and admire a large, ropy vine of California wild grape, perhaps more than 100 years old. Also here are two kinds of blackberry—California, a native, and Himalayan, and import from Europe.

### Mission Peak Regional Preserve

The final climb is on dirt and rock, past a clever observation device that allows you to identify more than two dozen Bay Area landmarks in a 360-degress circle around Mission Peak.

### Sunol Wilderness: Little Yosemite

Little Yosemite features in miniature some of the wonders of its Sierra Nevada namesake, including water rushing through a boulder-strewn gorge, sheer cliffs, forested hillsides, and towering rock formations. Stands of western sycamore add color in the fall.

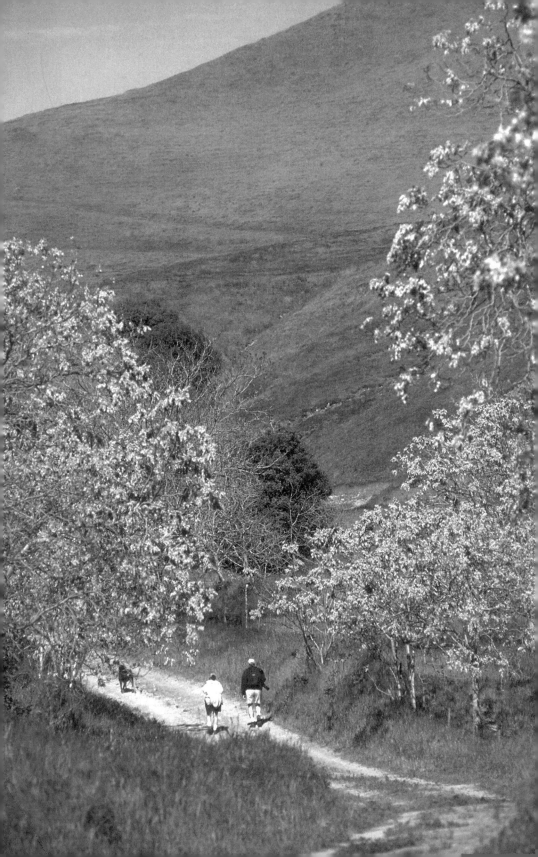

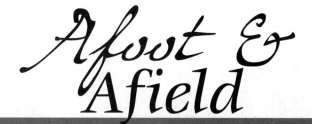

# Afoot & Afield

## San Francisco Bay Area
### A comprehensive hiking guide

David Weintraub

🐏 **WILDERNESS PRESS** · BERKELEY, CA

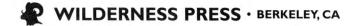

The Nortonville Trail climbs past Rose Hill Cemetery to Nortonville Pass

**Afoot & Afield San Francisco Bay Area: A Comprehensive Hiking Guide**

1st EDITION September 2004
**3rd printing 2010**

Copyright © 2004 by David Weintraub

Front cover photo copyright © 2004 by David Weintraub
Interior photos by David Weintraub
Maps: Ben Pease, Pease Press
Cover design: Andreas Schueller
Book design: Andreas Schueller
Book editor: Elaine Merrill

ISBN 978-0-89997-291-6

Manufactured in the United States of America

Published by:     **Wilderness Press**
                  **1345 8th Street**
                  **Berkeley, CA 94710**
                  **(800) 443-7227; FAX (510) 558-1696**
                  **info@wildernesspress.com**
                  **www.wildernesspress.com**

Visit our website for a complete listing of our books and for ordering information.

*Cover photo:*     Angel Island
*Frontispiece:*    Nortonville Trail, Black Diamond Mines

**SAFETY NOTICE:** Although Wilderness Press and the author have made every attempt to ensure that the information in this book is accurate at press time, they are not responsible for any loss, damage, injury, or inconvenience that may occur to anyone while using this book. You are responsible for your own safety and health. The fact that a trail is described in this book does not mean that it will be safe for you. Be aware that trail conditions can change from day to day. Always check local conditions and know your own limitations.

For all my Bay Area friends.

# Acknowledgments

First, I'd like to thank Tom Winnett, founder of Wilderness Press, for inviting me on this life-changing voyage. Without him, I'd still be just a photographer. Thanks also to all the other folks at Wilderness Press, current and former, including Caroline Winnett, Mike Jones, Jannie Dresser, Andreas Schueller, Larry Van Dyke, Roslyn Bullas, and Elaine Merrill.

Many people helped make this book by sharing their time, their information, and their expertise.

In the East Bay: Steve Fiala, Bert Johnson, Alan Kaplan, Juan Carlos Solis, Paul Ferreira, Anthony Fisher, Maryanne Canaparo, Bob Flasher, Pat Solo, John Steiner, Alvin Dockter, and Mike Koslosky.

In the North Bay: Ron Angier, Natalie Gates, Ane Rovetta, Denis Odion, Diana Roberts, Klytia Nelson, Ralph Ingols, Milan Pittman, Angela Nowicki, Lynda Doucette, Paul Larson, Al Vosher, Willard Wyman, Elizabeth Beale, Charles Potthast, Ronessa Duncan, Dawn Kemp, Marla Hastings, Cleve Dufer, Kevin McKay, Bill Cox, Patrick Robards, Gale Lester, Mia Monroe, Bill Michaels, Casey May, Scott Rasmussen, Glenn Ryburn, Fred Lew, Carlos Porrata, Landon Waggoner, Bill Grummer, Cheryl Lawton, Rich Lawton, Val Nixon, Greg Hayes, Bill Trunick, and Martha Wise.

On the Peninsula: Kristi Webb, Stephanie Jensen, John Kowaleski, John Escobar, Michael Newburn, Andrew Martin, Chris MacIntosh, Pete Siemens, Patrick Congdon, Deane Little, Tom Lausten, Lisa Zadek, Craig Britton, Kerry Carlson, Dennis Danielson, Ken Fisher, David Topley, Ward Paine, Larry Hassett, Mary Davey, Allan Lindh, Steve Tedesco, Mort Levine, Herb Grench, Jay Thorwaldson, Stephen Salveter, Elizabeth Salveter, Jane Huber, Janet Schwind, Elizabeth Dana, Rodger Alleman, Lorraine Alleman, Marc Auerbach, Nonette Hanko, Carrie Sparks-Hart, Ken Miller, Joyce Nicholas, Dave Knapp, Matt Freeman, Cindy Roessler, Paul McKowan, and David Sanguinetti.

Friends were enlisted (entrapped?) as photography models and sometimes as hiking companions. Thanks to Laura Wood, Paul Ash, Silvia Fernandez, Elena Ash, Jed Manwaring, Brenda Tharp, Steve Gregory, Vickie Vann, Ken Kobre, Betsy Brill, Mary Thorsby, John Macchia, Angela Macchia, Susan Rouder, George deTunq, Lea Redmond, Otto Schutt, Lee Eisman, Jay Tennenbaum, Jordan Tennenbaum, and Carla Palmer.

Enjoying the trails vicariously, Denise Rehse and Debi Devitt transcribed countless hours of taped notes. Ben Pease drew the excellent maps and made valuable comments and suggestions based on his extensive knowledge of Bay Area trails. Kate Hoffman and Jed Manwaring visited some of the East Bay parks included in this book and provided updated material.

On a sad note, two people involved with my first book, *East Bay Trails*, have since passed away. Dorothy L. Whitnah, a Wilderness Press author, reviewed my original outline and kept me informed of East Bay happenings. Galen Rowell, a great photographer and East Bay native, wrote the book's foreword.

Finally, thanks to my wife, Maggi, for her love and support.

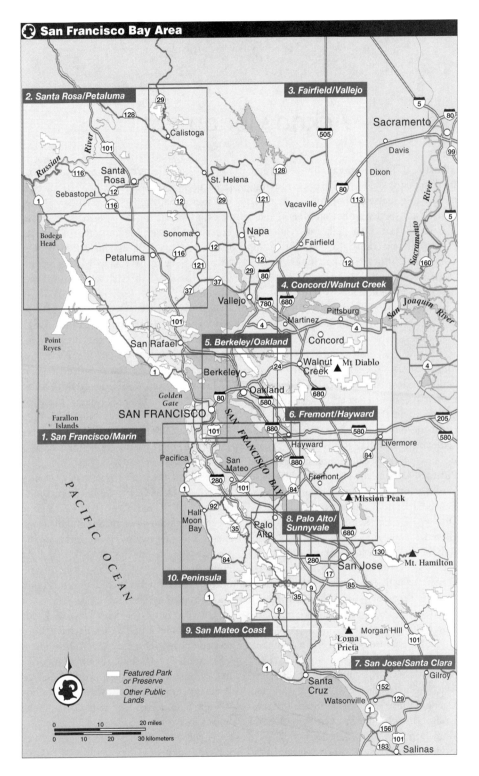

San Francisco Bay Area

2. Santa Rosa/Petaluma

3. Fairfield/Vallejo

4. Concord/Walnut Creek

5. Berkeley/Oakland

6. Fremont/Hayward

1. San Francisco/Marin

8. Palo Alto/Sunnyvale

10. Peninsula

9. San Mateo Coast

7. San Jose/Santa Clara

Sacramento
Davis
Dixon
Vacaville
Fairfield
Napa
St. Helena
Calistoga
Santa Rosa
Sebastopol
Sonoma
Petaluma
Vallejo
Pittsburg
Martinez
Concord
Walnut Creek
Mt Diablo
Berkeley
Oakland
SAN FRANCISCO
Golden Gate
Farallon Islands
Point Reyes
Bodega Head
Russian River
Sacramento River
San Joaquin River
Hayward
Livermore
Fremont
Mission Peak
Pacifica
San Mateo
Half Moon Bay
Palo Alto
San Jose
Mt. Hamilton
Loma Prieta
Morgan Hill
Santa Cruz
Watsonville
Gilroy
Salinas
San Rafael
PACIFIC OCEAN
SAN FRANCISCO BAY

Featured Park or Preserve
Other Public Lands

0      10      20 miles
0    10    20    30 kilometers

# Contents

# Preface

This book is the result of field work that began in 1996, when I started preparing my first book for Wilderness Press. Since then, I have logged countless miles, enjoying the beautiful Bay Area in every season, and traipsing from the Sonoma coast to Silicon Valley and beyond. The results of my wanderings appeared in three Wilderness Press trail guides, *East Bay Trails, North Bay Trails, Top Trails San Francisco Bay Area,* and also in *Peninsula Tales and Trails,* a history and guide commissioned by the Midpeninsula Regional Open Space District. Wilderness Press offers two other trail guides covering regions in the Bay Area, *Peninsula Trails* and *South Bay Trails.* So this book is a compendium of trips in the East Bay, North Bay, South Bay, and on the Peninsula.

My goal has always been to be a good guide, to share my love of the outdoors, and to show the importance of protecting Bay Area parklands. After all, a good guidebook should do more than get you from A to B. Through these pages, some of my personal predilections will no doubt come through: climbing high, enjoying native plants, looking at birds, and learning about Bay Area history.

I hiked all the trips described in this book, many more than once. I recorded all my observations on tape, and I have tried to be as accurate and as thorough as possible in both my observations and my writing. Keep in mind, though, that nature—not to mention various federal, state, and local agencies—equals change. So your experience on the trail, affected by season, weather, time of day, etc., will very likely be different from mine. I have tried to indicate this by liberally using the word "may," as in "Stow Lake is a favorite birding destination—from its shore you may spot great blue herons...." I hope you get to see the herons, but their appearance, like so many other things, is beyond my control.

If you have comments, corrections, and/or suggestions, please send them to mail@wildernesspress.com.

Ring Mountain: view northward from near the summit of Ring Mountain (chapter 1, trip 7).

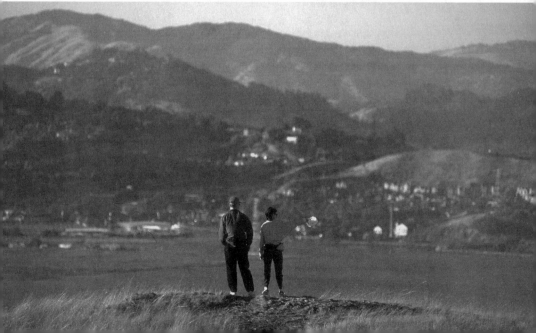

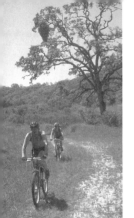
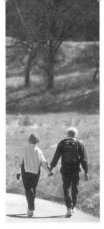
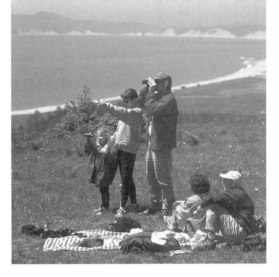

Clockwise from top left: Joseph D. Grant County Park (chapter 7, trip 3). Sonoma Valley Regional Park (chapter 2, trip 5). Mt. Wittenberg (chapter 1, trip 17). Russian Ridge OSP (chapter 10, trip 5). Mt. Burdell OSP (chapter 1, trip 14). Diablo Foothills Regional Park (chapter 4, trip 6).

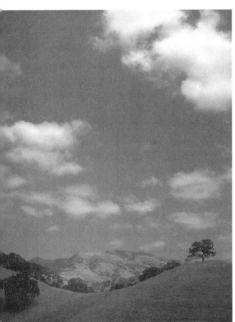
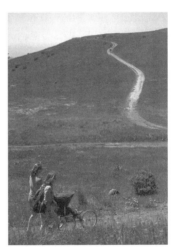
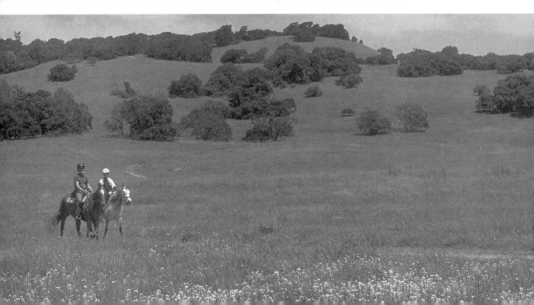

# Introducing the San Francisco Bay Area

**W**hatever your favorite outdoor activity, you're sure to find a place to pursue it in the Bay Area. There are about 1 million acres of public parklands within the nine counties that circle San Francisco Bay, featuring rugged coastlines, tree-filled canyons, cascading streams, grasslands sparkling with spring wildflowers, chaparral-cloaked ridges, and windy summits. No matter where you go, from Santa Rosa to San Jose, you are never far from a trailhead.

The Bay Area is usually divided into four regions—North Bay, East Bay, South Bay, and Peninsula. The North Bay includes Marin, Napa, Sonoma, and Solano counties; the East Bay consists of Alameda and Contra Costa counties; the South Bay takes in most of Santa Clara County; and the Peninsula covers San Francisco, San Mateo, and the northwestern part of Santa Clara County. Within these regions are bustling urban areas such as San Francisco, Oakland, San Jose, and the Silicon Valley, along with tranquil forests, mountains, beaches, marshes, and farmlands.

Bay Area parklands are administered by various federal, state, and local agencies, listed in Appendix 3.

## Climate

The Bay Area's climate is perfect for outdoor activities, with a dry season that lasts from May through October and a generally mild, if damp, winter. In summer, expect fog and cool temperatures near the coast, thanks to Pacific Ocean. Inland, temperatures can soar. The generally clear days of autumn are fine for hiking just about anywhere. The first rains turn hillsides green and fill seasonal creeks.

Winter storms from the Gulf of Alaska can drench the Bay Area and even bring snow to the highest peaks. Cold, clear weather usually follows—a great time to bundle up and visit high-elevation vantage points. Spring can be sunny, rainy, tranquil, or blustery—or a combination, sometimes on the same day! This is when the Bay Area's grasslands come alive with colorful displays of wildflowers.

The Pacific's moderating influence diminishes as you go inland. Temperature differences—the spread between the average highs and lows for any given location—widen as you leave the coast. Here's an example: The highest average high temperature for San Francisco is 68.5°F, whereas the same figure for St. Helena in Napa County—only about 65 miles away—is 89.2°F. But San Francisco's lowest average minimum, 45.7°F

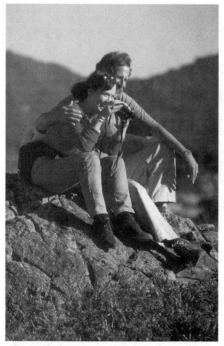

Hikers take a break just off Pine Mountain Road, with Mt. Tamalpais in the background.

(January), is about 10°F *warmer* than St. Helena's.

Yearly rainfall totals, too, change as you travel around the Bay Area. Each successive range of coastal hills blocks more and more Pacific moisture, creating a rain-shadow effect. Kentfield, in Marin County, receives about 48 inches (that's 4 feet!) of rain per year, whereas the town of Livermore, in eastern Alameda County, gets only about 15 inches. Yet the distance between these two towns is only about 55 miles.

Climate is one thing, but daily weather is another, so it's a good idea to check with a local source for current conditions and forecasts before heading out. You can use a weather radio, available at Radio Shack, outdoor stores, and other outlets, to receive broadcasts from the National Weather Service. You can also find up-to-the-minute weather information on the Weather Channel or on the Internet at www.weather.com.

## Geology

The Bay Area lies within a geological province called the Coast Ranges, a complex system of ridges and valleys that stretches from Arcata to near Santa Barbara, and inland to the edge of the Central Valley. The Coast Ranges were formed millions of years ago, as the floor of the Pacific Ocean was dragged under the western edge of North American continent. This process scraped material from the ocean floor and piled it

higher and higher on the continent's edge, in what is now California.

Within the Bay Area are sub-ranges such as the Sonoma, Mayacmas, and Vaca mountains in the North Bay; the Diablo Range in the East Bay and South Bay; and the Santa

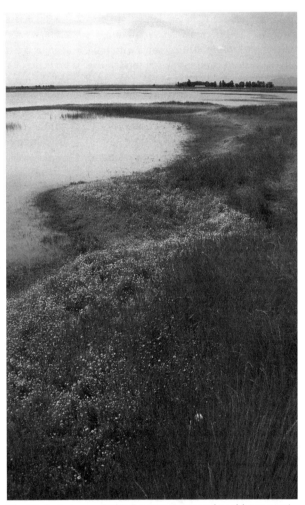

Olcott Lake in Jepson Prairie Preserve, a seasonal pool, hosts a variety of plants and animals, some quite rare.

Cruz Mountains on the Peninsula and in the South Bay. The tallest peak in the North Bay is Mt. St. Helena (4343'), at the corner of Sonoma, Napa, and Lake counties. Other prominent Bay Area summits include Mt. Hamilton (4213'), Mt. Diablo (3849'),

Loma Prieta (3806'), Mt. Tamalpais (2571'), and Sonoma Mountain (2295').

Most of the surface rock in the Bay Area is sedimentary, but volcanic activity has occurred here in the past. Young volcanic rock caps the Mayacmas and Vaca mountains bordering the Napa Valley, and there are four extinct volcanoes in the East Bay, including Round Top (1763'). California's state rock is serpentine (more properly, serpentinite), gray-green in color and often seen as outcrops beside the trail. Serpentine forms a soil that is toxic to many plant species, but some have adapted to it. Among these are Sargent cypress, leather oak, and a variety of uncommon wildflowers.

The San Andreas fault—which splits the Santa Cruz mountains and slices through Marin County—and a host of lesser faults crisscross the Bay Area. As the Pacific plate slides past the North American plate, tremendous bursts of energy are sometimes released in the form of earthquakes. Most of the time, however, the northward movement, which, over the last 25 million years has carried granite from southern California to Point Reyes, is imperceptible. Visit Point Reyes National Seashore in the North Bay, Sibley Volcanic Regional Preserve and Mt. Diablo State Park in the East Bay, and Los Trancos Open Space Preserve on the Peninsula to learn more about Bay Area geology.

## Plants

California has a rich diversity of plant life. Some species, like coast redwoods, date back to the dinosaurs, whereas others have evolved within the past several thousand years. Roughly 30 percent of the state's native plants grow nowhere else. These endemics, as they are called, include many types of manzanita (*Arctostaphylos*) and monkeyflower (*Mimulus*). Botanists divide the plant kingdom into several major groups: flowering plants, conifers, ferns and their allies, mosses, and algae. A plant community consists of species growing together in a distinct habitat. Here are the principal plant communities you will encounter along the trails.

### OAK WOODLAND

Inland from San Francisco Bay, the fog-free hills between 300 and 3500 feet host a generally open woodland, sometimes called a savanna. Species here include various oaks, California buckeye, gray pine, California bay, buckbrush, toyon, coffeeberry, snowberry, and poison oak. Examples of this community can be found in Sugarloaf Ridge State Park, Black Diamond Mines Regional Preserve, and Henry W. Coe State Park.

### RIPARIAN WOODLAND

Found beside creeks and rivers, these trees and shrubs provide the Bay Area's best hope for an autumn display of color.

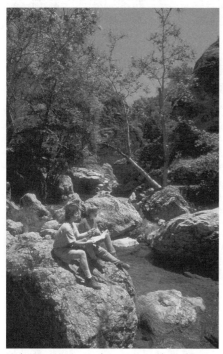

Little Yosemite is a rocky gorge on Alameda Creek, perfect for picnicking and nature study.

Common riparian species include bigleaf maple, white alder, red alder, California bay, various willows, California rose, poison oak, California wild grape, elk clover, and giant chain fern. Point Reyes National Seashore and Monte Bello Open Space Preserve give you opportunities to enjoy this community.

## REDWOOD FOREST

At one time, coast redwoods blanketed the Pacific coast from central California to southern Oregon. These giants are the world's tallest trees and are among the fastest-growing. Commercially valuable, they were heavily logged, especially in the Santa Cruz Mountains. The remaining old-growth coast redwoods in the Bay Area are confined a few areas, most notably Muir Woods National Monument in Marin County and Armstrong Redwoods State Reserve in Sonoma County.

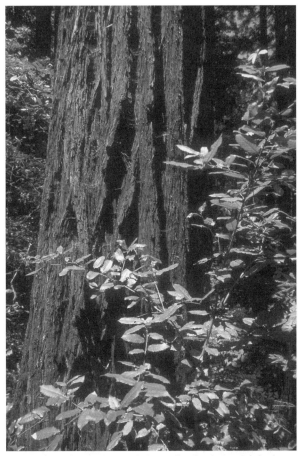

Coast redwoods grow in association wtih other trees and shrubs, creating a plant community.

Associated with redwoods are a number of plant species, including tanbark oak, California bay, hazelnut, evergreen huckleberry, wood rose, redwood sorrel, western sword fern, and evergreen violet. You can visit second-growth redwood forests and see a few old-growth giants at Muir Woods National Monument, Redwood Regional Park, and Purisima Creek Redwoods Open Space Preserve.

## DOUGLAS-FIR FOREST

These majestic trees often occupy similar habitats as coast redwoods, but thrive where soil conditions do not favor red-wood growth. In many parts of the Bay Area, Douglas-fir is the "default" evergreen, easily told by its distinctive cones, which have protruding, three-pointed bracts, sometimes called rats' tails. Like redwood, Douglas-fir is prized for its lumber. Some of the common plants associated with Douglas-fir are the same as those associated with coast redwood, namely California bay, tanbark oak, and western sword fern. Others include blue blossom, coffeeberry, and poison oak. Point Reyes National Seashore, Mt. Tamalpais State Park, and El Corte de Madera Creek Open Space Preserve have beautiful Douglas-fir forests.

## MIXED EVERGREEN FOREST

A mixture of evergreen trees, including California bay, canyon oak, coast live oak, and madrone, comprises this community. The understory often contains shrubs such as toyon, blue elderberry, hazelnut, buckbrush, snowberry, thimbleberry, oceanspray, and poison oak. Carpeting the forest floor may be an assortment of wildflowers, including milk maids, fairy bells, mission bells, hound's tongue, and western heart's-ease. Take a stroll through a mixed evergreen forest at China Camp State Park, Dry Creek Pioneer Regional Park, Sierra Azul Open Space Preserve, and Edgewood Park and Preserve.

## CHAPARRAL

This community is made up of hardy plants that thrive in poor soils under hot, dry conditions. Chaparral is very susceptible to fire, but some of its members, such as various species of manzanita, survive devastating blazes by sprouting new growth from ground-level burls. Although chaparral foliage is mostly drab, the flowers of many species are beautiful, with some blooming as early as December. The word chaparral comes from a Spanish term for dwarf or scrub oak, but in the Bay Area it is chamise, various manzanitas, and various species of ceanothus that dominate the community. Other chaparral plants include mountain mahogany, yerba santa, toyon, chaparral pea, and poison oak. You can study this fascinating assembly of plants on Pine Mountain, Mt. Diablo, and at Sierra Azul and Rancho San Antonio open space preserves.

## GRASSLANDS

Few if any grasslands in the Bay Area have retained their native character. Human intervention, in the form of fire suppression, farming, and livestock grazing, along with the invasion of nonnative plants, has significantly altered the landscape. Gone from most areas are the native bunchgrasses, perennial species that once dominated our area. Remaining, thankfully, are native wildflowers, which decorate the grasslands in spring and summer. Among the most common are bluedicks, California poppy, owl's-clover, checkerbloom, lupine, and blue-eyed grass. Look for these at Skyline Wilderness Park, Sunol Wilderness, Joseph D. Grant County Park, and Russian Ridge Open Space Preserve.

## COASTAL SCRUB

Also called soft chaparral, this community consists mostly of shrubs and grasses growing near the coast. Among the most common members are California sagebrush, coyote brush, toyon, bush monkeyflower, and various brooms. Point Reyes National Seashore, Tilden Regional Park, and San Bruno Mountain are all excellent places to find coastal scrub.

# Animals
## MAMMALS

It's always a thrill to see a coyote or a bobcat from the trail, but these sightings are uncommon. Glimpses of mountain lions are more rare still, but these large predators are present in the Bay Area, mostly in the more remote parks. Other, more common mammals in our area include squirrels, rabbits, deer, gray fox, raccoon, skunk, opossum, and chipmunk. Wild pigs have invaded some Bay Area parks and their rooting does extensive damage. Stay away from these dangerous animals.

## BIRDS

Located on the western edge of the Pacific Flyway, the Bay Area is a great place to go birding. The large variety of species results from the wide range of habitats—seashore to mountain—present here. Birders at Point Reyes National Seashore, the area with perhaps the greatest variety of birds, have logged an impressive 440 different species, or just under half of all bird species found in North America north of Mexico. Large numbers of individual birds reside in the Bay Area year-round, pass

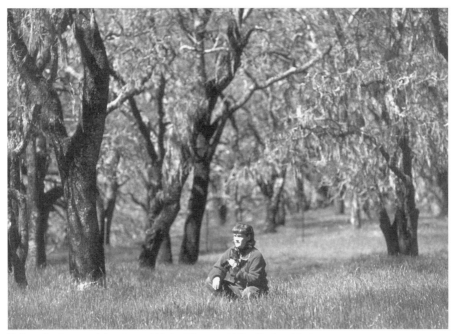

Early spring is a good time to spot birds at Sonoma Valley Regional Park.

through on migration, or winter here. For the common names of birds of the continental United States and Canada, the American Ornithologists' Union's (AOU) checklist is the authoritative resource. It can be found at www.aou.org/aou/birdlist.html.

Common birds seen from the trails include acorn woodpeckers, western scrub-jays, Steller's jays, spotted towhees, dark-eyed juncos, sparrows, and California quail, the state bird. Hawks, falcons, vultures, golden eagles, and kites soar above many Bay Area parks. If you learn to "bird by ear," identifying species by their distinctive notes, calls, and songs, you will quickly expand your list, because many birds are frustratingly hard to spot, especially in dense foliage. Birding with a group also improves your odds of seeing and identifying a large number of species, including rarities.

REPTILES AND AMPHIBIANS

A variety of snakes are present in the Bay Area, including California kingsnake, rubber boa, California whipsnake, yellow-bellied racer, garter snake, gopher snake, and western rattlesnake. Gopher snakes are often mistaken for rattlers, but a gopher snake has a slim head and a fat body, whereas a rattlesnake has a relatively thin body compared with its large, triangular head. Gopher snakes are common, but rattlers are seldom seen.

The ubiquitous western fence lizard is probably the Bay Area's most commonly seen reptile. Also here are the California whiptail, a lizard with a tail as long as its body, the alligator lizard, and the western skink. An animal resembling a lizard but actually an amphibian is the California newt, which spends the summer buried under the forest floor, then emerges with the first rains and migrates to breed in ponds and streams. Briones Regional Park and Monte Bello Open Space Preserve are among good places to witness these migrations. Other amphibians you might see or hear include western toad and Pacific tree frog.

# Comfort, Safety, and Etiquette

**M**ost of the routes in this book can be traveled with a minimum of preparation and equipment, calling for nothing more than sturdy footwear and a bottle of water. Probably the biggest safety concern is driving around the Bay Area. And trail etiquette means simply being considerate of others and picking up after yourself (and your pet). However, the more detailed information that follows may enhance your outdoor experience.

## Preparation and Equipment

A little common sense goes a long way when preparing for the outdoors. Be realistic about your level of physical conditioning—there are trips in this book to suit all abilities. None of the routes require anything more complicated than putting one

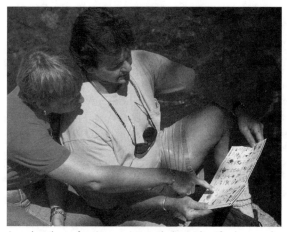

A pocket chart of native species can help to identify plants and animals you may encounter.

foot in front of the other. Some, however, require you to do this for several hours or more, uphill and down. In addition to terrain, weather conditions such as heat, cold, and wind can affect individual performance.

Good hiking boots are worth their weight in gold, and that weight is decreasing year by year. Many of today's light hiking boots combine running-shoe comfort with support, traction, and durability. Some are lined with Gore-Tex, making them waterproof yet breathable, helpful for rainy days and creek crossings. A good pair of hiking boots will protect your feet and ankles, and provide essential traction on steep slopes. Combine the boots with socks that wick moisture (avoid cotton) and cushion your feet, and you have a recipe for happy hiking.

Comfortable clothing will provide protection from sun, wind, cold, rain, poison oak, and ticks. Synthetic fabrics have the advantage over cotton because they wick moisture away from the skin and dry quickly when wet. Adjust easily to changing conditions by adding or removing an insulating layer. Hats, gloves, and insulating headbands are useful accessories. Carry a lightweight, waterproof/breathable jacket, and you'll be able to brave both rain and wind.

Other items to take along include plenty of water, snacks, sunglasses, sunscreen, insect repellent, map and compass, flashlight, knife, and basic first-aid supplies. Many hikers use a walking stick or trekking pole for stability and comfort. Binoculars, a handlens for plant study, and a pad and pencil are also useful. Try leaving your heavy field guides at home and instead make notes and sketches of birds or flowers you wish to identify. Please do not collect plant or flower specimens.

## Special Hazards

Outdoor travel in the Bay Area is relatively safe. Most of the trails covered by this book are well signed and easy to follow. Still, getting lost is possible, either by taking a wrong turn, venturing off the trail, or becoming disoriented. If you do lose your way, don't panic. Retrace your steps to a known point, use landmarks to get oriented, and refer to a map and compass if you have them. Altimeters are very useful if you have a map with elevation lines. A GPS (Global Positioning System) device may also be useful, but only if you have programmed the route in advance. Also, GPS devices vary in their ability to record an accurate position if the view skyward is obstructed.

Poison oak is a common Bay Area plant that comes in three forms—herb, shrub, and vine. Contact with any part of the plant produces an itchy rash in allergic individuals. "Leaflets three, let it be," is the rule. In fall the shrub's leaves turn yellow and red, adding color to the woods. In winter, upward-reaching clusters of bare branches identify the plant. Avoid contact with poison oak by staying on the trail and wearing protective clothing. Wash anything that touches poison oak—clothing, pets—in soap and water.

Western black-legged ticks carry the bacteria that causes Lyme disease, which, if left untreated, can cause serious health problems. These tiny insects are almost invisible, and often the victim doesn't know he or she has been bitten. The best protection against ticks is to wear long pants tucked into your socks and a long-sleeved shirt, use an insect repellent containing DEET on your clothes, stay on the trail, and shower and launder your clothes after your hike. If you find a tick attached, grasp it with a tweezers as close to your skin as possible and gently pull it straight out. Squeezing a tick that is attached may cause it to inject the bacteria. Wash the area, apply antiseptic, and call your doctor.

Western rattlesnakes are present in the Bay Area but seldom seen. Most of the time, the snake moves away when it senses humans. However, if a foot or hand lands in the snake's immediate vicinity, it may strike, sometimes without warning. If you do hear a rattling sound, stand still until you have located the snake, and then back slowly away. Protective clothing and boot material may absorb venom if the snake succeeds in biting. To avoid being bitten, stay on the trail, don't put your hands or feet beyond your range of vision, and don't handle snakes. If you are bitten, seek medical attention as quickly and effortlessly as possible, to avoid spreading the venom.

Mountain lions, though here, are rarely seen. These nocturnal hunters feed mostly on deer. If you do encounter a mountain lion, experts advise standing your ground, making loud noises, waving your arms to appear larger, and fighting back if attacked. Above all, never run. Report all mountain lion sightings to park personnel.

## Trail Etiquette

Public lands belong to everybody. Treat them as precious, and they will remain unspoiled for all to enjoy. Small, thoughtless acts can have unintended consequences, because everything in nature is interconnected. Effects of carelessness may be sudden and dramatic, such as fires, or they may not show up for years. The rules of trail etiquette are simple and based on common sense. Obey all posted restrictions. Stay on marked trails and do not cut switchbacks. Pack out all trash, and do not disturb the park's plants and animals. In short, tread lightly on the land.

The "trails" in the Bay Area are a combination of dirt roads, single tracks, and even paved paths. As you travel the routes described in this book, you will encounter other outdoor enthusiasts—hikers, runners, bicyclists, and equestrians. Most trails are open to hiking and equestrian use. In only a few cases are trails designated "hiking only," which means no bicycles or horses are allowed. Some parks and preserves allow bicycling, but generally only on dirt roads (Annadel and China Camp state parks in the North Bay are notable exceptions).

If you see or hear equestrians approaching, step off the trail to give them the right of way and remain motionless until they pass. Bicyclists should slow down and call out when approaching hikers, and dismount when near horses. Whenever possible, if a route described in this guide has a segment closed to bicycles, alternate trails are suggested. Some agencies close their trails to bicycles and horses during wet weather, often with special gates that allow hikers to pass through. Call ahead, and have an alternate route selected. (Agency phone numbers and their website addresses are listed in Appendix 3.)

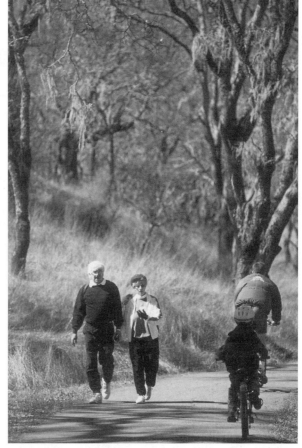

Hikers and bikers enjoy the multi-use path that wanders through Sonoma Valley Regional Park.

Dogs (and other pets) are not allowed on the trails in any Bay Area state park, and there are restrictions at other parks and open spaces as well. In areas where dogs are allowed, they generally must be on a leash no longer than 6 feet long. Some agencies allow dogs off-leash, but the dogs must be under *immediate* voice command of the person they are with, and must never be allowed to threaten or harm people or wildlife. People with dogs must clean up after their pets and obey all posted rules and regulations. Routes open to dogs are noted in this book.

# Using this Book

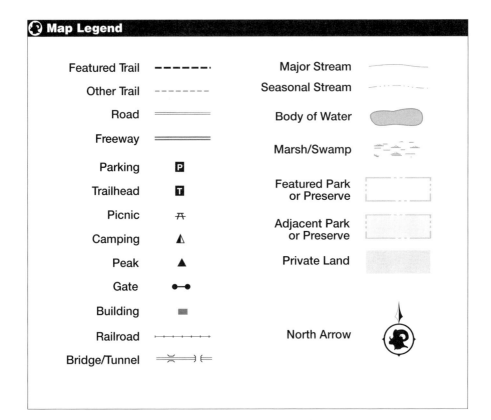

The trips in this book are organized in 10 chapters, with each chapter centered on a major population area. Chapter 1 is San Francisco/Marin, and from there the chapters (and trips) proceed roughly clockwise around the Bay Area, ending with the Peninsula. Thus the book reflects geography, and parklands that are neighbors will be found on neighboring pages. (Appendix 1 is a selection of highly recommended trips.)

In addition to the route description, each trip has highlights of the route, directions to the trailhead from the nearest major roadway, and what facilities, if any, are available at or near the trailhead. Each route has a map, along with symbols and capsulized summaries, which are explained below.

## Capsulized Summaries

### DISTANCE AND TRAIL TYPE

**DISTANCE** An estimate of the total mileage of the trip, exactly as described. Mileage for each out-and-back trip is the sum of its outbound and return legs.

**LOOP, SEMI-LOOP, OUT-AND-BACK** These designations identify the type of trip. Loop and semi-loop routes, the most common in this book, have been designed to minimize steep downhill sections whenever possible.

### HIKING TIME

An estimate of the time it takes an average hiker to complete the trip, including stops along the way.

## TOTAL ELEVATION GAIN/LOSS

Approximate sum of all the uphill and downhill segments of the trip (includes outbound and return legs for out-and-back trips).

## DIFFICULTY

A subjective rating based on distance, total elevation gain/loss, and terrain. Here is an explanation of the four categories:

**EASY** Short trips with little or no elevation gain.

**MODERATE** Trips of several hours or more, with some ups and downs but no significant elevation changes.

**DIFFICULT** Extended trips with significant elevation changes.

**VERY DIFFICULT** The longest, most rigorous trips in this book.

## TRAIL USE

**BACKPACKING OPTION** A few Bay Area parklands have campsites along or near the trip as described. Most of these require advance registration, as noted in the text.

**MOUNTAIN BIKING ALLOWED** Bicycling is allowed on the trip as described. Always check for seasonal closures and obey all posted restrictions. If a trip segment is closed to bicycles, and an alternate route is possible, this is noted in a footnote.

**LEASHED DOGS** In areas where dogs are allowed, they generally must be on a leash no longer than 6 feet.

**GOOD FOR KIDS** These are easy, short trips with not much total elevation gain, or longer trips that can be modified.

## BEST TIMES

Most Bay Area parks can be visited all year, but there are a few caveats to keep in mind. Summer brings fog and often wind to areas near the coast and along the crest of the Peninsula, but inland the heat can be extreme. Many trails may be muddy in wet weather, and there may be snow/ice on the highest peaks in winter. On the bright side, spring brings wildflower displays to Bay Area grasslands, and fall is usually perfect for enjoying the outdoors just about anywhere.

## AGENCY

This is almost always a government agency, either federal, state, or local. (Skyline Park Citizens Association, a volunteer group, runs Skyline Wilderness Park in Napa.) A listing of agencies, along with the abbreviations used in this book, is in Appendix 3.

## RECOMMENDED MAP(S)

Most agencies administering Bay Area parklands produce maps that cover the trips in this book. In many cases, these maps are available at the trailhead. Sometimes, however, maps are available only at entrance kiosks or visitor centers, and these may be closed when you visit. Some agencies have maps available by mail, by phone, or on the Web (agencies are listed in Appendix 3). There are also excellent, commercially available maps that cover some of the trips in this book.

Overleaf: A couple enjoys a quiet stroll on the Shoreline Trail in China Camp State Park.

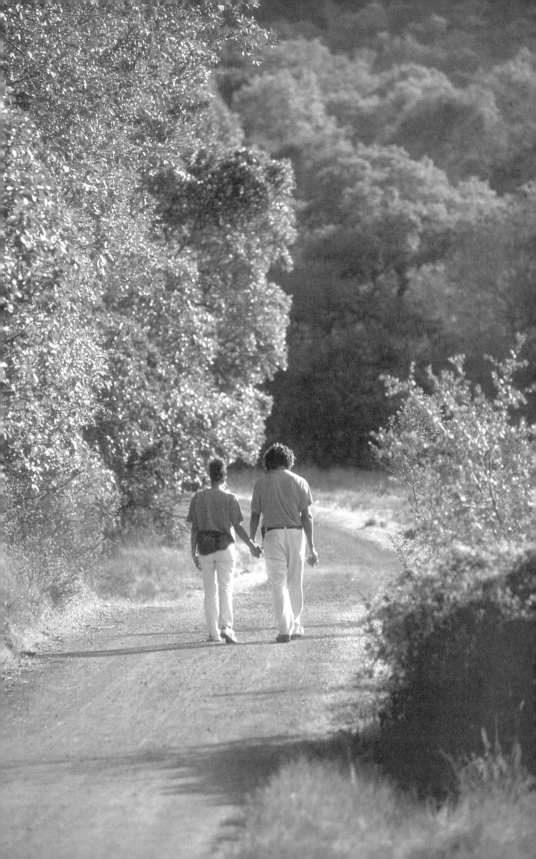

# Chapter 1
# San Francisco/Marin

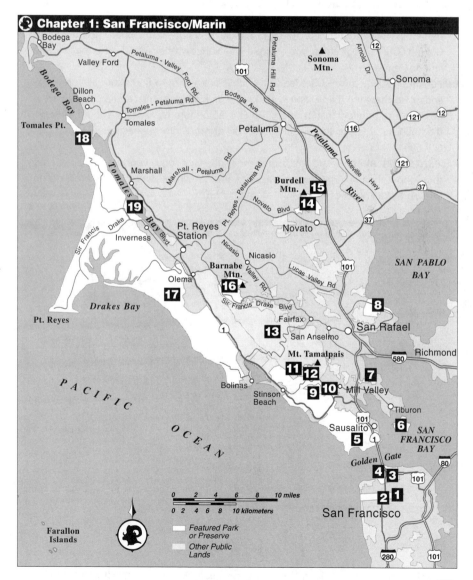

Chapter 1: San Francisco/Marin

Bodega Bay
Valley Ford
Dillon Beach
Tomales Pt.
Tomales
Marshall
Petaluma - Valley Ford Rd
Tomales - Petaluma Rd
Bodega Ave
Petaluma
Petaluma Hill Rd
101
Sonoma Mtn.
Arnold Dr
12
Sonoma
121
12
116
Petaluma River
Lakeville Hwy
121
37
Bodega Bay
Marshall - Petaluma Rd
Pt. Reyes - Petaluma Rd
18
Burdell Mtn. 15
14
Novato Blvd
Novato
37
19
Pt. Reyes Station
Inverness
Sir Francis Drake
Tomales Bay Blvd
Nicasio
Nicasio
SAN PABLO BAY
Barnabe Mtn.
16
Olema
17
Valley Rd
Lucas Valley Rd
101
8
Drakes Bay
Sir Francis Drake Blvd
13
Fairfax
San Anselmo
San Rafael
Pt. Reyes
580
Richmond
Mt. Tamalpais
11 12
7
Bolinas
Stinson Beach
9 10
Mill Valley
PACIFIC
Tiburon
6
Sausalito
5
SAN FRANCISCO BAY
80
OCEAN
Golden Gate
4 3
2 1
San Francisco
280
101

0   2   4   6   8   10 miles
0 2 4 6 8   10 kilometers

Farallon Islands

Featured Park or Preserve
Other Public Lands

# TRIP 1  Golden Gate Park: Native Oak Grove

| | |
|---|---|
| **Distance** | 1.5 miles, Loop |
| **Hiking Time** | 1 hour or less |
| **Difficulty** | Easy |
| **Trail Use** | Leashed dogs, Good for kids |
| **Best Times** | All year |
| **Agency** | SFR&PD |
| **Recommended Map** | *Map & Guide to Golden Gate Park* (Friends of Recreation and Parks) |

**HIGHLIGHTS** Tucked in the northeast corner of the park, this loop wanders through secluded groves of coast live oaks, but also joins joggers, skaters, and strollers beside busy John F. Kennedy Dr., as they zoom past the photogenic Conservatory of Flowers, reopened not long ago after years of repairs. It is hoped this brief introduction to Golden Gate Park will entice you to explore on your own, because there is much to see and do here.

**DIRECTIONS** Parking around Golden Gate Park is often hard to find, especially on weekends. Also, there are road closures within the park on weekends and most holidays. If possible, use public transportation. San Francisco Muni bus lines 5, 21, and 33 serve the trailhead at Fulton and Arguello streets. For more information, call SF Muni: (415) 673-6864.

**FACILITIES/TRAILHEAD** Restrooms, phones, and snack/food vendors are scattered throughout the park. There are no facilities at the trailhead, which is at Clark Gate, on the southeast corner of Arguello Blvd. and Fulton St.

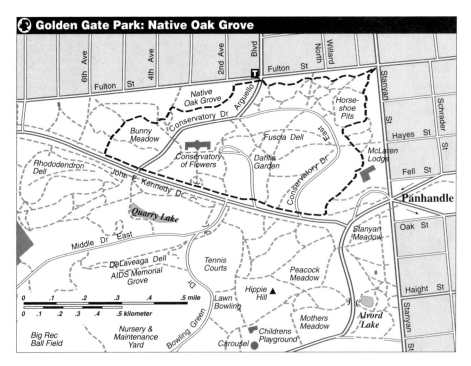

Opposite: Conservatory of Flowers is one of the park's best-loved and most-photographed buildings.

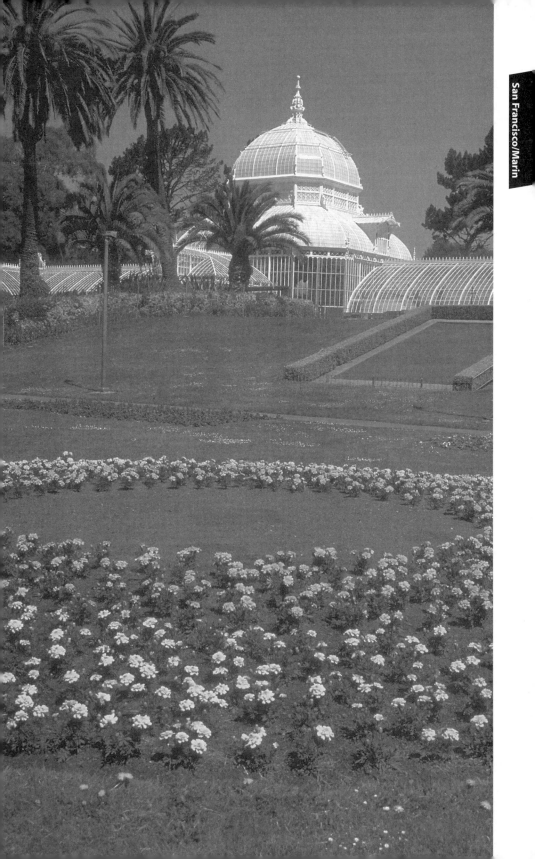

From the trailhead, you go through a gap in the stone wall, just left of the two pillars flanking the Arguello entrance to the park. Steps help you negotiate a steep uphill pitch that leads southeast, into a forest of ivy-draped coast live oaks. Passing a rest bench, you follow a single-track trail to a fork, where you bear left (the right-hand branch soon rejoins). Joining the native oaks in this part of the park are planted species such as eucalyptus, cypress, Monterey pine, acacia, and olive.

At the next fork, bear left and descend to a paved path, which you cross. The trail continues on the far side of the paved path, climbs moderately and then descends. At the next paved path, you turn left. After about 150 feet, just before you reach the corner of Fulton and Stanyan streets, turn right on a paved path that changes to dirt just beyond a rest bench.

Climbing gently on a single track, you soon merge with a wide dirt path by veering slightly left. Pass through a large clearing and then follow the path as it curves right and descends. At a T-junction, turn left on a wide dirt path, and then come to a paved path, where there is a water fountain. To your right is Conservatory Dr. East, a paved road.

Bear left on the paved path, then angle right at a fork. Rhododendrons line the path, ecologically at home beneath a large coast redwood. About 100 feet ahead, a paved path merges on your left. You continue straight, skirting a parking area, left, and then veer right to pass around McLaren Lodge.

Passing a couple of rest benches, right, your path bends left and meets a paved path that parallels Kennedy Dr. Here you turn right and soon cross Conservatory Dr. East. The paved path continues on the other side of Conservatory Dr., and you follow it past two well-known park attractions—the tennis courts, left, and the dahlia garden, right. The park's oldest building, the Conservatory of Flowers, is ahead and right.

---

**McLaren Lodge**

This picturesque stone building, which houses the San Francisco Recreation and Park Department headquarters, was built in 1896 and is named for the park's second, and most influential, manager, John McLaren.

---

The Conservatory was damaged in 1995 by a windstorm and was closed many years for repairs; it reopened in September 2003. It houses an extensive collection of tropical plants, including palms, orchids, bromeliads, and carnivorous species.

Just past the Conservatory, you cross Conservatory Dr. West, then resume your ramble along the north side of Kennedy Dr. To your right is the George Washington elm, planted here in 1952 by the San Francisco Chapter, Sons of the American Revolution. According to a plaque here, the parent of this tree spread its limbs over George Washington as he took command of the American Army on July 3, 1775.

Once common shade trees east of the Rockies, elms in the United States have been decimated by Dutch elm disease. This fungal disease, spread by beetles, was introduced by accident around 1930. It's good to see a healthy elm flourishing, especially one with so distinguished a past.

At about 1 mile, you come to a paved path on the right, the first since you crossed Conservatory Dr. West. Turning right, you climb moderately past several rest benches and dirt paths, all on your left. When you reach a chess-themed area—pedestals in the shape of knights and rooks supporting a covering that provides shade for tables and benches—bear left and follow a paved path through it.

With the chess area on your left, you merge with a paved path that joins from the right. Go about 75 feet to a junction, where you turn right onto a dirt path and stay left where it forks. Now you descend gently through a beautiful grove of coast live oak, traversing a hillside that drops left. At the next fork stay left again, and follow the path to a park entrance on Fulton St. across from 2nd Ave. Turn right and follow the sidewalk back to the trailhead.

# TRIP2 Golden Gate Park: Stow Lake

| | |
|---|---|
| **Distance** | 2.4 miles, Semi-loop |
| **Hiking Time** | 1 to 2 hours |
| **Difficulty** | Easy |
| **Trail Use** | Leashed dogs, Good for kids |
| **Best Times** | All year |
| **Agency** | SFR&PD |
| **Recommended Map** | Map: *Map & Guide to Golden Gate Park* (Friends of Recreation and Parks) |

**HIGHLIGHTS** Walking this charming semi-loop — which visits Stow Lake and also introduces you to the Rose Garden, the Japanese Tea Garden, and the Strybing Arboretum and Botanical Gardens — it's hard to imagine San Francisco's premier park as a bleak area of sand dunes, far removed from the city's population center, but that's what civil engineer William H. Hall had to work with when the park was created in the 1870s.

**DIRECTIONS** Parking around Golden Gate Park is often hard to find, especially on weekends. Also, there are road closures within the park on weekends and most holidays. If possible, use public transportation. San Francisco Muni bus lines 5 and 28 serve the trailhead at Presidio Blvd. and Fulton St. For more information, call SF Muni: (415) 673-6864.

**FACILITIES/TRAILHEAD** Restrooms, phones, and snack/food vendors are scattered throughout the park. There are no facilities at the trailhead, which is on the southeast corner of Presidio Blvd. and Fulton St. (The nearest restroom is just west of the Rose Garden.)

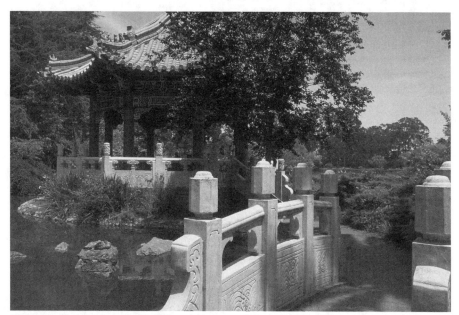

Chinese Pavilion, on the east side of Stow lake, was a gift from the city of Taipei.

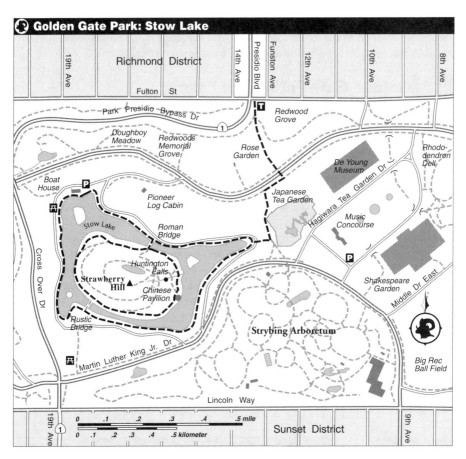

**Golden Gate Park: Stow Lake**

You follow a paved path beside noisy Presidio Blvd. into the park. After about 100 feet you reach a four-way junction, where you go straight through the park's lovely Rose Garden. Crossing John F. Kennedy Dr., you turn right on a paved path, and after about 150 feet veer left and climb past some tall eucalyptus trees. The path soon levels and curves left beside the Japanese Tea Garden, well worth a visit. Its entrance is ahead and then left about 100 yards on Hagiwara Tea Garden Dr.; there is a fee for admission.

Opposite the Tea Garden exit is a paved path going right and uphill to Stow Lake. Ahead, across Martin Luther King Jr. Dr., is Friend Gate and the entrance to the Strybing Arboretum and Botanical Gardens (free admission).

To visit Stow Lake, go uphill on the paved path and then climb a set of steps.

### The Arboretum

The 70-acre Strybing Arboretum and Botanical Gardens contains plants from around the world, including Asia, South America, Australia, New Zealand, South Africa, and, of course, California. You can explore the John Muir Nature Trail, walk through a garden with plants mentioned in the Bible, and experience the Garden of Fragrance. There is a small pond here, and the water, combined with the variety of flowering plants, attracts many species of birds. An information board near the entrance lists guided walks and classes that are available.

When you reach the lake, turn left and follow the paved path that circles the lake, which is actually a narrow body of water surrounding an island. Paddleboats ply the lake's placid waters, which are fringed by Monterey pine, eucalyptus, and Monterey cypress. On the southwest side is Rustic Bridge, an 1893 stone span that leads to the island. Continuing clockwise around the lake, you come to the Boathouse, where you can buy snacks and drinks and rent boats and bicycles. Restrooms are downhill and across a parking area, left.

Stow Lake is a favorite birding destination—from its shore you may spot great blue herons, black-crowned night herons, egrets, gulls, ducks, geese, and songbirds. Sometimes a rare bird shows up and creates a stir among local birders.

Passing the Boathouse and ambling beside the lake, you come to Roman Bridge. To visit the island, turn right and cross the bridge. At a four-way junction, you turn right again and now begin to circle the island counter clockwise on a dirt path. A hillside rises steeply left, and after about 100 yards you come to a fork; the branches soon rejoin, so you can take either. Passing Rustic Bridge, you soon come to the colorful and elaborate Chinese Pavilion, a gift from San Francisco's sister city, Taipei.

On the east side of the island is Huntington Falls, fed by the outflow from a reservoir atop the island. A series of stone steps allows you to cross the rushing water, which flows unimpeded into the lake. Just past the falls are steps leading to the reservoir. Now back at Roman Bridge, turn right to cross it, then right again when you reach the paved path to continue around the lake. At the northeast corner of the lake you close the loop. From here, retrace your route to the trailhead, or spend more time exploring the park and its many other attractions.

## TRIP3 Presidio of San Francisco: Ecology Trail

| | |
|---|---|
| **Distance** | 2.2 miles, Loop |
| **Hiking Time** | 1 to 2 hours |
| **Elevation Gain/Loss** | ±400 feet |
| **Difficulty** | Easy |
| **Trail Use** | Leashed dogs, Good for kids |
| **Best Times** | All year |
| **Agency** | GGNRA |
| **Recommended Map** | *Golden Gate National Recreation Area Presidio of San Francisco* (GGNRA) |

**HIGHLIGHTS** The Presidio was established in 1776 as a Spanish colonial outpost on a windy sand dune near San Francisco Bay. It later served as a Mexican fort and a U.S. military base before being turned over in 1994 to the National Park Service. The Americans built forts, housing, and coastal gun batteries, and planted trees that transformed the landscape. The Ecology Trail loops through the southeastern corner of the Presidio, providing a look at what human intervention has wrought, and also what conservation efforts have managed to preserve and restore, including native wildflowers and grasses, some of them rare, threatened, or endangered.

**DIRECTIONS** From the Presidio's Arguello Gate entrance, just north of Arguello Blvd. and Jackson St., go 0.1 mile northeast to the large paved parking area at Inspiration Point, on the right.

**FACILITIES/TRAILHEAD** There are no facilities at the trailhead, which is on the east side of the parking area.

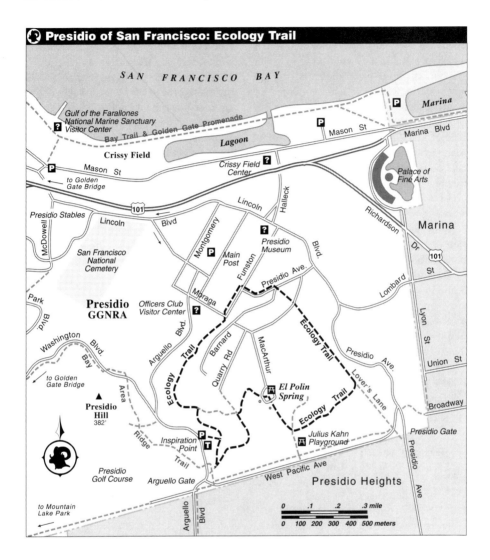

**Presidio of San Francisco: Ecology Trail**

**W**alk southeast down a set of wooden steps and after several hundred feet join the Ecology Trail, a wide, dirt path, by turning left. An outcrop of serpentine rock in the midst of a grassy, wildflower-filled meadow is right, behind a fence, in an area that is being restored.

The trail skirts Inspiration Point and descends on a gentle grade. At a junction with a trail heading right, you continue straight, now in forest. Several unofficial trails branch right and left; ignore them. Soon the red brick buildings of the

**Presidio Flora**

Grasslands are a threatened ecosystem, and this serpentine grassland is unique in the Golden Gate National Recreation Area. Serpentine soil, high in magnesium and low in calcium, is toxic to many plants, but some have adapted to it, including ones that are rare, threatened, or endangered.

Among the wildflowers that grow beside the trail are goldfields, coastal tidytips, California buttercups, blue-eyed grass, and California poppies.

Presidio's Main Post are visible ahead. Now on a paved path, you descend to a gate, and pass it on the left. With Pershing Hall on your left, you follow a sidewalk to Moraga Ave., which you cross. A sidewalk along Funston Ave. takes you past part of Officers Row, built in 1862 to house commissioned officers and their families.

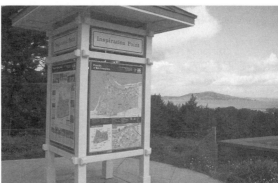

Inspiration Point is the trailhead for the Ecology Trail, a loop through the Presidio.

At the corner of Funston Ave. and Presidio Blvd., get on the left side of Presidio and follow the sidewalk gently downhill to a crosswalk just past Barnard Ave. Turn right, cross Presidio, and then follow a paved path through a corridor of eucalyptus trees and berry vines. A footbridge, built around 1865, takes you over a watercourse. When you reach MacArthur Ave., cross it and continue on Lovers' Lane, a paved path that is part of the Ecology Trail.

You walk moderately uphill, past stands of Monterey cypress and eucalyptus. At the intersection of Liggett Ave. and Clarke St., you continue straight, now on a sidewalk. Passing a row of brick houses, you turn right onto a dirt path, which almost immediately merges with another coming sharply from the left. Now you pass a fenced area that has been planted with trees, and soon reach a four-way junction, not shown on the park map.

Here you turn right and descend over loose sand to a fork, where you bear right. With Paul Goode Field on your right, you come to a large dirt parking area and a junction with a trail going left. Turn right, cross the parking area, and then follow a trail past some white buildings with red roofs. The trail bends left and descends steeply into forest.

Rare, threatened, or endangered plants are found in the Presidio, and, at the time of research, there was a controversial plan in the works to remove some of the Presidio's planted trees, such as eucalyptus, Monterey pine, and Monterey cypress, and to restore the original dune habitat.

When you reach a loop of paved road with a grassy area in its middle, go straight across, passing El Polin Spring. Your trail continues from the northwest side of the loop and climbs moderately to a four-way junction at the base of Inspiration Point. Turn left, pass an unsigned trail, left, and climb to the next junction, also four-way. Here you turn right and follow a mostly level path to close the loop. Here, turn left and retrace your route to the parking area.

---

**Lovers' Lane**

According to a sign, Lovers' Lane

> ...has witnessed the passing of Spanish soldiers, Franciscan missionaries, and American soldiers of two centuries. It is perhaps the oldest travel corridor in San Francisco. In 1776 this path connected the Spanish Presidio with the Mission 3 miles to the southeast. During the 1860s it became the main route used by off-duty soldiers to walk into San Francisco. Many of those men made the trip into town to meet their sweethearts, and the trail became known as Lovers' Lane.

# TRIP4 Presidio of San Francisco: Fort Winfield Scott Loop

| | |
|---:|:---|
| **Distance** | 2.6 miles, Loop |
| **Hiking Time** | 1 to 2 hours |
| **Elevation Gain/Loss** | ±300 feet |
| **Difficulty** | Easy |
| **Trail Use** | Leashed dogs, Good for kids |
| **Best Times** | All year |
| **Agency** | GGNRA |
| **Recommended Map** | *Golden Gate National Recreation Area Presidio of San Francisco* (GGNPC) |

**HIGHLIGHTS** This loop through the northwest corner of the Presidio is both an enjoyable walk back in time — the Spanish built a fort here shortly after the Declaration of Independence was signed — and a hopeful look forward at the effort to reclaim and restore developed lands for public enjoyment. After more than 200 years of military use, the Presidio was turned over to the National Park Service in 1994. Along the way you pass military buildings from the late 19th and early 20th centuries; vantage points with views of the Golden Gate, San Francisco Bay, and beyond; and a warming hut where food, drinks, books, maps, and other information are available.

**DIRECTIONS** From the Presidio's Marina Gate entrance at the west end of Marina Blvd., go west on Mason St. 1 mile to a paved parking area, left.

**FACILITIES/TRAILHEAD** A visitor center with food, restrooms, phone, and water is on the southwest corner of Mason and Halleck streets, about 0.6 mile east of the parking area. The center is open Wednesday through Sunday, 9 A.M. to 5 P.M. There are no facilities at the trailhead, which is on the west end of the parking area. Some of this route follows streets used by cars: if there is no sidewalk, walk on the left side of the street, facing traffic.

From the west end of the parking area, go west several hundred feet on Mason Ave. to its junction with Crissy Field Ave. Turn sharply left and follow Crissy Field Ave. uphill, passing under Doyle Dr., to a junction with McDowell Ave. Here you angle right and climb moderately past the Presidio stables and the park's archives and records center. You can visit the Presidio San Francisco Pet Cemetery, an unusual landmark, under Doyle Dr., on the southwest side of Crissy Field Ave.

Carefully crossing Lincoln Blvd., you take Park Blvd. gently uphill to a junction. Here you angle left on a dirt path, which rises steadily through a forest of Monterey cypress and eucalyptus, both planted here. Meeting Park again and crossing it, you follow Kobbe Ave. past Officers Row, a set of beautiful homes built in 1912. Climbing gently, you pass Barnard Hall, an imposing brick building named for an Army chief engineer.

At a four-way junction, you turn right on Upton Ave., following a sidewalk on its left side. Some of the officer's homes in the Presidio are quite lavish, with spacious

> **Fort Winfield Scott**
> The fort is named for Winfield Scott, who served in the army from before the War of 1812 until the Civil War. He is best known for his command of U.S. troops during the Mexican-American War. Completed in 1915, the fort was the headquarters for the artillery designed to protect the Bay Area.

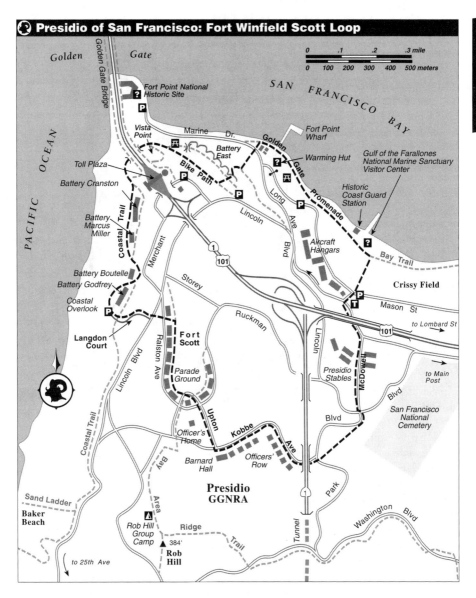

**Presidio of San Francisco: Fort Winfield Scott Loop**

Golden Gate

Golden Gate Bridge

PACIFIC OCEAN

SAN FRANCISCO BAY

0 .1 .2 .3 mile
0 100 200 300 400 500 meters

Fort Point National Historic Site

Vista Point

Marine Dr.

Battery East

Fort Point Wharf

Golden

Warming Hut

Gulf of the Farallones National Marine Sanctuary Visitor Center

Toll Plaza

Bike Path

Gate

Battery Cranston

Long Ave

Promenade

Historic Coast Guard Station

Lincoln

Battery Marcus Miller

Coastal Trail

Merchant

Aircraft Hangars

Bay Trail

Crissy Field

Battery Boutelle
Battery Godfrey

Storey

Lincoln

Mason St

to Lombard St

Coastal Overlook

Ruckman

101

Langdon Court

Ralston Ave

Lincoln Blvd

Fort Scott

Parade Ground

Lincoln

McDowell

Presidio Stables

to Main Post

Coastal Trail

Upton

Kobbe

Blvd

San Francisco National Cemetery

Officer's Home

Barnard Hall

Officers' Row

Ave

Blvd

Bay Area

**Presidio GGNRA**

Sand Ladder

Baker Beach

Rob Hill Group Camp

Ridge

Park

Washington Blvd

384'
**Rob Hill**

Trail

Tunnel

to 25th Ave

lawns and exotic landscaping. Where Upton veers right, you continue straight across Ralston Ave., and then enter Fort Winfield Scott. Turn left and keep the parade ground on your right.

You walk along the left side of the parade ground, where views stretch to the Golden Gate Bridge, Angel Island, and Mt. Diablo. With a sports field on your right, you turn left on the Juan Bautista de Anza National

Historic Trail, part of the Bay Area Ridge Trail. You walk on pavement between two buildings (numbers 1207 and 1208), cross Ralston, and then come to Lincoln. Cross carefully, and then follow Langdon Court about 50 feet to a trail post. You jog left, then veer right through a parking area, heading toward the Pacific Ocean.

At the west end of the parking area, follow a paved road that soon changes to dirt and gravel. Turning right at a trail post, you get on the Coastal Trail, a wide dirt-and-gravel path that is part of the Anza/Bay Area Ridge Trail. Near the bunkers the trail forks: hikers stay left, bicyclists stay right. You follow the rocky and eroded hiking trail to another fork, where the left branch is signed for the Anza/Bay Area Ridge Trail. The low concrete bunkers beside the trail were built from 1891 to 1900 for coastal defense. At the end of World War II, the guns in these bunkers were removed.

Staying left here, and right at the next fork, where a trail goes left to a viewpoint, you skirt the coastal cliffs and descend via wooden steps. Now on level ground, you merge with the trail for bicyclists, which joins sharply from the right.

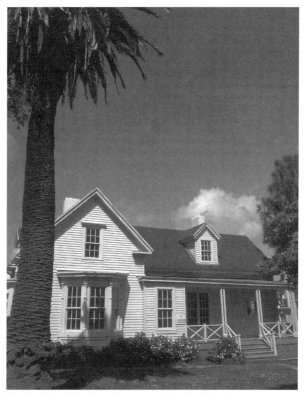

The Presidio of San Francisco is noted for its distinctive architecture and military history.

Ahead is a paved path which goes under the Golden Gate Bridge. You get on it and angle left, watching out for bicyclists and joggers.

Beyond the bridge the trail forks, and you stay left. You pass a trail, left to Battery East, which dates from 1876, and a picnic area. A brick path goes right and uphill to the Golden Gate Bridge gift shop. You descend to a junction with a trail, left, signed for Fort Point. Here you turn left and come to a four-way junction. Continue straight and descend steeply over rough ground, passing a trail, right. Aided by steps, you soon reach Marine Dr., a paved road.

Cross the road, and when you reach a seawall, turn right on a paved path, part of the Golden Gate Promenade and the San Francisco Bay Trail. Nearby are restrooms, water, and a warming hut with food, drinks, books, maps, and other information. The hut is open daily, 9 A.M. to 5 P.M. Beyond the warming hut, the path changes to dirt and gravel. A path cuts sharply right, going back to the warming hut. You pass a picnic area, right, and then reach a five-way junction beside Long Ave.

Here you continue straight on the dirt-and-gravel path. A historic Coast Guard station and the Gulf of the Farallones National Marine Sanctuary visitor center are left. You are passing through an area that has been extensively restored and landscaped with native plants. Several hundred feet past the visitor center, you turn right, climb a few steps, and then cross Crissy Field, formerly a landing strip for planes. After about 100 yards you reach Mason St., which you cross to return to the parking area.

# *TRIP5* Marin Headlands

|  |  |
|---|---|
| **Distance** | 5.4 miles, Loop |
| **Hiking Time** | 3 to 4 hours |
| **Elevation Gain/Loss** | ±1100 feet |
| **Difficulty** | Moderate |
| **Trail Use** | Backpacking option, Mountain biking allowed[1] |
| **Best Times** | All year |
| **Agency** | GGNRA |
| **Recommended Maps** | *Marin Headlands Trail Map* (GGNPC), *Trails of Mt. Tamalpais and the Marin Headlands* (Olmsted) |
| **Notes** | [1]Bicycles are not allowed on the northern half of the Miwok Trail, and must instead use the Old Springs and Marincello trails to complete the trip |

**HIGHLIGHTS** This scenic loop uses the Miwok and Bobcat trails to circle Gerbode Valley, an area slated in the 1960s for urban development but later protected as part of the Golden Gate National Recreation Area (GGNRA). The hills surrounding Gerbode Valley, part of the Marin Headlands, are vibrant in the spring with wildflowers, and alive with birdsong and avian acrobatics most of the year, but especially during the fall raptor migration. Views of San Francisco, Marin, and the Pacific coast from the high points along this loop are superb.

**DIRECTIONS** From Highway 101 northbound, just north of the Golden Gate Bridge, take the Alexander Ave. exit, go north 0.2 mile, and turn left on Bunker Road. After 0.1 mile you reach a one-direction-only tunnel where traffic is controlled by a stoplight. At 2.5 miles from Alexander Ave. there is roadside parking on the right. Additional parking is available at the Marin Headlands visitor center (see below).

From Highway 101 southbound, just south of the Waldo Tunnel, take the Sausalito exit, which is also signed for the GGNRA. Bear right (despite the left-pointing GGNRA sign) and go 0.25 mile to Bunker Road Turn left, and follow the directions above.

**FACILITIES/TRAILHEAD** The Marin Headlands visitor center — which has interpretive displays, books and maps for sale, helpful rangers, restrooms, and water — is on Field Road, which is 0.2 mile past the roadside parking area. Turn left onto Field Road and go 0.1 to the visitor center. There are no facilities at the trailhead, which is on the north side of the roadside parking area near its midpoint.

**W**alk north on a dirt-and-gravel path, cross a bridged creek, and reach a T-junction with the Miwok Trail, a dirt road. An information board here describes the fight to save Gerbode Valley from development. On your right is a low-lying marsh, formed by the creek that drains the valley and empties into Rodeo Lagoon. At the next junction, where the Bobcat Trail goes right, you continue straight.

In fall, the Marin Headlands is one of the best places on the West Coast to observe hawks and falcons in migration. These southward-bound raptors take advantage of rising air currents, called thermals, to gain elevation for their crossing of the Golden Gate.

Soon the trail begins a moderate but relentless and unshaded climb toward the east end of Wolf Ridge. Finally, just past 1 mile, you reach a notch with views northwest to Mt. Tamalpais, and west, over a declivity in a neighboring ridge, to the Pacific Ocean. A few paces ahead is a junction with the Wolf Ridge Trail, left. This

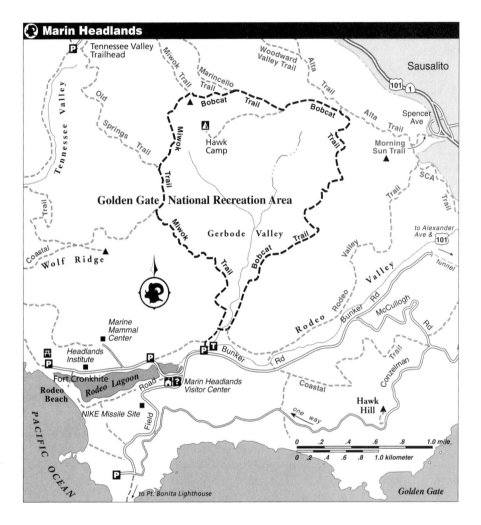

**Marin Headlands**

Tennessee Valley Trailhead

Woodward Valley Trail

Sausalito

Miwok Trail

Marincello Trail

Old

Springs Trail

Bobcat Trail

Alta Trail

Bobcat Trail

Alta Trail

Spencer Ave

Miwok Trail

Hawk Camp

Morning Sun Trail

Tennessee Valley

SCA

Trail

Golden Gate National Recreation Area

Miwok Trail

Gerbode Valley Trail

to Alexander Ave & 101

Coastal Trail

Wolf Ridge

Valley Trail

Bobcat Trail

Rodeo Valley

tunnel

Marine Mammal Center

Rodeo Rodeo Rd

Bunker Rd

McCullogh Rd

Headlands Institute

Bunker Rd

Conzelman Trail

Fort Cronkhite

Rodeo Lagoon

Road

Marin Headlands Visitor Center

Coastal

Hawk Hill

Rodeo Beach

NIKE Missile Site

Field

one way

PACIFIC OCEAN

| 0 | .2 | .4 | .6 | .8 | 1.0 mile |
| 0 | .2 | .4 | .6 | .8 | 1.0 kilometer |

to Pt. Bonita Lighthouse

Golden Gate

trail is for hiking only, and dogs must be leashed. Your route, which from here on is closed to dogs, continues straight.

At a four-way junction, you meet the Old Springs Trail, left, open to hikers, horses, and bicycles. Your route, from here on closed to bicycles, continues straight and begins to climb over severely eroded ground that alternates between moderate and steep.

In addition to the ever-present turkey vultures, you may see another large black bird, the common raven. These relatives of jays, crows, and magpies are able to make an astounding variety of sounds. And while

Poe's "Nevermore" may not truly be part of their vocabulary, other weirdly human sounds certainly are. Ravens are also great

**Wild for Flowers**

In spring, especially after a wet winter, the hills are decorated with a dazzling display of California poppy, mule ears, paintbrush, Ithuriel's spear, yarrow, blow wives, and blue-eyed grass. Nearly 50 species are listed in the pamphlet *Frequently Seen Wildflowers of the Marin Headlands,* available at the visitor center.

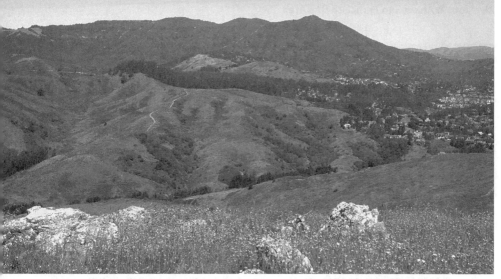

View northwest of Mt. Tamalpais from a high point on the Miwok Trail in the Marin Headlands.

aerial acrobats, and seem to enjoy chasing each other in frenzied pursuit.

A single-track trail, right, climbs to a vantage point beside a fenced-in communication facility, used by the FAA to direct commercial aircraft. Just left of this junction are a few large rocks, a convenient place to sit and rest. After enjoying the scenery, continue uphill on a gentle grade, and then begin a moderate descent. The 1041-foot high point on the ridge dividing Tennessee and Gerbode valleys, home of the FAA facility, is uphill and right.

Where a dirt road goes right to the FAA facility, you bear left and descend to a junction. Here the Miwok Trail turns left, but you go straight, now on the Bobcat Trail. Soon the Marincello Trail, part of the Bay Area Ridge Trail, joins from the left. This trail is open to hikers, horses, and bicycles. Continuing straight and passing several unsigned dirt roads, you come to a junction with the road to Hawk Camp, right.

Passing the road to Hawk Camp at about 3 miles, your route continues downhill on a gentle and then moderate grade, then follows a rolling course to a junction. Here, a short connector goes left to the Alta Trail, closed to bicycles, but you continue straight on the multi-use Bobcat Trail. Soon your

route makes a sweeping right-hand bend and passes the Rodeo Valley Cutoff, a hiking-only trail veering left.

The Bobcat Trail now zigzags gently down into Gerbode Valley. After passing through a eucalyptus grove, you enjoy a level walk parallel to the creek, which remains hidden from view behind a screen of willow thickets. You pass the Rodeo Valley Trail, left, then cross the creek, which passes under the road through a culvert. In about 50 feet, you close the loop at the Miwok Trail. Here you turn left and retrace your route to the parking area.

### Hawk Camp

Hawk Camp is the most primitive of the three walk-in campgrounds in the Marin Headlands. It has three sites that can each hold up to four people. There are picnic tables and a toilet, but no water. No fires are allowed, so if you want to cook, you need a camp stove. For reservations, call (415) 331-1540 between 9:30 A.M. and 4:30 P.M. You must pick up your permit at the visitor center during the above hours. Reservations may be made up to 90 days in advance.

# TRIP6 Angel Island State Park

|  |  |
|---|---|
| **Distance** | 4.5 miles, Loop |
| **Hiking Time** | 2 to 3 hours |
| **Elevation Gain/Loss** | ±800 feet |
| **Difficulty** | Moderate |
| **Trail Use** | Good for kids |
| **Best Times** | All year |
| **Agency** | CSP |
| **Recommended Map** | *Angel Island State Park* (CSP) |
| **Notes** | Bicycles are not allowed on the trails described below, but can be used on the island-circling system of main roads, and can be brought to the island on ferries |

**HIGHLIGHTS**  Angel Island is a sentinel, guarding the entrance to San Francisco Bay. This route uses the Northridge and Sunset trails to circle the island, and also visits its highest point, Mt. Caroline Livermore (781'), a superb vantage point from which all the familiar landmarks in the Bay Area are revealed. There is much historic interest to the island as well, and an outing here can easily include a tour by bicycle or tram.

**DIRECTIONS**  The most frequent ferry service to Angel Island leaves from Tiburon, (415) 435-2131, www.angelislandferry.com. There is also ferry service from San Francisco, (415) 773-1188, www.blueandgoldfleet.com; and from Oakland/Alameda, (510) 522-3300, www.eastbayferry.com. There is no weekday ferry service to Angel Island during the winter; be sure to check for the most current schedule before departing. There are fees for ferry service and park entrance (the CSP annual day-use pass is not accepted here).

**FACILITIES/TRAILHEAD**  Near the ferry landing are a visitor center, café, picnic tables, restrooms, water, phone, lockers, bike rentals, and tour trams. State park volunteers provide interpretive programs at the island's historic sites on weekends and holidays from May through October. For tram tours, call (415) 897-0715. For camping and group picnicking reservations, call (800) 444-7275. The trailhead is on the northeast side of the ferry landing, to the left of the restrooms and phone.

Angel Island, the largest island in San Francisco Bay, has played a role in the area's history for thousands of years. Coast Miwok Indians used the island as a fishing and hunting site. In August 1775, the first European to enter the bay, Juan Manuel de Ayala, anchored his ship San Carlos in a cove on the island's northwest side that now bears his name.

During both world wars, Angel Island served the U.S. military as an embarkation/debarkation point and also as a prison for enemy aliens and prisoners of war. Following World War II, the island was declared surplus property, and a campaign was started to make it a state park. Mt. Caroline Livermore, the island's 781-foot high point, honors a leading Marin County conservationist who spearheaded the campaign.

A little-known aspect of the island is its history as a detention center for immigrants, 97 percent of them Chinese, from 1910 to 1940. The detainees, who were held from two weeks to six months, faced tough questioning about their family and village background. Thanks to the efforts of the late Paul Chow, head of the foundation to restore

## Angel Island State Park

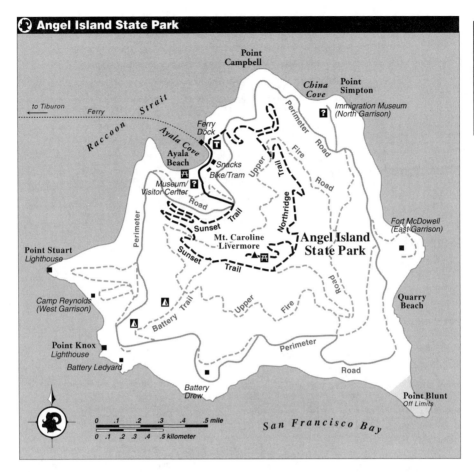

Angel Island, the Immigration Station on the island's northeast side is now a museum.

Climb steeply on the Northridge Trail past several picnic areas to Perimeter Road, the island's main paved thoroughfare. Cross the road, turn right, and in about 50 feet find the continuation of the Northridge Trail. A dramatic view extends west from here to Tiburon, the Marin Headlands, and Mt. Tamalpais. Now the grade eases to a gentle uphill as you alternate between forest and clearings full of wildflowers.

As the trail curves around the north side of the island, you encounter a densely overgrown area where California bays rise above a shrubby understory. Carpets of forget-me-nots, abundant in the island's shady enclaves, put on a fabulous spring and sum-

mer display of light blue flowers. Suddenly the terrain opens, and you cross a sandy, rocky area dominated by manzanita.

As the trail curves right, you enjoy a ridgetop walk and then reenter dense forest. Just shy of 1 mile, you reach a dirt fire road which, like Perimeter Road, circles the

### Alien Trees

The state park has cleared many eucalyptuses and a lesser number of Monterey pines, both nonnative, from the island in an effort to prevent their spread and encourage native plants. Stumps beside the trail are evidence of this project.

island. Here you turn left, and about 75 feet ahead find the continuation of the Northridge Trail on your right. Now circling the island's east side, the route switchbacks right and climbs into a large wildflower meadow, and soon offers views of Mt. Livermore, the island's summit.

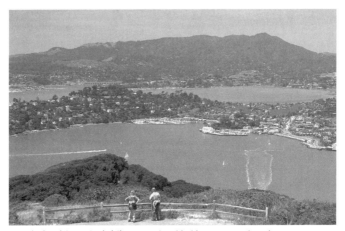

Angel Island State Park: hikers nearing Mt. Livermore enjoy view across Raccoon Strait.

At a Y-junction you leave the Northridge Trail and turn sharply right to contour across a grassy slope dotted with coyote brush and other native shrubs. The single-track trail switchbacks twice, then ascends west along a ridgeline. Nearing the summit, you pass two sets of picnic tables set on concrete platforms (the platforms are remnants of a Nike missle radar site). The very top of Mt. Livermore has been restored and revegetated, based on historical photographs.

Atop the summit are more picnic tables, from which you can enjoy fine views of San Francisco, the Golden Gate Bridge, the Pacific Ocean, and some of the Bay Area's tallest peaks — Mt. St. Helena, Mt. Hamilton, Mt. Diablo, and Mt. Tamalpais. From here the trail descends to a vantage point on the west side of the peak and dead-ends. When you have finished enjoying Mt. Livermore, retrace your route to the junction with the Northridge Trail at the previously mentioned Y-junction.

From here, angle right and soon reach a paved road. (The old paved route to the summit, right, has been regraded and replanted, and soon it will disappear.) You turn left and, after about 50 feet, swing sharply right on the Sunset Trail.

The Sunset Trail, which traverses the south flank of Mt. Livermore, one of the best places on the island for spring wildflowers. After crossing a closed trail, your route curves right and, at about 3 miles, enters forest. When you reach the dirt fire road, bear right and find the continuation of the Sunset Trail about 75 feet ahead and on your left.

---

**Raccoon Strait**

Depending on the tide, Raccoon Strait, named for a 19th century British warship that was repaired in Ayala Cove, may be blue-green with water from the Pacific, or muddy brown with runoff from the Sacramento and San Joaquin rivers.

---

The trail turns left and begins a series of switchbacks (please stay on the trail). You descend through a wooded area to Perimeter Road, where you also meet a paved road rising from Ayala Cove. Cross Perimeter Road and descend the paved road to Ayala Cove, past a bike trail, right, and another paved road, left. Continuing straight, you follow the paved road as it passes the visitor center and lawn, soon arriving at the ferry loading dock. (There are different waiting areas for each ferry, so be sure to get in the right one.)

# *TRIP7* Ring Mountain Open Space Preserve

| | |
|---|---|
| **Distance** | 3.3 miles, Semi-loop |
| **Hiking Time** | 2 to 3 hours |
| **Elevation Gain/Loss** | ±650 feet |
| **Difficulty** | Moderate |
| **Trail Use** | Leashed dogs |
| **Best Times** | All year |
| **Agency** | MCOSD |
| **Recommended Map** | *Southern Preserves* (MCOSD) |

**HIGHLIGHTS** Ring Mountain Open Space Preserve, surrounded by residential development near busy Corte Madera, perfectly demonstrates the value of land conservation and protection. Its slopes are home to a wonderful array of trees, shrubs, and wildflowers, some quite rare, and one, the Tiburon Mariposa lily, is found nowhere else in the world. As a vantage point with great views, Ring Mountain's summit rivals better-known Bay Area peaks. This route uses the Loop and Phyllis Ellman trails, along with the Taylor Ridge Fire Road, to explore the mountain's slopes and summit.

   **Boldface** numbers in the route description below refer to numbered markers along the trail, which are keyed to an MCOSD brochure that is no longer available. Some text from the brochure is summarized below and appears as part of the trail description.

**DIRECTIONS** From Highway 101 in Corte Madera, take the Paradise Dr./Tamalpais Dr. exit and go east on Tamalpais Dr., staying in the right lane, which becomes San Clemente Dr. After 0.1 mile, San Clemente Dr. bends right; follow it and go another 0.5 mile to a stoplight at Paradise Dr. Turn left onto Paradise Dr., go 0.9 mile, and park in a turnout on the right, near a gated dirt road.

**FACILITIES/TRAILHEAD** There are no facilities at the trailhead, which is on the south side of Paradise Dr., at a gated dirt road.

Head south on a dirt trail, with a seasonal creek in a gully on your right. After about 100 feet, where a faint trail continues straight, you turn right and cross a bridge over the creek. Climb on the Phyllis Ellman Trail past an information board detailing the history of the fight to save Ring Mountain. Shortly after a leftward bend, the trail reaches a junction. Here your route, the Loop Trail, goes straight, and the Phyllis Ellman Trail, which you rejoin later, veers right.

   About 75 feet past the junction is marker **2**, right, which calls attention to soil differences between the mountain's upper and lower reaches. Sandstone soil, lower down, is perfect for a wide variety of plants, including wildflowers such as Ithuriel's spear, blue-eyed grass, false lupine, suncup, wild iris, and miniature lupine. Serpentine soil, higher up, is toxic to most plant species, but tolerated by a few, including the preserve's rarities.

   A line of California bay and coast live oak, left, borders a seasonal creek that flows through a ravine and into the marsh, saturating it with water during the rainy season. Just before you reach the ravine, you pass a trail, right. Your trail dips down to cross the ravine, and once across, turns sharply left to marker **3**, right. The large boulders seen from here are schists, composed of 12 to 15 different types of minerals—a relatively large number. (In comparison, Sierra granite contains only three to five different minerals.) The colored blotches on the boulders

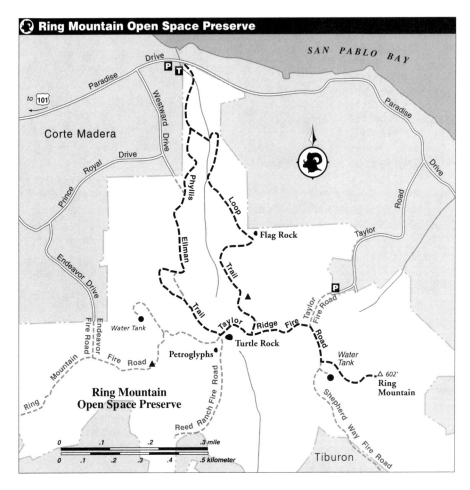

are lichens, composite plants containing both a fungus and an alga.

Out in the open, you reach marker **4**. Just beyond it, at an unsigned junction, the trail forks. Here you stay right and climb over rocky ground. Nearing the seasonal creek, you come to marker **5**.

At a T-junction just ahead, you turn left and climb to a junction, where the trail that forked left just beyond marker **4** rejoins your route. Ahead on the right is marker **6**, which refers to birds found in the preserve, including raptors and songbirds, and also to the large rock formation, described as "a gigantic Indian warrior" standing guard on the hill to your left.

Now you climb gently across an open hillside, heading for an obvious watercourse

and marker **7**. Growing here are moisture-loving plants such as giant chain fern, rushes, and wax myrtle.

The source of Ring Mountain's creeks and wet areas is rainwater that cannot penetrate deeply into the rocky soil on the mountain's upper reaches, and instead emerges as seeps and springs.

Turning left, you cross a wet area via two plank bridges, and then climb a set of wooden steps that take you out of the watercourse. At an unsigned T-junction you turn right, soon reaching a fork, where you bear left and continue climbing. About 100 feet past the fork is marker **8**, for an oak grove on the right.

Continuing straight on the main trail, you pass a four-way junction and then

---

**Oaks — How Mighty?**

Oaks may seem invincible, but practices such as land clearing, firewood cutting, and over-grazing are threatening California's oak woodlands. Restoration projects, combined with public awareness, may help reverse this trend.

---

reach a junction marked by a blank trail post. Here a trail continues straight, but you turn right, into a grotto of bay trees strewn with rock boulders, where marker **9** awaits. This grotto is called a tree island, and like a real island it stands in marked contrast to its surroundings — a shady shelter for birds, small mammals, and insects in the midst of wind-swept, sun-baked fields. Within the grotto, the trail becomes indistinct, but keeping marker **9** on your left, you go about 30 feet past it, turn left, and continue uphill.

Leaving the grotto behind, you merge with the trail that went straight at the blank trail post. About 75 feet ahead, you pass a trail on the right, and your route bends left. At a fork marked by a trail post, you bear left, pass marker **10**, left, and continue winding your way uphill toward a grove of bay and coast live oak. When you reach the grove, turn right.

As you emerge from the grove, a fabulous scene greets you — the San Francisco skyline, the Marin Headlands, Sausalito, Richardson Bay, and the towers of the Golden Gate Bridge. Before the glaciers melted at the end of the last Ice Age, San Francisco Bay and San Pablo bays, also visible from the mountain, were a river valley, and the coastline was 20 to 30 miles farther west. As you walk downhill, passing marker **11**, right, the view improves, as Alcatraz and the Bay Bridge come into view.

About 75 feet past marker **11**, you reach a four-way junction at the Taylor Ridge Fire Road, around the 1-mile point. Ahead is a short path leading to a boulder sometimes used by rock climbers for practice. Turning left onto the fire road, you begin to gain elevation as you near the mountain's summit, a high point to the southeast.

At a T-junction with a paved road, you turn right, following this road for about 150 yards and then bearing left onto a dirt-and-gravel road interrupted by stretches of broken pavement. The summit of Ring Mountain (602') is in a grove of trees just left of the road, which dead-ends in a broad, gravelly area. From this dead end, a path heads south to a viewpoint. When you are ready, retrace your route to the junction of the Loop Trail and the Taylor Ridge Fire Road.

Continuing west on the fire road, you drop steeply over rough ground and then reach a junction where a road branches left. Here you continue straight, and in about 75 feet come to a four-way junction marked by a trail post missing its number — it should be marker **12**. From this junction, the Phyllis Ellman Trail, your return route, goes right, and a trail to a rock inscribed with petroglyphs heads left. Turtle Rock, just east

---

**Survivor Tactics**

Plants, being fixed in one place, use a variety of strategies to disperse their seeds. For example, birds eat berries and then deposit the seeds after digestion. Other animals that depend on seeds for food often drop some during transport. The wind also spreads the seeds of many plants. To survive, plants must develop defenses against being eaten by insects, birds, and other animals. These defenses can involve toxic chemical agents, like tannins, and physical barriers, like spines. Oaks are well defended, but their seeds, acorns, are eagerly consumed by mammals and birds.

Plants use chemical inhibitors to prevent premature sprouting: only when enough rain falls will the inhibitors leach out, thereby allowing the seed to sprout at the right time.

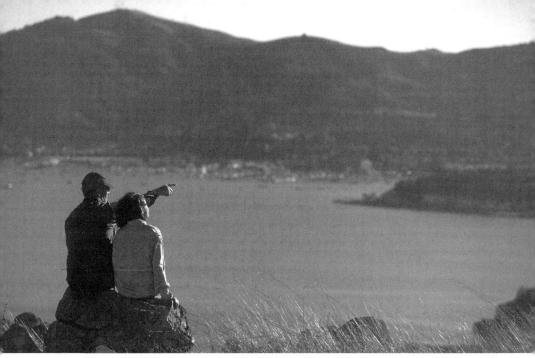

Ring Mountain: view south across Richardson Bay to the Marin Headlands.

of the junction, looks like it has a turtle crawling up it. The exact age of the ancient petroglyphs is uncertain, but they resemble ones in the Sierra that are two to three thousand years old.

From the four-way junction, descend the Phyllis Ellman Trail, a single track heading northwest. In about 100 yards, you come to marker **13**, right, indicating the tree island ahead and right. Trees can grow on this site because the rock is fractured, allowing roots to penetrate until they find water.

About 100 feet ahead, at a trail post, you turn left. The trail gains a little elevation and then levels, taking you across a rocky hillside in the heart of the serpentine belt. Now descending, you pick your way over rocky ground to marker **14**. This is the area to look for rare plants, such as Marin dwarf flax, Tiburon paintbrush, serpentine reedgrass, and the Tiburon Mariposa lily, a late-May bloomer that grows nowhere else in the world.

Level for a while, the trail curves right and then drops on a moderate grade. At a junction where a trail merges from the right, you bear left and continue downhill. In about 100 yards, at the next junction, a sign with an arrow prompts you to turn right.

Marker **15**, right, refers to soap plant, identified by its long, wavy leaves. The bulb of soap plant had several uses for Native Americans: it yields a cleansing substance when crushed; it contains toxins that stun fish; and, when detoxified by cooking, it can be eaten. Soap plant, which blooms from May through July, carries its flowers aloft on tall stalks, but these don't open until shade falls in the late afternoon.

Before you reach the next line of vegetation, turn sharply left at a junction, where a path goes straight to the creek bed. After a leftward bend, the trail reaches a four-way junction just shy of a tree-lined ravine. Here you make a hard right and then work your way downhill on a moderate grade, aided in places by steps, to marker **16**, right.

Nearing the seasonal creek again, your route bends left, winding downhill over rocky ground and passing a trail, right. Close the loop where the Loop Trail heads right, then retrace your route to the parking area.

# TRIP8 China Camp State Park

| | |
|---|---|
| **Distance** | 4.9 miles, Semi-loop |
| **Hiking Time** | 2 to 3 hours |
| **Elevation Gain/Loss** | ±400 feet |
| **Difficulty** | Moderate |
| **Trail Use** | Mountain biking allowed |
| **Best Times** | All year |
| **Agency** | CSP |
| **Recommended Map** | *China Camp State Park* (CSP) |

**HIGHLIGHTS** This semi-loop starts at China Camp Point and uses the Village, Shoreline, Oak Ridge, and Peacock Gap trails, and the Miwok Fire Trail, to explore the western part of this fine park. Except for a short but rigorous climb up the Miwok Fire Trail, most of the route is in the shade, making it pleasant on a warm day. Most of the park's signed and maintained trails are open to hikers, bicyclists, and equestrians. Be sure not to miss the visitor center, open daily 10 A.M. to 5 P.M., in the village just downhill from China Camp Point.

**DIRECTIONS** From Highway 101 northbound in San Rafael, take the N. San Pedro Road exit, which is also signed for the Marin County Civic Center and China Camp State Park. After exiting, bear right, following the lane marked EAST. After 0.3 mile you join N. San Pedro Road.

Go another 5.1 miles to the China Camp Village entrance, left, and a large paved parking area. If this parking area is full, continue downhill 0.1 mile into the village, which has a large dirt parking area and a self-registration station.

From Highway 101 southbound in San Rafael, take the N. San Pedro Road exit, which is also signed for the Marin County Civic Center and China Camp State Park. After 0.2 mile, you come to a stop sign. Turn left, go 0.1 mile to a stoplight, and turn left again, onto N. San Pedro Road. At 0.3 mile, the exit ramp from Highway 101 northbound joins on your right. From here, follow the directions from the second paragraph, above.

**FACILITIES/TRAILHEAD** A visitor center with displays on the Chinese shrimp industry is in the village, along with picnic tables, restrooms, phone, and water. The snack bar and fishing pier here are open weekends only. Maps are for sale from a coin-operated machine at the visitor center. There are restrooms near the trailhead, which is on the northwest corner of the upper parking area.

China Camp State Park takes its name from a Chinese fishing village that flourished here during the late 1800s, one of 26 on San Francisco Bay. The early 1900s saw the passage of a series of restrictive laws, including bans on bag nets, peak-sea-

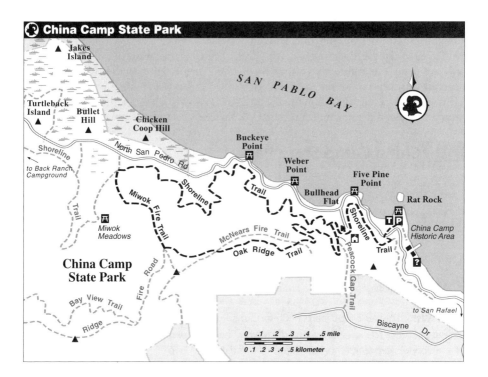

China Camp State Park

**Songbirds**

Some of the songbirds found in the park's wooded areas include dark-eyed juncos, warblers, kinglets, chickadees, and towhees. These, in turn, may attract predators such as Cooper's and sharp-shinned hawks.

son fishing, and even possessing dried shrimp. These laws effectively shut down the Chinese shrimping industry, and the village soon suffered a precipitous decline.

Take the Village Trail about 100 feet to a fork and bear left. When you reach North San Pedro Road, cross it and regain the Village Trail, which soon merges with the Shoreline Trail. Coast live oak, madrone, black oak, and California bay grow along here.

The trail follows a mostly level track until it descends to park headquarters, where you will find a ranger station, picnic tables, and water. Maps are usually available from a self-serve bin at the ranger station.

From the ranger station, cross a paved road and continue on the Shoreline Trail, climbing gently via several switchbacks. Meeting the Peacock Gap Trail, left, your route continues straight on the Shoreline Trail, then zigzags through the forest. Around 1 mile, the route rounds the end of a ridge and begins a gentle descent, soon reaching level ground.

Near the head of a gully spanned by a bridge, you pass an unofficial trail going uphill and left. Your route swings right, crosses the bridge, and jogs left. At the next gully, you cross another bridge, turn right, and begin to climb on a gentle grade. Breaking out of the trees, you have the best views yet of San Pablo Bay.

**Burning as Stimulus**

Park personnel use prescribed burns to remove nonnative plants such as French broom and star thistle, and to stimulate native grasses and other native plants.

Leaving the clearing and returning briefly to forest, you cross another bridge over a deep gully, and then, in a few paces, come into the open again.

Nearly at sea level, with a marsh sporting cattails just ahead, you reach a fork and bear left. Ahead is a four-way junction, where you turn left on the Miwok Fire Trail, a dirt road. Climb steadily for about 0.5 mile—the first part steep, the rest moderate and gentle—over eroded ground, with only patches of shade. Watch for bicycles careening downhill!

Around 3 miles, turn left on the Oak Ridge Trail, entering a cool, shady forest. Uphill and right is a ridge that slopes gradually down to meet your trail. Soon you merge with the McNears Fire Trail and in about 60 feet reach a fork. Here, at a low point on the ridge, the McNears Fire Trail veers left, but you bear right, still on the Oak Ridge Trail.

Now on the south side of the ridge, the vista expands dramatically, taking in San Francisco, Angel Island, and Mt. Diablo.

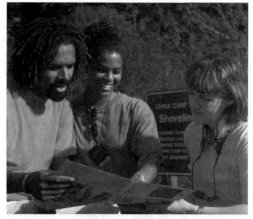

Hikers check map near the junction of the Miwok Fire Trail and the Shoreline Trail.

Descend on a gentle grade to cross the McNears Fire Trail again and continue straight, still on the Oak Ridge Trail. A switchbacking descent in dense forest brings you to the end of the Oak Ridge Trail. Here you continue straight, now on the Peacock Gap Trail. Close the loop at the Shoreline Trail, turn right, and retrace your route to the parking area.

# TRIP9 Muir Woods National Monument: Redwood Creek

| | |
|---|---|
| **Distance** | 1.9 miles, Loop |
| **Hiking Time** | 1 to 2 hours |
| **Difficulty** | Easy |
| **Trail Use** | Good for kids |
| **Best Times** | All year |
| **Agency** | GGNRA |
| **Recommended Maps** | Muir Woods (GGNPC), Trails of Mt. Tamalpais and the Marin Headlands (Olmsted) |

**HIGHLIGHTS**  Muir Woods, one of the last remaining stands of old-growth coast redwoods anywhere in the world, is a treasure not to be missed. This loop, using the paved Main Trail and the Hillside Trail, takes you among the giant redwoods on both sides of Redwood Creek, the monument's central watercourse, where you will also find other trees, shrubs, and wildflowers associated with a redwood forest. The parking areas and trails are usually crowded on weekends, especially during summer, so visit midweek if you can.

**DIRECTIONS**  From Highway 101 northbound in Mill Valley, take the Highway 1/Mill Valley/Stinson Beach exit. After exiting, stay in the right lane as you go under Highway 101. You are now on Shoreline Highway (Highway 1). About 1 mile from Highway 101, get in the left lane, and, at a stoplight, follow Shoreline Highway as it turns left.

Continue another 2.7 miles to Panoramic Highway and turn right. After 0.8 mile, turn left onto Muir Woods Road. After 1.6 miles, turn right into the main parking area for Muir Woods. If this area is full, there is another about 100 yards southeast on Muir Woods Road.

From Highway 101 southbound in Mill Valley, take the Highway 1 North/Stinson Beach exit. After exiting, bear right, go 0.1 mile to a stop sign, and turn left. You are now on Shoreline Highway (Highway 1). Go 0.5 mile to a stoplight, turn left, and follow the directions in the second paragraph, above.

**FACILITIES/TRAILHEAD**  Just beyond the entrance station are a visitor center with books, maps, and helpful staff, as well as a cafe, a gift shop, restrooms, phone, and water. The trailhead is on the northwest end of the main parking area, just left of the entrance station and visitor center.

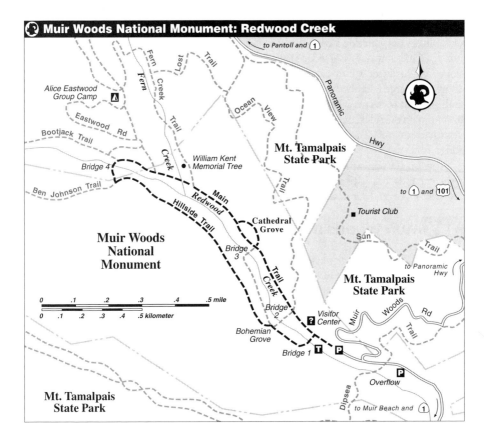

After paying a small entrance fee, head northwest on a level, paved path, passing an information board with history of the park and of the redwood-conservation movement. This path is commonly called the Main Trail, but it is also the continuation of the Bootjack Trail from Mt. Tamalpais State Park.

About 100 feet from the trailhead, you pass a path, right, to the gift shop and the cafe, which are open 9 A.M. to 5 P.M. Redwood Creek, which gathers water from several tributaries cascading down the south side of Mt. Tamalpais, is on your left.

Approaching Bridge 1, you get your first look at the giant coast redwoods that fill the valley, making this such a special place. Beyond Bridge 1, you stay on the east side of Redwood Creek. Rest benches here and there invite you to sit and contemplate the sights and sounds of this ancient forest, which, on weekends, may be full of visitors. On a quiet, fog-shrouded mornings, however, your only companions may be feathered ones. About 70 species of birds, including the secretive spotted owl, have been observed in Muir Woods.

A junction with the Ocean View Trail, right, serves as a meeting place for ranger-led walks; times for these are posted near the entrance station. Continuing straight, you enter a realm dominated by giants. Dense stands of redwoods create a shady environment suited to only certain other types of plants, and the thick carpet of needles and twigs deposited each winter, called duff, makes it hard for seeds to sprout. Coast redwoods are often joined by other plants suited to the damp, shady environment. Among these are California bay, tanbark oak, hazelnut, thimbleberry, evergreen huckleberry, and western sword fern.

When you reach Bridge 2, where a vending machine has maps for sale, look across the creek: there stands the monument's tallest tree—253 feet—and, at 13 feet in

---

### Redwood Creek

Redwood Creek has runs of coho salmon and steelhead trout, both listed as threatened species under federal law. Channeled in the 1930s to prevent flooding, the creek is now being allowed to resume its winding course.

---

diameter, its most stout. Stay on the east side of the creek for now; you'll visit the west side later. Beyond the bridge, the canyon holding Redwood Creek narrows, with steep hillsides rising both left and right.

Passing Bridge 3, left, you enter Cathedral Grove, where the path divides around this fantastic stand of trees. Here, on May 19, 1945, delegates who came to San Francisco to form the United Nations met to honor Franklin Roosevelt, who had just died. Some of the trees here show scars from fire; others have large, grotesque lumps called burls.

The coast redwood, a species that first appeared some 250 million years ago, has developed strategies to withstand natural disasters, including fire. These include thick, insulating bark, and sprouting from burls, or clusters of dormant buds.

Passing the Fern Creek Trail, right, you cross a stone bridge over Fern Creek, and then, in a couple of hundred feet, pass the Camp Eastwood Trail, right. Several hundred yards ahead, your path curves left, and a single-track trail, the Bootjack Trail, heads right, into Mt. Tamalpais State Park. After about 100 feet, you come to Bridge 4, which takes you across Redwood Creek.

Climb moderately on the rocky trail to a T-junction, where you turn left on the Hillside Trail and continue to climb, aided now by wooden steps. The grade soon eases, and you follow a narrow trail, sliced from a steep hillside, into a ravine that holds a tributary of Redwood Creek. After crossing a plank bridge, the route swings sharply left, finds a short stretch of level ground, and then descends on a gentle grade.

---

### Fallen Giant

Near the end of your hike, when you reach a fallen tree, sawed to clear a path for the trail, take a minute to imagine yourself nearby on April 6, 1993, when this 419-year-old giant, its roots loosened by winter rains, came crashing down. Actually, the tree had begun to lean several centuries ago, but it responded by growing more wood on the supporting side. Thus its cross-section is an oval instead of a circle.

In places, parts of the complex, but shallow, root system underlying a redwood-forest floor are exposed. Redwoods lack a main tap root, and instead stabilize themselves by interlocking their roots with those of other trees.

Your route stays well above Redwood Creek, in places squeezing between two or more giant trees, then descends to a four-way junction and, just beyond it, Bridge 2. Here you turn right, staying on the west side of the creek and walking through Bohemian Grove, another stand of extraordinary trees, some of them fire-scarred. Fire is part of the natural cycle, and is often beneficial. The National Park Service now recognizes the importance of fire and since 1997 has conducted prescribed burns in Muir Woods.

At Bridge 1 the route crosses the creek and closes the loop. Here you turn right and retrace your route to the parking area.

# TRIP 10 Muir Woods National Monument: Tourist Club

|  |  |
|---|---|
| **Distance** | 3.8 miles, Loop |
| **Hiking Time** | 2 to 4 hours |
| **Elevation Gain/Loss** | ±1250 feet |
| **Difficulty** | Moderate |
| **Best Times** | All year |
| **Agency** | CSP, GGNRA |
| **Recommended Map** | *Trails of Mt. Tamalpais and the Marin Headlands* (Olmsted) |

**HIGHLIGHTS** This loop, which uses the Main, Fern Creek, Lost, Ocean View, Panoramic, Redwood, Sun, and Dipsea trails, climbs high above Redwood Creek, visiting Mt. Tamalpais State Park and also the grounds of the Bavarian-style Tourist Club before plunging back into the redwoods. Congressman William Kent and his wife, Elizabeth, purchased the large grove of redwoods bordering Redwood Creek in 1905, and then granted it to the federal government with the understanding that it be named after John Muir.

Along the way you will walk beside giant redwoods, enjoy views of the Pacific Ocean — or the fog bank that shrouds it — and test your mettle on a stretch of a famous footrace route from Mill Valley to Stinson Beach.

**DIRECTIONS** From Highway 101 northbound in Mill Valley, take the Highway 1/Mill Valley/Stinson Beach exit. After exiting, stay in the right lane as you go under Highway 101. You are now on Shoreline Highway (Highway 1). About 1 mile from Highway 101, get in the left lane, and, at a stoplight, follow Shoreline Highway as it turns left.

Continue another 2.7 miles to Panoramic Highway and turn right. After 0.8 mile, turn left onto Muir Woods Road. After 1.6 miles, turn right into the main parking area for Muir Woods. If this area is full, there is another about 100 yards southeast on Muir Woods Road.

From Highway 101 southbound in Mill Valley, take the Highway 1 North/Stinson Beach exit. After exiting, bear right, go 0.1 mile to a stop sign, and turn left. You are now on Shoreline Highway (Highway 1). Go 0.5 mile to a stoplight, turn left, and follow the directions in the second paragraph, above.

**FACILITIES/TRAILHEAD** Just beyond the entrance station are a visitor center with books, maps, and helpful staff, as well as a cafe, a gift shop, restrooms, phone, and water. The trailhead is on the northwest end of the main parking area, just left of the entrance station and visitor center.

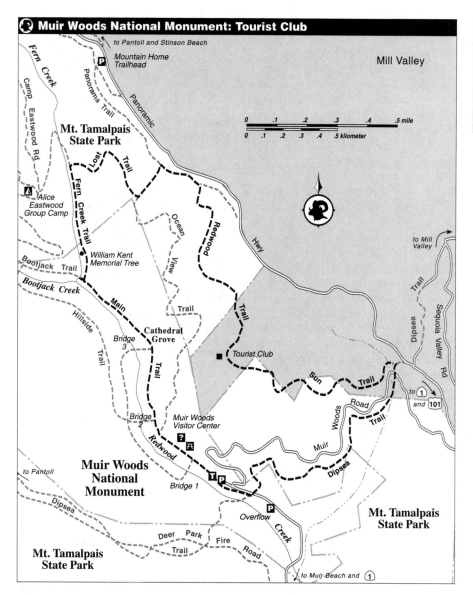

## Muir Woods National Monument: Tourist Club

to Pantoll and Stinson Beach

Mountain Home
Trailhead

Mill Valley

Fern Creek

Camp Eastwood Rd.

Panorama Trail

Panoramic

Mt. Tamalpais
State Park

Lost Trail

Fern Creek Trail

Alice
Eastwood
Group Camp

William Kent
Memorial Tree

Bootjack Trail

Bootjack Creek

Main

Hillside

Ocean View

Redwood

Trail

Hwy

Trail

to Mill
Valley

Dipsea Trail

Sequoia Valley Rd

Trail

Cathedral
Grove

Bridge
3

Trail

Tourist Club

Sun Trail

Trail

to ① and ⑩①

Bridge
2

Muir Woods
Visitor Center

Redwood

Road

Woods Trail

Muir

to Pantoll

Muir Woods
National
Monument

Bridge 1

Dipsea

Dipsea

Overflow

Creek

Mt. Tamalpais
State Park

Mt. Tamalpais
State Park

Deer Park

Fire

Trail

Road

to Muir Beach and ①

0   .1   .2   .3   .4   .5 mile
0   .1   .2   .3   .4   .5 kilometer

After paying a small entrance fee, head northwest on a level, paved path, passing an information board with history of the park and of the redwood-conservation movement. This path is commonly called the Main Trail, but it is also the continuation of the Bootjack Trail from Mt. Tamalpais State Park.

About 100 feet from the trailhead, you pass a path, right, to the gift shop and the cafe, which are open 9 A.M. to 5 P.M. Redwood Creek, which gathers water from several tributaries cascading down the south side of Mt. Tamalpais, is on your left.

Approaching Bridge 1, you get your first look at the giant coast redwoods that fill the valley, making this such a special place. Beyond Bridge 1, you stay on the east side of Redwood Creek. Rest benches here and there invite you to sit and contemplate the sights and sounds of this ancient forest, which, on weekends, may be full of visitors.

A junction with the Ocean View Trail, right, serves as a meeting place for ranger-led walks; times for these are posted near the entrance station. Continuing straight, you enter a realm dominated by giants. Dense stands of redwoods create a shady environment suited to only certain other types of plants, and the thick carpet of needles and twigs deposited each winter, called duff, makes it hard for seeds to sprout.

When you reach Bridge 2, where a vending machine has maps for sale, look across the creek: there stands the monument's tallest tree—253 feet—and, at 13 feet in diameter, its most stout. Stay on the east side of the creek. Beyond the bridge, the canyon holding Redwood Creek narrows, with steep hillsides rising both left and right.

Passing Bridge 3, left, you enter Cathedral Grove, where the path divides around this fantastic stand of trees. You come to the Fern Creek Trail, where you turn right, leave the paved path, and get on a dirt trail. With Fern Creek in a narrow canyon on your left, you enter Mt. Tamalpais State Park. A wooden bridge takes you across Fern Creek, and then the trail bends right, passing a set of steps leading down to the creek. The next bridge takes you back across Fern Creek, and a third, parallel to the creek, crosses a gully which holds a seasonal stream.

Soon the trail makes a sharp right-hand switchback and begins to climb. Where the Fern Creek Trail continues straight across a plank bridge nailed to a fallen redwood, at about 1 mile, you go straight on the Lost Trail. After a set of wooden steps, the trail bends left, still rising on a moderate grade. A dramatic change in vegetation marks a transition out of the redwood forest and into the realm of Douglas-fir, canyon oak, and fragrant California bay.

After following a winding course, the trail meets the Ocean View Trail at a T-junction. Turn left and continue climbing on a

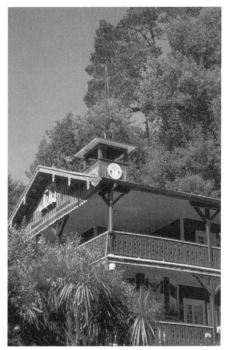

Tourist Club, with Bavarian-style architecture, is on the Redwood Trail, east of Muir Woods.

long, steady grade that changes from gentle to moderate. From the base of a large boulder, a rough path leads uphill and right, but your route curves left, then straightens. After a rising traverse across a steep, open hillside that drops left, you come to a four-way junction.

Turn right onto the Panoramic Trail, which heads southeast just beneath Panoramic Highway. Coming around a bend, you pass a rough path, right, and a trail merging sharply from the left—both unsigned. Ahead, at a signed fork, you veer right on the Redwood Trail and descend. After passing a wet area and negotiating a steep, rocky downhill pitch, you are back among the redwoods, which are smaller, though, than the giants beside Redwood Creek.

A sign marks the boundary of Mt. Tamalpais State Park, and you are now on land owned by the Tourist Club.

**Tourist Club**

The Tourist Club is part of an international conservation organization, founded in 1895 in Vienna, which has approximately 600,000 members in the U.S. and Europe. Immigrants from Germany and Austria founded the club's Bay Area branch in the early 1900s and bought several acres of land next to Muir Woods. The club's collection of colorful Bavarian-style buildings, set amid a Pacific-coastal forest, with a bandstand, a dance floor, and a few palm trees thrown in for good measure, is remarkable. The club is open on weekends year-round, and during the week if the caretaker is available. Hikers are welcome.

The Redwood Trail skirts the upper edge of the club's grounds and joins a dirt access road just past a small shed. Bearing left, you meet the Sun Trail after several hundred feet. Here you turn right and wander through open terrain with great views of the often fog-shrouded ridges and ravines sloping down toward the Pacific Ocean.

The Sun Trail ends at a junction with the Dipsea Trail, which goes straight and also sharply right. Stretching from Mill Valley to Stinson Beach, the Dipsea Trail is the route of a rugged footrace, famous for its pulse-pounding uphills and knee-jarring descents, which has been held nearly every year since 1905. For more information on the race, see the website www.dipsea.org.

Here you turn right and descend over rocky ground, finally reaching Muir Woods Road via several sets of wooden steps. A trail post at about 3 miles directs you across the road to the continuation of the Dipsea Trail. Follow the trail downhill, crossing Camino del Canyon, a dirt road, and then finally meeting Muir Woods Road, which you carefully cross. From here, at the entrance to the overflow parking area, turn right and follow a dirt trail for about 100 yards to the main parking area.

## TRIP 11  Mt. Tamalpais: High Marsh Loop

| | |
|---|---|
| **Distance** | 5.8 miles, Loop |
| **Hiking Time** | 4 to 5 hours |
| **Elevation Gain/Loss** | ±1400 feet |
| **Difficulty** | Difficult |
| **Trail Use** | Leashed dogs |
| **Best Times** | All year |
| **Agency** | Parking, CSP; trails, MMWD |
| **Recommended Map** | *Trails of Mt. Tamalpais and the Marin Headlands* (Olmsted) |

**HIGHLIGHTS** This beautiful and strenuous loop, using the Cataract, High Marsh, Kent, Benstein, and Simmons trails, takes you past a scenic waterfall, beside a freshwater marsh, through areas of chaparral, and into groves of Sargent cypress and forests of Douglas-fir and oak as it explores the rugged canyons and ridges of MMWD lands above Alpine Lake on the north side of Mt. Tamalpais. Cataract Falls are best in winter and early spring

**DIRECTIONS** From Highway 101 northbound in Mill Valley, take the Highway 1/Mill Valley/Stinson Beach exit. After exiting, stay in the right lane as you go under Highway 101. You are now on Shoreline Highway (Highway 1). About 1 mile from Highway 101, get in the left lane, and, at a stoplight, follow Shoreline Highway as it turns left.

Continue another 2.7 miles to Panoramic Highway and turn right. Go 5.4 miles to Pantoll Road, right (across from the Pantoll Campground and Ranger Station). Turn right, and go 1.4 miles to a T-intersection with East Ridgecrest Blvd. and West Ridgecrest Blvd. Across the intersection is a large paved parking area.

From Highway 101 southbound in Mill Valley, take the Highway 1 North/Stinson Beach exit. After exiting, bear right, go 0.1 mile to a stop sign, and turn left. You are now on Shoreline Highway (Highway 1). Go 0.5 mile to a stoplight, turn left, and follow the directions in the second paragraph, above.

**FACILITIES/TRAILHEAD**  There are toilets near the trailhead, which is on the north side of the parking area, near its midpoint.

**Mt. Tamalpais: High Marsh Loop**

**H**ead north on the Cataract Trail, a wide dirt-and-gravel path, passing a faint trail heading right. The large, grassy meadow ahead and right is called Serpentine Swale, named for California's state rock, which is found on the upper reaches of Mt. Tamalpais and elsewhere throughout the state. Serpentine soil, rich in magnesium, makes life difficult for many plants, but some have adapted to it and others thrive in it. Later today, you will pass through a grove of Sargent cypress, a serpentine lover.

The trail descends gently about 100 yards to a fork. Here, the Simmons Trail, used later, goes right, but your route, the Cataract Trail, bends left and crosses a bridge over Cataract Creek, which drains Serpentine Swale and flows into Alpine Lake. Several hundred feet downstream from the bridge, you come to a jumble of big, moss-covered boulders. Although you may see a trail across the creek, stay on the creek's right side and follow the trail through the boulders.

Soon you reach a clearing and another wood bridge, this one over Ziesche Creek, named for Edward Ziesche, secretary of the Tamalpais Club, a hiking group founded around 1880. The route turns left, descends a few wooden steps, and then crosses a bridge over Cataract Creek. Just before you reach a large wood bridge over Cataract Creek, you pass a great tangle of evergreen huckleberry that hangs over the creek.

Passing a trail, left, that crosses Cataract Creek via a large wood bridge, you continue straight. At the edge of a clearing, you meet the Mickey O'Brien Trail, heading sharply right. O'Brien was president of the Tamalpais Conservation Club in the 1920s. Here the you turn right, as the Cataract and Mickey O'Brien trails join for a short distance. Then you follow the Cataract Trail as it branches left and crosses a bridge over a stream.

Skirting a large meadow, left, you soon reach Laurel Dell Road and the Laurel Dell picnic area. Here there are restrooms, a watering trough, and a place to hitch horses. Crossing the road, you pass through the scenic picnic area, located at a bend in Cataract Creek.

The Cataract Trail leaves the picnic area from its west side, with the creek on your left. During winter and spring, a waterfall cascades over the ledge of a rocky cliff, downhill and left. The hillside drops steeply

---

**Two Blues**

The Bay Area has two common "blue" jays, the western scrub-jay and the Steller's jay. A bird of the forest, Steller's jay is a dark bird identified by its black crested head and harsh call. The scrub jay, light blue and gray, favors more open country. Both are often called blue jays, but this name is properly reserved for an Eastern species that is only rarely seen on the West Coast.

---

here, so use caution: you will have a much better and safer view in a few minutes.

At a T-junction, the Cataract Trail turns left, and the High Marsh Trail goes right. Although you will be following the High Marsh Trail from here, you can get a fine view of the waterfall by turning left on the Cataract Trail and walking several hundred feet to a level area near the base of the falls. This route is well shaded, thanks to stands of Douglas-fir, coast live oak, canyon oak, tanbark oak, and California bay.

Now return to the T-junction and go north on the High Marsh Trail, a narrow, single track. Soon you reach a fork where the trail splits temporarily: stay right. At the head of a narrow ravine, the trail turns left, breaks out of the trees, and traverses a steep, grassy hillside beautifully decorated in spring with California poppies, bluedicks, lupine, and mule ears.

A steep climb at about 2 miles brings you to a junction with a short trail to Laurel Dell Road, right. The route now alternates between wooded and open areas, and from one of these clearings, a superb view extends northeast to San Pablo Bay and beyond. Beyond this clearing, the trail descends in a narrow corridor through chaparral, in some places via wooden steps. When the manzanita has berries, you can see why it was given a name that, in Spanish, means "little apples."

You cross a creek bed, which may be dry, and then begin a steep climb, passing an unsigned trail heading uphill and right. Giving up hard-won elevation, you drop steeply into a ravine that holds a seasonal creek. The trail fights to maintain a contour, but soon plunges steeply among rocks and small boulders to Swede George Creek, named for a mountain man who once had a cabin in the area.

Now you cross the creek on rocks and follow a rolling course past an unsigned trail, right. About 100 yards from the unsigned trail, you reach an unsigned fork. The Willow Trail descends left, but you stay right and climb on a moderate grade. After topping a ridge, the trail descends to a T-junction. Here, the Cross Country Boys Trail goes right, and your route turns left. High Marsh, a seasonal wetland that may contain a lovely shallow pond, is left.

The route skirts the marsh and soon reaches a four-way junction, at about 4 miles. You turn right on the Kent Trail and begin climbing. As you gain elevation via steps and nicely graded switchbacks, the hodge-podge of trees and shrubs gives way to a forest of Douglas-fir. Now the trail, rocky and in places indistinct, runs parallel to a stream bed, which is downhill and left.

After more climbing, the Cross Country Boys Trail, unsigned here, merges from the right, as does another, fainter trail a few paces ahead. Out of the trees once again, you cross a manzanita barren.

Crossing a rocky rib, you descend moderately to a lovely stream, the headwaters of Swede George Creek. Reaching a T-junction at Potrero Meadows, you turn right, cross the bridged stream, and arrive at a picnic area. Here you turn left and follow a dirt-and-gravel road steeply uphill about 100 yards to a T-junction with Laurel Dell Road.

Turn left and descend gently for about 150 feet to a junction with the Benstein Trail. Here you turn right and climb steeply on a single track. Soon you are climbing almost entirely on serpentine (which can be slippery when wet), interspersed with dirt and gravel sections. The trees here, which appear stunted and spindly, are Sargent cypress, lovers of serpentine soil. Sargent cypress, found in the Coast Ranges of California, was

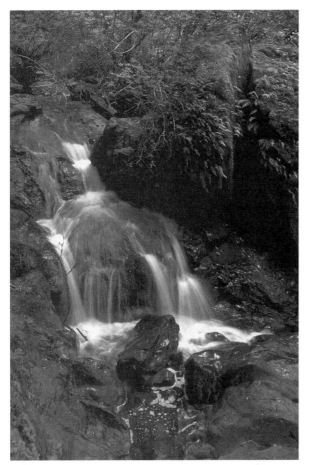

Cataract Falls, best in winter and spring, is near junction of Cataract and High Marsh trails.

---

**The Oakland Star Tulip**

The manzanita barren is a good place to look for the Oakland star tulip, which has upright bowls of white, three-petaled flowers with lavender points between the petals. This wildflower, a serpentine lover, is on a watch list for plants of limited distribution.

---

named for Charles Sprague Sargent, who founded the Arnold Arboretum at Harvard and also wrote 14 volumes on the trees of North America.

At a fork in the route, you turn sharply right, head for open ground, and then climb through forest to a ridgetop. The moderate grade changes to steep as you near the top of a ridge, but once across it, the trail descends gently to a junction with Rock Spring–Lagunitas Road. Bear right on the road and follow it downhill about 100 yards to a junction beside the upper reaches of Ziesche Creek.

Veer right on the single-track Benstein Trail and follow it to a junction marked by a trail post. Stay on the Benstein Trail by turning right, then descending some wooden steps. The trail skirts Serpentine Swale, and after a few switchbacks reaches a T-junction with the Simmons Trail. Turn left, cross the headwaters of Cataract Creek, and about 100 feet from the creek, you reach the Cataract Trail. Here you bear left and retrace your route to the parking area.

## TRIP 12 Mt. Tamalpais: South Side Ramble

| | |
|---|---|
| **Distance** | 7.1 miles, Semi-loop |
| **Hiking Time** | 4 to 5 hours |
| **Elevation Gain/Loss** | ±1100 feet |
| **Difficulty** | Difficult |
| **Best Times** | All year |
| **Agency** | Parking, CSP; trails CSP, MMWD |
| **Recommended Map** | *Trails of Mt. Tamalpais and the Marin Headlands* (Olmsted) |

**HIGHLIGHTS** This semi-loop route, using the Hogback, Matt Davis, Nora, Rock Spring, and Bootjack trails, starts across Panoramic Highway from Mountain Home and takes you past two other Mt. Tamalpais landmarks, West Point Inn and Mountain Theater. Along the way, you will explore the mountain's south side, which alternates between chaparral and forest, with some attractive stands of coast redwoods. Although the fire roads on this side of the mountain are popular with mountain bicyclists, this route stays mostly on single-track trails, which are closed to bicycles.

**DIRECTIONS** From Highway 101 northbound in Mill Valley, take the Highway 1/Mill Valley/Stinson Beach exit. After exiting, stay in the right lane as you go under Highway 101. You are now on Shoreline Highway (Highway 1). About 1 mile from Highway 101, get in the left lane, and, at a stoplight, follow Shoreline Highway as it turns left.

Continue another 2.7 miles to Panoramic Highway and turn right. Go 2.6 miles to a parking area, left, just opposite the Mountain Home Inn. If this lot is full, as it may be on nice weekends, there is an overflow parking area 0.1 mile back (southeast) on Panoramic Highway

From Highway 101 southbound in Mill Valley, take the Highway 1 North/Stinson Beach exit. After exiting, bear right, go 0.1 mile to a stop sign, and turn left. You are now on Shoreline Highway (Highway 1). Go 0.5 mile to a stoplight, turn left, and follow the directions in the second paragraph, above.

It is also possible to park along the start of Gravity Car Grade, just north of the main parking area, but this dirt road is often deeply rutted and may damage your car. To find Gravity Car Grade, continue northwest on Panoramic Highway about 60 feet past the entrance to the main parking area. Turn right, go 75 feet, passing a private gravel driveway, right. At a fork, bear right again, onto Gravity Car Grade, a dirt road. (The left-hand fork is a fire-station access road: do not block it!) Park along the side of the road.

**FACILITIES/TRAILHEAD** There are water, phone, and toilets in the parking area. Food and lodging are available at Mountain Home Inn, just across Panoramic Highway from the parking area. The trailhead is on the north end of the main parking area.

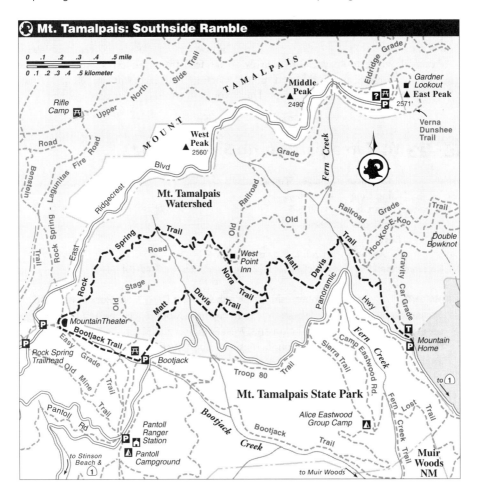

Carefully cross Panoramic Highway, turn left, and continue north for about 60 feet to a paved road that branches right. This is the access road to the Throckmorton Ridge fire station. Follow this road uphill, veering left as you pass first a private driveway and then the start of Gravity Car Grade, a dirt road, both right.

Continuing uphill toward the fire station on a gentle grade, you enter MMWD lands. When you reach the station, you go around its left side and begin a moderate climb on a dirt road, called the Hogback Trail on the Olmsted map and the Throckmorton Trail on an upcoming trail post. This area contains a preview of some of the trees and shrubs commonly found on Mt. Tamalpais, including Douglas-fir, California bay, madrone, chamise, coyote brush, evergreen huckleberry, bush poppy, and several varieties of manzanita.

Passing a dirt-and-gravel road that joins from the left, you soon circle around the right side of a water tank and then reach a junction. Here the Hogback (Throckmorton) Trail continues steeply uphill, but your route, the single-track Matt Davis Trail, named for an early Mt. Tam trail builder and member of the Tamalpais Conservation Club, veers left and climbs a set of wooden steps.

Now you enter a brushy, overgrown area of trees and shrubs. These thickets soon give way to a forest of mostly tanbark oak and madrone. The trail now maintains a contour on the edge of a canyon, left. After a wet winter, this canyon, which holds Fern Creek, may be filled with rushing water, its sound a pleasant accompaniment to your footfalls. Coast redwoods rise from the canyon.

Soon you reach an unsigned junction, right, with the Hoo-Koo-E-Koo Trail. This odd name was bestowed by a member of the Tamalpais Conservation Club to honor an Indian tribe that was supposed to have lived nearby. Here you continue straight, and after about 150 feet reach a wood bridge that crosses Fern Creek. After crossing the bridge, you turn left and begin a moderate climb that soon eases and then levels. Areas of chaparral give you the chance to study plants such as chinquapin, manzanita, chaparral pea, yerba santa, and dwarf interior live oak.

Gaining elevation again and crossing a few seasonal creeks which may dampen the trail, you can just barely see the buildings of West Point Inn through the trees uphill and

left. With Laguna Creek left and downhill, you come to a junction marked by a trail post, where the route forks. The Matt Davis Trail heads left across a bridge over the creek, but your route, the Nora Trail, goes straight and begins a relentless climb via switchbacks to West Point Inn.

Soon the trail turns left, crosses Laguna Creek on a wooden bridge, and then veers right and resumes its uphill course, steep in places, through a forest of spindly redwoods. As you get farther from the creek, the redwoods give way to tanbark oak, toyon, huckleberry, and poison oak. Dark-eyed juncos—small black-headed birds with a pink bill and white along the sides of their tails—may be flitting through the trees in noisy flocks.

A clearing with picnic tables and a water fountain signals your arrival at West Point Inn, a wonderful place to stop, rest, and enjoy the view. Restrooms are on the Inn's east side; find them by walking through the covered deck area.

**West Point Inn**

From the deck West Point Inn, you have fine views that range from Mt. Diablo to the Pacific Ocean. Drinks and snacks are available when the Inn is open. Rustic overnight accommodations are available here at $25 per person per night for adults, $12 for children under 18, free for children under 5. For reservations, call (415) 646-0702, Tuesday through Friday, 11 A.M. to 7 P.M.

To resume hiking, follow Old Railroad Grade uphill, around the west side of the inn. After about 125 feet, turn left onto the Rock Spring Trail, a single track, and follow it on a level grade through a corridor of chaparral. At about 2 miles, you step across Spike Buck Creek, only a foot or so wide, and then begin to gain elevation over rocky, eroded ground.

Soon you reach a junction, right, with the Alice Eastwood Trail. The trail name honors noted botanist Alice Eastwood

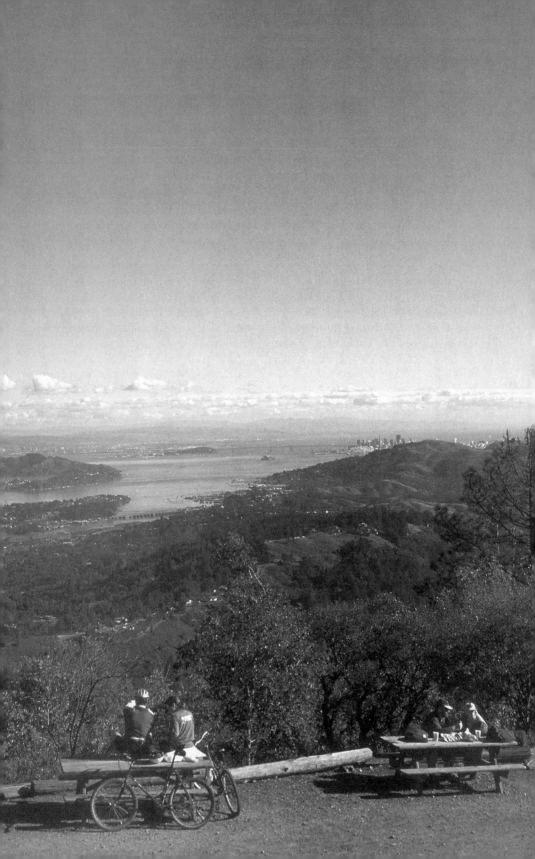

(1859–1953), who for 57 years was curator of botany at the California Academy of Sciences. The naming of Eastwood manzanita, a local species, and the designation of Camp Alice Eastwood, which lies just north of Muir Woods, were two more honors bestowed upon the woman whom author Dorothy L. Whitnah called "the patron saint" of Mt. Tamalpais.

Continuing straight on the Rock Spring Trail, you walk on the edge of a steep drop-off, left, high above Old Stage Road. After crossing Rattlesnake Creek on rocks, you follow the trail as it bends left and begins a gentle, then moderate, ascent. (Rattlesnakes are found on Mt. Tamalpais and have been seen in this area.)

The route traverses an outcrop of gray-green serpentine, then passes a seasonal creek, bends left, and enters a wooded area. Just as you emerge from the trees, you may notice a rock bearing a plaque with the inscription: TO JOHN M. COLIER, A LOVER OF NATURE. Colier, an eccentric Scot and one of the early Mt. Tam trail builders, has two features on the mountain's north side named for him, a spring and a trail.

The trail descends, crosses more seasonal creeks, and then climbs past a rest bench to a fork. Here the Rock Spring Trail goes right, but you continue straight, passing two water fountains, left, at the edge of the Mountain Theater.

Just past the fountains, turn left and walk down a series of stone steps, toward the stage area. Once at the level of the stage, continue behind it. When you are directly behind the center of the stage, you turn left and descend a few more steps and then walk down a path that connects to the Bootjack Trail. About 150 feet from the back of the stage, you reach a T-junction with the Bootjack Trail. (Restrooms are about 100 yards uphill and right.)

Here you turn left and follow the Bootjack Trail as it switchbacks downhill on

### Mountain Theater

Dramatic productions have been given almost every summer since 1913 on Mt. Tamalpais, except during wartime, most of them at Mountain Theater, a large amphitheater with stone seats. Most of the construction on this impressive venue, involving about 5000 massive stones moved into position by cranes and derricks, was done during the 1930s by the Civilian Conservation Corps.

a moderate grade, past little streams that gather to form the headwaters of Redwood Creek. Continuing downhill through a small ravine, you finally emerge from the forest into a grassy area dotted with California poppies, blue-eyed grass, and false lupine. A final descent on wooden steps brings you to a T-junction with Old Stage Road, at about 4 miles.

Here you turn right, walk about 40 feet to a paved road, and then turn left. After 50 feet or so, you turn right onto the continuation of the Bootjack Trail, a single track. Now, at first with the aid of a few wooden steps, you pursue a moderate downhill grade through forest, with the creek you have been following since just below the Mountain Theater on your right. A short descent puts you at the Bootjack picnic area, where trails sprout in all directions.

From here, both the Bootjack Trail to Muir Woods and the Matt Davis Trail to the Pantoll Campground head right. Your route, the Matt Davis Trail to Mountain Home, a single track, goes sharply left. Alternating between sun and shade, the trail finds a rolling course over ridges and into gullies, including one that holds bridged Rattlesnake Creek. Crossing Spike Buck Creek via a bridge, you contour across a ridge and then enter the canyon holding Laguna Creek. Close the loop at a T-junction with the Nora Trail, then turn right and retrace your route to the parking area.

West Point Inn is a popular spot on the south side of Mt. Tamalpais.

# TRIP **13** Pine Mountain

| | |
|---:|:---|
| **Distance** | 4.7 miles, Out-and-back |
| **Hiking Time** | 2 to 3 hours |
| **Elevation Gain/Loss** | ±1000 feet |
| **Difficulty** | Moderate |
| **Trail Use** | Mountain biking allowed, Leashed dogs |
| **Best Times** | All year |
| **Agency** | MMWD |
| **Recommended Map** | *Trail Map of Mt. Tamalpais and the Marin Headlands* (Olmsted) |

**HIGHLIGHTS**  This out-and-back route, using Pine Mountain Road and a short trail atop Pine Mountain to its summit, takes you to one of the best vantage points in the Bay Area, where your efforts on a clear day will be rewarded by fantastic views. Pine Mountain's name refers to a nearby grove of bishop pines — a coastal, two-needled species.

Along the way, plant lovers will stay busy identifying a variety of trees and shrubs, some found only on the locally prevalent serpentine soil. This area is also a favorite with mountain bikers.

**DIRECTIONS**  From Highway 101 northbound, take the San Anselmo exit, also signed for San Quentin, Sir Francis Drake Blvd., and the Richmond Bridge. Stay in the left lane as you exit, toward San Anselmo, crossing over Highway 101. After 0.4 mile you join Sir Francis Drake Blvd., with traffic from Highway 101 southbound merging on your right. From here, it is 3.6 miles to a stoplight at the intersection with Red Hill Ave. From the intersection, stay on Sir Francis Drake Blvd. as it goes straight and then immediately bends left.

At 5.5 miles from Highway 101, in Fairfax, turn left at a stoplight onto Claus Dr., jog left onto Broadway and right onto Bolinas Road, which is heavily used by bicyclists. After 0.4 mile, you pass an intersection with Cascade Dr., where you bear left. (Bolinas Road soon becomes Fairfax – Bolinas Road.) At 3.9 miles, turn left into a gravel parking area. (Fairfax – Bolinas Road to the Azalea Hill parking area may be closed because of high fire danger.)

From Highway 101 southbound, take the Sir Francis Drake/Kentfield exit and follow the directions above.

**FACILITIES/TRAILHEAD**  There are no facilities at the trailhead, which is on the west side of Fairfax–Bolinas Road, about 50 feet north of the parking area.

After carefully crossing Fairfax–Bolinas Road, you walk north about 50 feet from the parking area to a gated dirt road. This is Pine Mountain Road, which brings you, in about 2.3 miles, to within 100 yards or so of the mountain's summit; a short, narrow trail covers the remaining ground. Passing an information board and an old wooden sign, right, you follow the dirt road as it climbs, bends right, and then follows a rolling course atop a broad ridge.

### Serpentine Soil

The underlying rock in this area, serpentine, creates a soil that gives rise to a number of unusual plants. Among these are leather oak, a shrub, and Sargent cypress, an evergreen tree growing here in a stunted form. Leather oak grows in low clumps, its dull green, oval leaves curled under and often spiny. Sargent cypress, found farther up the road, has round, gray-brown cones, and angled strips of gray bark.

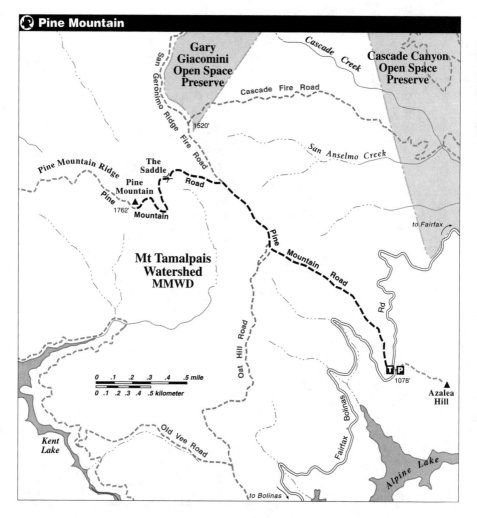

## Pine Mountain

Gary Giacomini Open Space Preserve

Cascade Creek

Cascade Canyon Open Space Preserve

Cascade Fire Road

San Geronimo Ridge Fire Road

1520'

San Anselmo Creek

Pine Mountain Ridge

The Saddle

Pine Mountain

Pine

1762'  Mountain

Road

to Fairfax

Pine

Mountain  Road

Mt Tamalpais Watershed MMWD

Oat Hill Road

Rd

0  .1  .2  .3  .4  .5 mile
0  .1  .2  .3  .4  .5 kilometer

T P

1078'

Azalea Hill

Fairfax–Bolinas

Old Vee Road

Kent Lake

Alpine Lake

to Bolinas

Now on rocky ground, you climb on a gentle and then moderate grade past a few pines, stands of manzanita, chinquapin, and chaparral pea, and a dense thicket of oak—some of the trees are the dwarf form of interior live oak, and others are a hybrid variety. The grade eases, and as you crest a high point, you can see The Saddle, a windy gap between Pine Mountain and an unnamed peak to its northeast.

Dropping slightly, you soon pass Oat Hill Road, left, at about 1 mile. Now on a moderate descent, you may just be able to make out the summit of Mt. St. Helena, perched on the border of Sonoma, Napa,

and Lake counties, to the north. Gaining elevation once again, you begin to see a few Sargent cypress trees, the advance guard of a large forest that blankets a flat expanse to the north of Pine Mountain.

Now you reach a junction where Pine Mountain Road turns sharply left, and San Geronimo Ridge Road goes straight. (To extend the trip, follow San Geronimo Ridge Road northeast through a dwarf Sargent cypress forest to Gary Giacomini Open Space Preserve.)

Following Pine Mountain Road, here a rocky track, you begin a moderate ascent. As you near The Saddle, flattened grasses

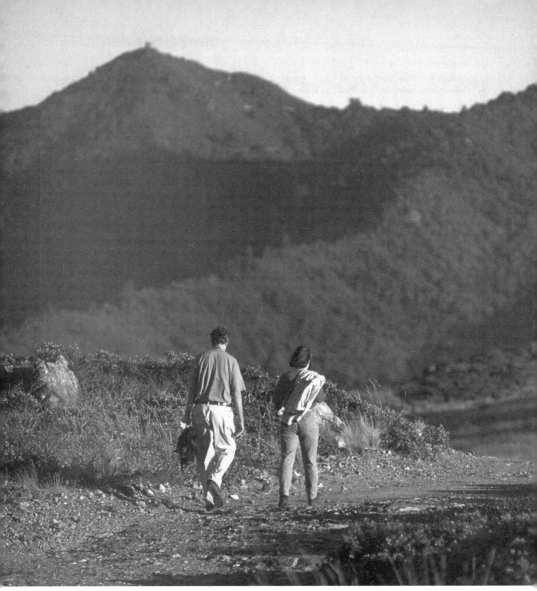

Hikers returning to trailhead along Pine Mountain Road enjoy view of Mt. Tamalpais.

downhill and left attest to the wind's power as it rushes through the gap. From The Saddle, the road swings left and rises on a moderate grade, which soon becomes steep.

The rough and rocky road eventually levels, and now you find a single-track trail, right, signed PINE MOUNTAIN SUMMIT. Turning right, you begin the final push, hemmed in on both sides by chaparral shrubs, among them chamise and silk tassel. Passing a large boulder sporting a metal spike, right, you continue for another 100 feet or so, to where a jumble of rocks forms the summit of Pine Mountain.

From here, the 360-degree panorama may keep you busy for a while, identifying such landmarks as Mt. Tamalpais, Mt. Diablo, the East Bay hills, San Pablo Bay, Big Rock Ridge, Bolinas Ridge, Tomales Bay, and Kent Lake. Without a doubt, this is one of the best vantage points in the Bay Area. After you've enjoyed the scenery, retrace your route to the parking area.

# TRIP 14 Mt. Burdell Open Space Preserve

| | |
|---:|:---|
| **Distance** | 5.6 miles, Semi-loop |
| **Hiking Time** | 3 to 4 hours |
| **Elevation Gain/Loss** | ±1200 feet |
| **Difficulty** | Moderate |
| **Trail Use** | Mountain biking allowed[1], Leashed Dogs |
| **Best Times** | Fall through spring |
| **Agency** | MCOSD |
| **Notes** | [1]Bicycles are not allowed on the Michako Trail, and must instead use the San Carlos, San Marin, and Big Tank fire roads to complete the trip |

**HIGHLIGHTS** This trip, using the San Andreas, Middle Burdell, Cobblestone, San Carlos, and Big Tank fire roads, and the Michako Trail, explores the open grasslands, groves, and high ground of Burdell Mountain, a bulky ridge that rises to 1558 feet and dominates the northeast corner of Marin County. The mountain's southern flank is designated Mt. Burdell Open Space Preserve, and in spring its grassy slopes and oak woodlands come alive with carpets of wildflowers and a chorus of birdsong.

**DIRECTIONS** From Highway 101 in Novato, take the Atherton Ave./San Marin Dr. exit. Go west 2.2 miles on San Marin Dr., turn right onto San Andreas Dr., and go 0.6 mile to where the road makes a sweeping bend to the left. Park on the shoulder and observe the NO PARKING signs.

**FACILITIES/TRAILHEAD** There are no facilities at the trailhead, which is located at the foot of the San Andreas Fire Road, just northeast of the parking area.

At the foot of the San Andreas Fire Road, which is gated and locked, head east on a dirt path and, in about 50 feet, go through a gate and then turn sharply left. After 100 feet or so, you merge with the San Andreas Fire Road, which climbs on a gentle grade. About 75 feet ahead, you pass the Big Tank Fire Road, signed BIG TANK FIRE TRAIL, which you will use on your return. Your route here is part of the Bay Area Ridge Trail, and it is popular with local residents, their horses, and their dogs.

Soon you pass a single-track trail heading left through an opening in a barbed-wire fence. The area behind the fence, also part of Mt. Burdell Open Space Preserve, is designated a Sensitive Wildlife Area, where dogs are not allowed. Now climbing on a moderate grade, you pass another trail, left, signed TO LITTLE TANK FIRE ROAD. About 75 feet farther, you pass through an opening in a fence.

Passing a concrete wall, right, you come to a clearing that affords a view of Burdell Mountain's summit ridge and the communication tower perched just below it. The middle ground of this beautiful scene is composed of rolling hills studded with oaks. The foreground, in spring, may be carpeted with California buttercup and owl's-clover.

Soon you meet a junction, left, with the Dwarf Oak Trail. During and just after the rainy season, the open ground surrounding the junction is a marshy area, home to red-winged blackbirds, western bluebirds, and a wildflower called Douglas meadowfoam, which sports five yellow petals tipped with white. A few hundred feet farther, you pass two unofficial trails, right.

As you continue walking on a gentle downhill course, you are surrounded by open, grassy fields, and rising, rolling hills. The main ridge of Burdell Mountain trends east–west, and is topped with many rounded summits.

Soon the road reaches a low point, then bends left and begins to climb. In a shady

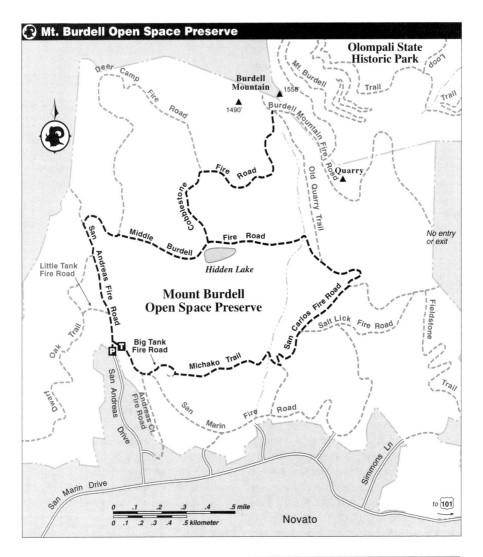

**Mt. Burdell Open Space Preserve**

grove of valley oak, an unofficial trail departs uphill and right, but you continue straight. In about 50 feet, you come to a junction marked by a trail post. Here, the San Andreas Fire Road heads left, and your route, the Middle Burdell Fire Road, also part of the Bay Area Ridge Trail, goes straight.

Now the road, still rising, splits at a fork and then rejoins. In a grove of oak and buckeye, you pass the Deer Camp Fire Road, left. Your route follows a barbed-wire fence and a streambed, both right. Passing a single-track trail, right, you reach level

**Mountain Moniker**

The mountain was named for Galen Burdell, one of the first dentists in San Francisco, who lived with his wife, Mary, just north of here, in what is now Olompali State Park. The couple received the land in 1863 as a wedding present from Mary's father, James Black, one of Marin County's largest landowners.

ground and a T-junction. Here, at about 1.5 miles, the Middle Burdell Fire Road turns right, and the Cobblestone Fire Road, the way to the top of Burdell Mountain, heads left. (If you do not wish to make the approximately 700-foot, 1-mile climb, turn right and pick up the directions below to complete the trip.)

Turning left, you begin climbing on a moderate grade, past grassy fields full of California poppies and bluedicks. The route gets steeper and rockier, but you are rewarded by terrific views west toward Bolinas Ridge, and southeast to San Pablo Bay and the peninsula that holds China Camp State Park. As the grade eases somewhat, you pass through groves of coast live oak and bay, offering welcome shade on a warm day.

Soon you come to a fork where the Deer Camp Fire Road branches left and the Cobblestone Fire Road veers right. Stay right, and as you gain elevation, the communication tower near the summit of Burdell Mountain comes into view. The upper slopes of the mountain host dramatic displays of wildflowers in spring, and this area may be full of wild irises.

Now the road turns north, trying to find the easiest way up Burdell Mountain. The climbing is moderate, with a few level areas to ease your efforts, and some groves of bay and coast live oak for shade. Your view extends south, across the housing developments of Novato, all the way to triple-peaked Mt. Tamalpais.

As you climb, ignore the faint trails that diverge from the main route. The communication tower, once a distant feature, is now to the left and just slightly uphill. There is higher ground ahead, but the true

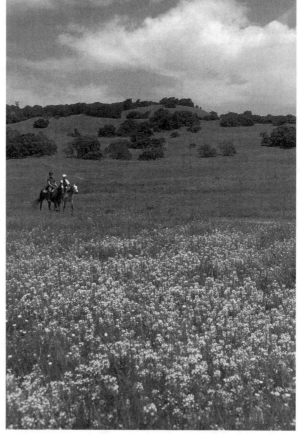

Equestrians ride on the San Andreas Fire Road at Mt. Burdell Open Space Preserve.

summit of Burdell Mountain (1558') is just beyond the preserve boundary, unreachable, on private land.

Nearing the end of the climb, you come to a junction with the Old Quarry Trail, right, and, almost immediately, a T-junction with the Burdell Mountain Ridge Fire Road, a paved road. The preserve's high point lies just ahead, across the road and at

---

**Burdell Mountain Rocks**

A rock wall, reminiscent of New England but actually built by Chinese laborers who worked in a nearby quarry, marks the preserve boundary. The quarry, which produced rocks used for cobblestone streets, is about 0.25 mile southeast on the Burdell Mountain Ridge Fire Road. A rough path heads left from the road, through trees and brush, to the quarry.

**Birds in the Bush**

Passing through a wooded area, you may be startled by a flock of band-tailed pigeons taking flight. These cousins of the urban pigeon are large, beautifully marked birds that favor forested areas, where they often gather in large flocks. When disturbed, they leave their perches singly at first, and then in increasingly larger groups until the whole flock has departed.

the end of a faint single-track trail that heads north and uphill through the grass, which is dotted blue with larkspur.

After exploring Burdell Mountain's high ground, retrace your route to the junction of the Cobblestone and Middle Burdell fire roads. Here, about 3.5 miles, you continue straight, now back on the Middle Burdell Fire Road, and pass Hidden Lake, a large vernal pool on your right, which may hold ducks, egrets, and other water-loving birds. Growing around the lake are at least 10 species of rare plants, including white water-buttercup, pale navarretia, and yellow linanthus.

Your route now heads east over level ground, with open, grassy slopes sweeping uphill on your left. Dipping into and then out of a small wooded ravine, you soon pass a junction, left, with the Old Quarry Trail. Several hundred feet past this junction, the continuation of the Old Quarry Trail heads right, but you continue straight.

Soon you reach a junction and a watering trough for animals, where the Middle Burdell Fire Road continues straight, and your route, the San Carlos Fire Road, turns right. Descending gently for about 75 feet, you come to a gated fence. After passing through the gate, you descend past the Old Quarry Trail, right, and, about 350 feet ahead, pass the Salt Lick Fire Road, left.

Continuing straight and downhill on the San Carlos Fire Road, your route soon veers right, and then makes a sharp left-hand bend. At a four-way junction, where the San Carlos Fire Road continues straight and a faint trace heads left, you turn right onto the Michako Trail, a single track, which is closed to bicycles. Still descending, you pass through an opening in a fence, cross a seasonal creek via some rocks, and then find level ground.

Just past the creek, a faint trail heads left, but you continue straight and soon begin a gentle climb. Now a trail joins sharply from the left, and then you cross another seasonal creek. In about 100 feet, the route forks and you bear left, soon crossing yet another creek, this one the site of a stone hut, once used to protect a freshwater spring. After another 150 feet or so, your route is joined by a trail, right, coming from the previous fork.

Soon you come to a four-way junction, where the Big Tank Fire Road crosses the Michako Trail. Here you continue straight across a grassy field, and, in about 200 feet, come to a watercourse that, when flowing, has a series of delightful miniature waterfalls. Once across this watercourse, you soon reach the next junction, where the Michako Trail merges with the San Marin Fire Road, coming from the left. About 25 feet past this spot, you reach a junction with the Big Tank Fire Road, joining from the right.

From here, you continue straight, now on the Big Tank Fire Road. Now the route forks, with the main road bending left and descending, and a single-track heading right. You bear left, passing a few homes and the San Andreas Court Fire Road, left. Your route now swings right, climbs, and is soon joined by the single-track trail coming from the previous fork.

Now on an easy descent, you pass a landslide area where the road may have disappeared. If so, follow a narrow path next to the embankment, where a creek flows under the roadbed through a culvert. About 100 feet ahead is the junction with the San Andreas Fire Road you passed at the start of this loop. Turn left here and retrace your route to the parking area.

# TRIP 15 Olompali State Historic Park

| | |
|---|---|
| **Distance** | 2.7 miles, Loop |
| **Hiking Time** | 1 to 2 hours |
| **Elevation Gain/Loss** | ±900 feet |
| **Difficulty** | Moderate |
| **Trail Use** | Good for kids |
| **Best Times** | All year |
| **Agency** | CSP |
| **Recommended Map** | *Olompali State Historic Park* (CSP) |

**HIGHLIGHTS** Where else can you walk in the footsteps of Coast Miwok Indians, Jesuit seminarians, and the Grateful Dead rock band? This historic state park sits on the northeastern side of Burdell Mountain, a high ridge of rolling, grassy slopes graced with majestic oaks, and furrowed with deep, densely forested ravines. The Loop Trail, though short, gives you a fine introduction to the landscape, flora, and fauna of Marin County's northeast corner. The south side of Burdell Mountain, a Marin County open space preserve, can be explored by following the description for Trip 14, Mt. Burdell Open Space Preserve on pages 55–58. You can also make a traverse of Burdell Mountain from Olompali to the open space preserve on a trail that connects with the route described below.

**DIRECTIONS** From Highway 101 northbound, north of Novato, go 2.4 miles past the park entrance, which has no access from the northbound lane. At San Antonio Road, carefully turn left, across the southbound lane. Swing into a wide turnout, where San Antonio Road joins Highway 101. Now merge into the southbound lane, go south on Highway 101 for 2.4 miles, and, at the signed entrance road, turn right. Go 0.2 mile to the parking area and a self-registration station.

From Highway 101 southbound, south of Petaluma, go 2.4 miles past San Antonio Rd, turn right at the signed entrance road, and go 0.2 mile to the parking area.

**FACILITIES/TRAILHEAD** A visitor center is in the Burdell Frame House north of parking area. Water and a toilet are available here. Picnic tables and a toilet are beside the parking area and in the garden area. The trailhead is on the west side of the parking area. Learn more about the park's fascinating history at the visitor center, or through the park's educational programs. For more information call (415) 892-3383.

Climb an overgrown dirt road to a T-junction in a grove of California bay. To the right is a 50-foot bridge that crosses Olompali Creek; you will use this later. Turn left and continue uphill on a gentle grade. Where the road bends sharply right, you have a fine view east over the marshy confluence of San Antonio Creek and the Petaluma River, and out across San Pablo Bay. Now your route, the Loop Trail, changes from dirt road to single-track trail and swings left.

**Park Flora**

Olompali State Historic Park has showy displays of spring wildflowers, including blue-eyed grass, winecup clarkia, and Ithuriel's spear. The park's trees include coast live oak, valley oak, blue oak, black locust, madrone, and California buckeye.

The trail continues to zigzag uphill, alternating between gentle and moderate grades. Just shy of 2 miles, you reach a four-way

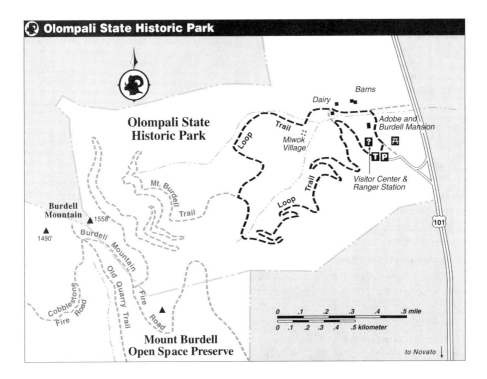

**Olompali State Historic Park**

Olompali State
Historic Park

Barns

Dairy

Trail

Miwok
Village

Loop

Mt. Burdell

Trail

Loop

Trail

Adobe and
Burdell Mansion

Visitor Center &
Ranger Station

Burdell
Mountain   ▲ 1558'

▲
1490'

Burdell

Mountain

Old Quarry Trail

Cobblestone
Fire   Road

Fire   Road

101

Mount Burdell
Open Space Preserve

0    .1    .2    .3    .4    .5 mile

0   .1   .2   .3   .4   .5 kilometer

to Novato

junction. From here, a trail opened in the fall of 1999 leads over Burdell Mountain to Mt. Burdell Open Space Preserve. Your route, the Loop Trail, goes right and begins to descend. After the descent eases and you reach a flat spot in the midst of a dense forest, the trail makes a 90-degree right turn and then continues on a gentle downhill grade.

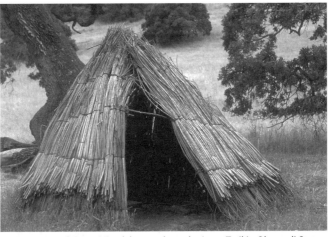

A reconstructed Coast Miwok house along the Loop Trail in Olompali State Historic Park.

Nearing Olompali Creek, the grade steepens. A set of wooden steps brings you to a junction, where a wide dirt path merges from the left, and your route, now a dirt road, swings right. Olompali Creek is in a deep ravine, left, and the road, which may be muddy in places, heads downstream, soon passing a reservoir made by damming the creek.

You pass through an open, grassy area, and nearby is a reconstructed Coast Miwok village consisting of two typical houses, one made from tule reeds, the other from redwood bark. After passing several picnic tables, the road swings left, crosses Olompali Creek, which flows through a culvert, and then veers right.

The Burdell Barns, part of the historic ranch complex, are just ahead. Just ahead of the first barn—one with a corrugated metal roof—leave the dirt road by veering right. Go about 200 feet, across a weedy field, to a bridge over Olompali Creek. Once across, close the loop, turn left, and retrace your route to the parking area.

## TRIP 16 Samuel P. Taylor State Park: Barnabe Mountain

| | |
|---|---|
| **Distance** | 6.3 miles, Semi-loop |
| **Hiking Time** | 3 to 4 hours |
| **Elevation Gain/Loss** | ±1900 |
| **Difficulty** | Difficult |
| **Best Times** | All year |
| **Agency** | CSP |
| **Recommended Map** | *Samuel P. Taylor State Park* (CSP) |

**HIGHLIGHTS** This semi-loop, using Devils Gulch Creek, Bill's, and the Riding and Hiking trails, and the Barnabe Fire Road, climbs gently through mixed forest, alive with birdsong and brightened by wildflowers, struggles steeply to high ground just below the summit of Barnabe Mountain (1466'), and then descends through open country with wonderful views of west Marin, Point Reyes, and the Tomales Bay area. Near the end of the loop, before heading back into the forest, you can visit the grave site of Samuel P. Taylor (1827–1896), who established the West Coast's first paper mill, on the banks of nearby Lagunitas Creek.

Barnabe Mountain, named for a retired army mule once belonging to John C. Frémont and purchased by Taylor at the Presidio in San Francisco, is called Barnabe Peak on the state park map.

**DIRECTIONS** From Highway 101 northbound, take the San Anselmo exit, also signed for San Quentin, Sir Francis Drake Blvd., and the Richmond Bridge. Stay in the left lane as you exit, toward San Anselmo, crossing over Highway 101. After 0.4 mile you join Sir Francis Drake Blvd., with traffic from Highway 101 southbound merging on your right. From here, it is 3.6 miles to a stoplight at the intersection with Red Hill Ave. Stay on Sir Francis Drake Blvd. as it first goes straight and then immediately bends left.

At 15.5 miles on Sir Francis Drake Blvd., you pass the main entrance to Samuel P. Taylor State Park. At 16.5 miles you reach a wide turnout, left, at Devil's Gulch. Park here.

From Highway 101 southbound, take the Sir Francis Drake/Kentfield exit and follow the directions above.

**FACILITIES/TRAILHEAD** Picnic tables, restrooms, phone, and water are just inside the state park's main entrance. There are no facilities at the trailhead, which is across Sir Francis Drake Blvd. from the parking area.

Carefully cross Sir Francis Drake Blvd. and follow a paved road about 0.1 mile to unsigned Devils Gulch Creek Trail. Bear right toward the creek, go past a set of wooden steps, left, that climb to a picnic area with toilets, and reach a four-way junction at

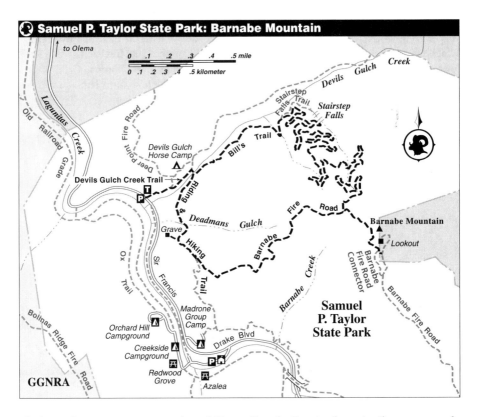

**Samuel P. Taylor State Park: Barnabe Mountain**

the base of an enormous coast redwood. You turn right and cross a long bridge spanning the creek.

Once across, you arrive at a T-junction, drawn incorrectly on the state park map. Here the Riding and Hiking Trail to the Barnabe Trail, which you will use later, goes right. Your route, Bill's Trail, heads left and begins a long, gentle climb. Just shy of the 1-mile point, you reach a junction with the Stairstep Falls Trail, left, a short trail to a vantage point where you can view the falls.

From this junction, your route turns right and uphill, its course etched out of a steep hillside that drops left. In places, your ascent is aided by a series of switchbacks. Two bridges, separated by a twisted stretch of trail, get you across a single deep ravine.

Finally leaving most of the trees behind, you reach a superb vantage point where the view extends west to the lands of Point Reyes National Seashore, and northwest to

Tomales Bay. At about 4 miles, you meet the Barnabe Fire Road. Once on the road, you can turn left to continue the ascent of Barnabe Mountain, a climb of about 200 feet in 0.3 mile. Or you can turn right to begin the descent to Sir Francis Drake Blvd.

If you choose to climb, follow a moderate and then steep course, passing the Barnabe Fire Road Connector, to a T-junction at the

**Trees and Birds**
The forest cloaking Barnabe Mountain includes Douglas-fir, bigleaf maple, California bay, California buckeye, white alder, and California nutmeg. Dark-eyed juncos and spotted towhees, both lovers of forest and dense cover, may be seen and heard here. Both species show white along the tail in flight, but the towhee is a larger, more dramatically patterned bird, colored black, white, and orange.

state park boundary. From here, a dirt road goes left and uphill to a fire lookout, and also right. (Please respect all private property postings.)

When you have finished enjoying this wonderful vantage point, retrace your route to the junction with Bill's Trail. From here, continue on the dirt road, descending over rocky ground that alternates between moderate and steep. The grasslands beside the trail may contain bluedicks, blue-eyed grass, paintbrush, and bellardia.

Around 5.5 miles, you pass the Riding and Hiking Trail to the Madrone picnic area, left, and then reach a junction. To visit the nearby Taylor grave site, go straight. Otherwise, turn right on the Riding and Hiking Trail to Devil's Gulch.

Heading into forest, you follow a rough, eroded road steeply downhill into Deadman's Gulch. Now the road narrows, veers left, and then skirts a hillside. With Devil's Gulch Creek downhill and left, you make a steep descent and soon close the loop at the junction with Bill's Trail, beside the bridge. Here you turn left, cross the bridge, turn left again, and retrace your route to the parking area.

# TRIP 17 Point Reyes National Seashore: Mt. Wittenberg

| | |
|---|---|
| **Distance** | 5.1 miles, Semi-loop |
| **Hiking Time** | 2 to 3 hours |
| **Elevation Gain/Loss** | ±1300 feet |
| **Difficulty** | Moderate |
| **Trail Use** | Backpacking option[1] |
| **Best Times** | All year |
| **Agency** | NPS |
| **Recommended Map** | *Point Reyes National Seashore South District Trail Map* (NPS) |
| **Notes** | [1]Sky Camp, a hike-in campground, is on the Sky Trail, northwest of its junction with the Mt. Wittenberg Trail. For reservations, call (415) 663-8054 weekdays from 9 A.M. to 2 P.M. |

**HIGHLIGHTS**  Using the Bear Valley, Mt. Wittenberg, Sky, and Meadow trails, this athletic loop takes you up Inverness Ridge to the summit of Mt. Wittenberg, the highest point in Point Reyes National Seashore. No reason other than the joy of hiking is needed to try this route, but further inducements include a wonderful variety of plant and bird life, and great views. Be sure to check with rangers at the visitor center for the latest trail conditions and closures.

**DIRECTIONS**  From Highway 1 northbound in Olema, just north of the junction with Sir Francis Drake Blvd., turn left onto Bear Valley Road and go 0.5 mile to the visitor-center entrance road. Turn left and go 0.2 mile to a large paved parking area in front of the visitor center. If this area is full, there is a dirt parking area ahead and left.

From Highway 1 southbound in Point Reyes Station, go 0.2 mile from the end of the town's main street to Sir Francis Drake Blvd. and turn right. Go 0.7 mile and turn left onto Bear Valley Road. At 1.7 miles you reach the visitor-center entrance road; turn right and follow the directions above.

**FACILITIES/TRAILHEAD**  A visitor center with displays, books, maps, and helpful staff is located next to the parking area, along with picnic tables, restrooms, phone, and water.

The Bear Valley trailhead is at the end of the paved entrance road, about 150 feet south of the paved parking area.

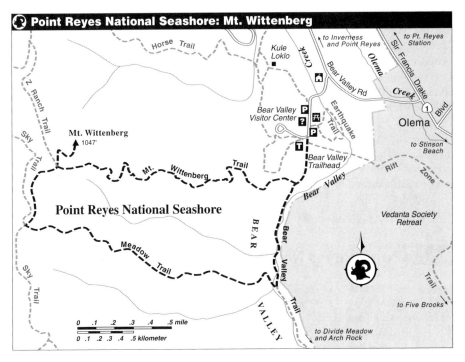

**Point Reyes National Seashore: Mt. Wittenberg**

The Bear Valley trailhead is one of the busiest in Point Reyes National Seashore, giving visitors access to the heart of this wonderful area. Hikers, bikers, and equestrians share the main thoroughfare, a dirt road called the Bear Valley Trail, for most of its length; but bicycles are not allowed past its junction with the Glen Trail, about 0.8 mile short of the coast, and horses are not allowed on weekends and holidays.

After walking through a gap in a wooden fence that marks the trailhead, you pass the Rift Zone Trail, left, and the Woodpecker Trail, right. Coming over a low rise, you make a gentle descent to a junction with the Mt. Wittenberg Trail, a single track. Here you turn right, walking under the outstretched limbs of a large, lichen-draped California bay tree. The trail, now rough and rocky, widens and steepens, taking you uphill on a moderate grade.

Short level stretches relieve the otherwise constant climbing, and the variety of plants provides ample reason to stop often

### The Birds and the Trees

Acorn woodpeckers are common here — a good place to spot them is in the oak-shaded picnic area, just east of the visitor center. Look for a robin-sized bird, black with white wing patches, a white rump, and a red cap on its head. These busy birds collect fallen acorns and then stuff them one by one into holes they have drilled in the trunk of a tree.

The forest here, with bay, tanbark oak, hazelnut, evergreen huckleberry, and western sword fern, resembles a coast redwood forest with one exception — no coast redwoods. The San Andreas fault defines the western limit of these trees in Marin County, perhaps because the granitic soil on the Point Reyes peninsula is unsuitable for them. Instead of redwoods, there are tall Douglas-firs.

and study your surroundings. After several switchbacks, you come to a clearing filled with young Douglas-firs. Before long, this

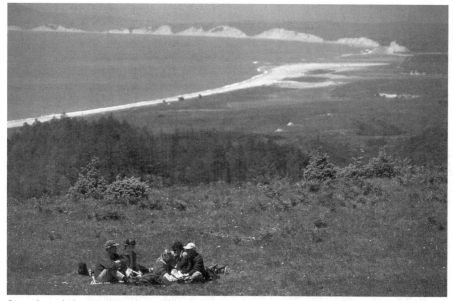

Open slopes below Mt. Wittenberg offer great picnicking spots with superb views.

clearing, and others like it, may be indistinguishable from the mature forest that blankets Inverness Ridge. Narrowing to singletrack width, the trail leads uphill on a moderate grade and returns to dense forest.

Now the trail makes a series of switchbacks to gain the crest of a ridge. You break out of the forest at last and cross an open field, with Mt. Wittenberg rising to the right. At about 2 miles, you reach a junction, where a short trail to Mt. Wittenberg's summit, which is closed to horses, goes sharply right and uphill. Here too is the Z Ranch Trail, going right on a level grade. Also from this junction, the continuation of the Mt. Wittenberg Trail veers slightly left. The mountain is named for a rancher who once lived nearby, not for Hamlet's alma mater.

To reach the summit of Mt. Wittenberg, at 1407 feet the highest point on Inverness Ridge, turn sharply right and begin a moderate climb. After about 0.2 mile you arrive at the summit, where you have fine views of the Point Reyes peninsula, the Olema Valley, Mt. Tamalpais, and, on a clear day, other landmarks to the east, south, and

southwest. The summit is a broad clearing bordered by an arc of trees that stretches from north to west, blocking views in those directions.

After enjoying the summit, return to the junction and continue on the Mt. Wittenberg Trail, now descending on a gentle and then moderate grade, with a steep hillside dropping right. The view here extends west and southwest into the zone blackened by the October 1995 Vision Fire, where the once-dominant bishop-pine forest is reestablishing itself. Beyond are Limantour Estero, Drakes Beach, and the great curving arm of the Pt. Reyes peninsula itself.

After a pleasant downhill ramble, the Mt. Wittenberg Trail ends, and you merge with the Sky Trail by bearing left. It was this trail, a dirt road, that finally blocked the fire's path after it had burned for three days and charred more than 12,000 acres. About 50 feet past the junction, you leave the Sky Trail and turn left onto the Meadow Trail, a single track. At first on a level course, the trail soon begins a descent that alternates between gentle and moderate. The route suddenly breaks out of the trees and crosses a wide meadow, with a lovely view straight ahead of Mt. Tamalpais.

At the end of the meadow, the route returns to forest and begins a winding descent, often steep, over eroded, root-crossed ground. The trail levels when it reaches a low divide, and then resumes its plunge off Inverness Ridge into Bear Valley. The sound of running water indicates Bear Valley Creek, which you cross via a wooden bridge. Just ahead is a junction with the Bear Valley Trail, where you turn left. Passing a rest bench, right, you soon arrive at the junction with the Mt. Wittenberg Trail. Continue straight and retrace your route to the parking area.

## TRIP 18 Point Reyes National Seashore: Tomales Point

| | |
|---|---|
| **Distance** | 9.4 miles, Out-and-back |
| **Hiking Time** | 4 to 5 hours |
| **Elevation Gain/Loss** | ±900 feet |
| **Difficulty** | Moderate |
| **Trail Use** | Good for kids |
| **Best Times** | All year |
| **Agency** | NPS |
| **Recommended Map** | *Point Reyes National Seashore North District Trail Map* (NPS) |

**HIGHLIGHTS**  One of the premier hikes in the North Bay, this out-and-back trip over rolling terrain uses the Tomales Point Trail to reach Tomales Bluff, the northwest tip of Tomales Point. Starting from historic Pierce Point Ranch, the trail takes you through a tule-elk preserve, where sometimes you can see these magnificent creatures at close range. Exposed as this area is to the wind, this hike is best on a warm day.

**DIRECTIONS**  From Highway 1 just south of Point Reyes Station, turn southwest onto Sir Francis Drake Blvd. and, as the road swings toward the northwest, follow it for 6.5 miles to a fork, where you bear right onto Pierce Point Road. At 9.2 miles from the fork, where Pierce Point Road bends sharply left toward McClures Beach, there is parking on the right for the Pierce Point Ranch and Tomales Point. If the parking area is full, park on the east side of Pierce Point Road, just before the bend.

**FACILITIES/TRAILHEAD**  There are restrooms at nearby McClures Beach. The trailhead is on the west side of the parking area.

Point Reyes was, and still is, a prime area for dairy ranching. The ranch buildings adjacent to the parking area were part of a 2200-acre spread purchased in 1858 by Solomon Pierce and later owned by his son Abram. Pierce Point Ranch, which is on the National Register of Historic Places, is being restored and serves as a museum of ranching history. A path through the ranch complex starts on the north side of the parking area.

The Tomales Point Trail leaves from the west side of the parking area and passes an information board displaying a short history of the Point Reyes dairies. Other than a line of tall Monterey cypress and a few eucalyptus trees, the terrain is treeless— just rolling, grassy hills and fields.

Rounding a large barn, right, the trail begins climbing on a gentle grade. On your left, several hundred feet below, are the Pacific Ocean and wave-washed McClures Beach. If you look south, you may be able to see the tip of Point Reyes, where the light-house is. To the north lie Bodega Bay, Bodega Head, and the Sonoma County coast. As the trail swings right, you have a great view of

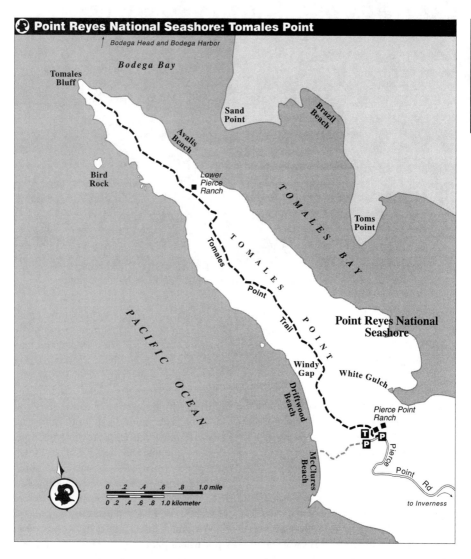

**Point Reyes National Seashore: Tomales Point**

Bodega Head and Bodega Harbor

*Bodega Bay*

Tomales Bluff

Sand Point

Brazil Beach

Avalis Beach

Bird Rock

Lower Pierce Ranch

Toms Point

*TOMALES BAY*

Tomales Point Trail

*TOMALES POINT*

*PACIFIC OCEAN*

**Point Reyes National Seashore**

Windy Gap

White Gulch

Driftwood Beach

Pierce Point Ranch

McClures Beach

Pierce Point Rd

*to Inverness*

0  .2  .4  .6  .8  1.0 mile

0  .2  .4  .6  .8  1.0 kilometer

the steep, eroded cliffs that form the southwest rampart of Tomales Point, a long finger of land jutting northwest and separating the outer reaches of Tomales Bay from the ocean. The name "Tomales" refers to a tribe of Indians called Tamal, which is Coast Miwok for "west" or "west coast." Mt. Tamalpais was also named for this tribe.

The trail now descends to a flat spot at the head of White Gulch, a valley heading down to Tomales Bay. This is a good place to glimpse tule elk, if you haven't already

seen them. Now on a moderate and then steep uphill, you reach the top of a rocky bluff, a vantage point with views, on a clear day, of some North Bay landmarks, including the hulking outlines of Mt. St. Helena and Mt. Tamalpais. From this high point, at about 2 miles, the route begins to descend toward the site of Lower Pierce Ranch, devoid of buildings but marked by a grove of Monterey cypress and eucalyptus.

Following the rough and rocky trail as it bends right, you pass a pond, right, that is a

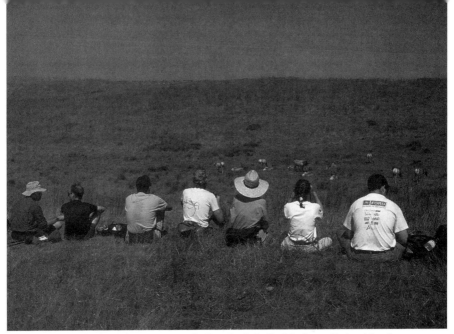
Observing tule elk is a popular pastime on the Tomales Point Trail, Pt. Reyes National Seashore.

favorite elk hang-out. Hikers often gather here in large groups, conversing in hushed tones, to watch the elk. These beasts are used to people, and as long as you keep a safe distance, it is possible to observe them at your leisure. Males use the pond to bathe by splashing water over themselves with their antlers. Lounging females, if startled, rise and run, but their guardian and protector usually stays put until he can catch the intruder's scent and determine the level of threat.

**Tule Elk**

If you hear eerie, high-pitched calling, don't be alarmed. You are in a tule-elk preserve, and the male elk uses these weird vocalizations to assemble his harems of females and to announce his territorial intentions to competing males. During the fall rutting season, a male tule elk with a large harem is often challenged by a younger upstart, and will defend his turf by charging the outsider, locking antlers with him, and pushing him back across an unmarked, but very real, territorial limit. Once thought to be extinct, tule elk in California now number about 3200 in 22 herds, thanks to active management by the Department of Fish and Game.

After a final, steep descent to the ranch site, you cross a gully that may be seasonally wet, home to ferns, rushes, sedges, and tangles of blackberry vines. Now the trail climbs moderately to a signed junction, where a faint trace veers left. You continue straight, climbing on soft sand. This soil seems to favor yellow bush lupine above all else—it is everywhere, growing in large, shrubby clumps. On warm fall days, lupine seed pods open with a startling "pop!" During winter months, gray whales pass by Point Reyes on their journey from the Bering Sea to Baja and back.

Around 4 miles, you reach a wide, level spot where paths seem to lead in all directions. Continue straight, finding your way into a large, open, sandy area. Descending now over loose sand, you may hear the metallic clanging of the Tomales Bay entrance buoy. The trail takes you very close to the sheer cliffs fronting the Pacific, where a signed warning, TRAIL CLOSED, DANGEROUS CONDITIONS, should be heeded. The view does not improve beyond this point, but your risk of injury certainly does. When you've had your fill of this remote and wonderful place, called Tomales Bluff, retrace your route to the parking area.

# TRIP19 Tomales Bay State Park

| | |
|---|---|
| **Distance** | 2.5 miles, Loop; with out-and back option to Shell Beach, 7 miles |
| **Hiking Time** | 1 to 2 hours; with out-and-back option, 3 to 4 hours |
| **Elevation Gain/Loss** | ±600 feet; with out and back option, ±1500 feet |
| **Difficulty** | Easy; with out-and-back option, difficult |
| **Best Times** | All year |
| **Agency** | CSP |
| **Recommended Map** | *Tomales Bay State Park* (CSP) |

**HIGHLIGHTS**  This easy loop, using the Jepson and Johnstone trails, takes you through a wonderful grove of rare bishop pines and then to Pebble Beach, a secluded cove on Tomales Bay with not a golf course in sight. The variety of plant life along the way is stunning, and it is no wonder the pine grove and one of the trails are named in honor of California's premier botanist, Willis Linn Jepson (1867-1946). The 4.5-mile out-and-back option on the Johnstone Trail takes you to Shell Beach, and the extended route gives you further evidence, if needed, of the wisdom of including this stretch of valuable beachfront property in the state park system.

**DIRECTIONS**  From Highway 1 just south of Point Reyes Station, turn southwest onto Sir Francis Drake Blvd. and, as the road swings toward the northwest, follow it for 6.5 miles to a fork, where you bear right onto Pierce Point Road. Go 1.2 miles to the state park entrance road and turn right. At 0.7 mile you come to the entrance station, where you pay a day-use fee. If no ranger is on duty, pay at the self-registration station here. At 1.2 miles you pass the turnoff to Hearts Desire Beach. Continue another 0.1 mile to a fork, the start of a one-way loop leading to parking areas for the picnic grounds. Park in the upper area, along the left side of the road, before it makes a 180-degree bend to the left.

**FACILITIES/TRAILHEAD**  There are picnic tables, restrooms, and water near the parking area. The trailhead is on the southwest side of the upper parking area, near its midpoint.

Your route, a single-track trail climbing on a moderate grade, honors the late Willis Linn Jepson, a University of California botanist who wrote the definitive guide to California plants. This state park encloses a grove of rare bishop pines, also named for Dr. Jepson, which lies a short distance ahead.

Soon you reach a junction where a branch of the Jepson Trail turns right to an overnight-parking area beside Pierce Point Road. Here you continue straight, still on the main branch of the Jepson Trail, and in about 100 yards cross a paved road that winds downhill. After crossing the road, you descend a few wooden steps and then enjoy a gentle downhill ramble. The Jepson Trail ends at a T-junction with the Johnstone Trail, a single track named for Bruce and Elsie Johnstone, who helped with efforts to create this park.

To visit Shell Beach, turn right and go a little more than 2 miles on a shaded, rolling trail that eventually drops to the shore of Tomales Bay. Don't be surprised when you get there to find the beach crowded: this scenic spot can also be reached via a short trail from the end of Camino Del Mar. If you elect to skip Shell Beach, turn left at the T-junction, follow a level course, then cross the paved road you met earlier and begin winding downhill.

The large, oak-like trees beside the trail here are chinquapin, a chestnut relative, often found as a small shrub associated with manzanita and evergreen huckleberry.

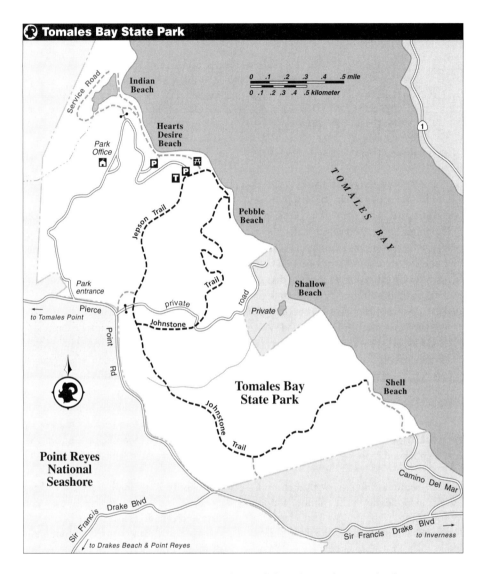

## Tomales Bay State Park

Chinquapin's dark green leaves are coated on the underside with golden scales, making it easy to confuse with canyon oak. This golden coloration is alluded to in the scientific names of both chinquapin (*Chrysolepis chrysophylla*) and canyon oak (*Quercus chrysolepis*)— "chrysolepis" is Greek for "golden scale."

Making several sharp switchbacks, the route descends to the floor of a small valley, a wet and muddy area that you cross via raised boardwalks. Rising from the valley,

and then descending gently, the route soon reaches a T-junction, where a short trail, right, takes you to Pebble Beach, a secluded spot on Tomales Bay enjoyed by swimmers, picnickers, sunbathers, and boaters. At either end of the cove, a rugged coastline drops steeply to meet the bay. Behind the beach is a little marsh with cattails and sedges.

After visiting the beach, retrace your steps to the previous junction, and then continue straight on the Johnstone Trail,

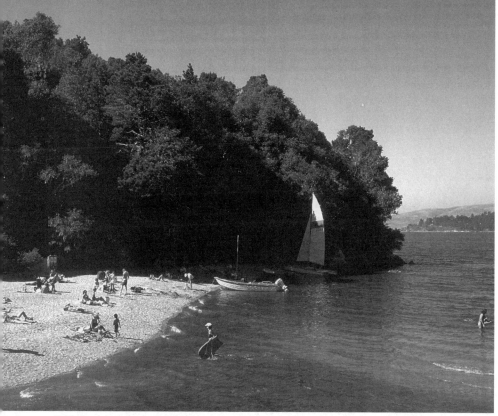

Shell Beach is at the end of the Johnstone Trail, but also has easy access from a road.

### Trees Abounding

Bishop pine, restricted to coastal California and a few locations in Mexico, has thick, deeply furrowed gray bark, spiny cones that remain closed and attached to the tree for many years, and needles in bundles of two. As an adaptation to fire, the cones open and release their seeds after a blaze, allowing the forest to renew itself. The tree's common name apparently comes from the place of its 1835 discovery, near the mission of San Luis Obispo — which was named for Saint Louis, Bishop of Toulouse.

In addition to bishop pines, the park has a rich abundance of other trees, including coast live oak, California bay, and madrone, along with common shrubs such as hazelnut, coffeeberry, bush monkeyflower, toyon, thimbleberry, evergreen huckleberry, and several varieties of ceanothus.

climbing on a moderate grade. Cresting a low rise, you follow a rolling course on a winding trail, passing a path to a viewpoint, right. Soon you come to a picnic area and a large sign that lists distances on the Johnstone Trail to various points, including Hearts Desire Beach, which is 0.2 mile ahead. Once past the sign, you leave the Johnstone Trail, bearing left through the picnic area until you reach the restrooms and then, in about 100 feet, the lower parking area. From here, turn left and follow the paved road to the upper parking area.

# Chapter 2
# *Santa Rosa/Petaluma*

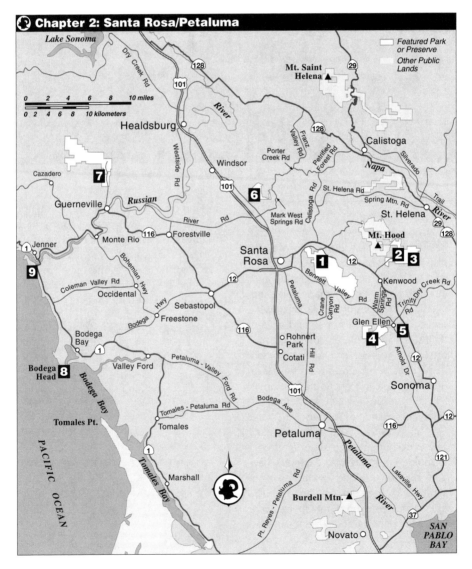

Featured Park or Preserve

Other Public Lands

Lake Sonoma

Dry Creek Rd

128

101

River

0 2 4 6 8 10 miles
0 2 4 6 8 10 kilometers

Healdsburg

Mt. Saint Helena ▲

29

128

Calistoga

Westside Rd

Windsor

101

Porter Creek Rd

Franz Valley Rd

Petrified Forest Rd

*Napa*

Silverado Trail

Cazadero

**7**

**6**

Calistoga Rd

St. Helena Rd

Spring Mtn. Rd

St. Helena

29

*River*

Guerneville

*Russian*

River

Rd

Mark West Springs Rd

Mt. Hood ▲

**2** **3**

128

Jenner

**1**

**9**

Monte Rio

116

Forestville

Santa Rosa

12

**1**

12

Kenwood

Bennett

Valley

Warm Springs Rd

Trinity Rd

Dry Creek Rd

Bohemian Hwy

Coleman Valley Rd

Occidental

Hwy

Sebastopol

Freestone

Bodega

12

Crane Canyon Rd

Petaluma

Glen Ellen

**4** **5**

Bodega Bay

1

116

Rohnert Park

Cotati

Hill Rd

Sonoma

Arnold Dr

12

Bodega Head **8**

Bodega Bay

Valley Ford

Petaluma - Valley Ford Rd

101

Bodega Ave

116

12

*Petaluma*

121

Tomales Pt.

Tomales - Petaluma Rd

Tomales

1

Petaluma

*River*

Lakeville Hwy

P A C I F I C   O C E A N

Tomales Bay

Marshall

Pt. Reyes - Petaluma Rd

Burdell Mtn. ▲

37

Novato

SAN PABLO BAY

# TRIP 1 Annadel State Park

|  |  |
|---|---|
| **Distance** | 8.8 miles, Semi-loop |
| **Hiking Time** | 5 to 6 hours |
| **Elevation Gain/Loss** | ±1600 feet |
| **Difficulty** | Difficult |
| **Trail Use** | Mountain biking allowed |
| **Best Times** | Spring and fall |
| **Agency** | CSP |
| **Recommended Map** | *Annadel State Park* (CSP) |

**HIGHLIGHTS**  Length, not terrain, earns this trip its difficult rating. Using the Cobblestone, Orchard, Rough Go, Canyon, and Spring Creek trails, this semi-loop route encounters dense forest, oak savanna, and a wonderful, albeit artificial, lake during its tour of the northwestern part of Annadel State Park. A massive and ongoing restoration effort, begun in 1998, has completely transformed many of the park's eroded dirt roads into winding, multi-use paths shared by hikers, equestrians, and bicyclists. Many of the trails are subject to seasonal closure during wet weather. Please observe all closure signs, and use only named and maintained trails.

**DIRECTIONS**  From Highway 101 in Santa Rosa, take the Sebastopol/Sonoma/Highway 12 exit and follow Highway 12 east toward Sonoma. At 1.4 miles, turn left onto Farmers Lane, go 0.8 mile, and turn right onto Montgomery Dr. Go 2.7 miles and turn right onto Channel Dr., signed for Annadel State Park and Spring Lake. Go 0.6 mile to a large dirt-and-gravel parking area, left.

From Highway 12 going northwest from Kenwood to Santa Rosa, turn left on Los Alamos Road and go 0.2 mile to Melita Road. Turn right on Melita Road and then immediately left onto Montgomery Dr. Go 0.5 mile to Channel Dr., turn left, and go 0.6 mile to a large, dirt-and-gravel parking area, left.

Please obey signs in the parking area, which is not part of the state park.

**FACILITIES/TRAILHEAD**  There are no facilities at the trailhead, but inside the park are a ranger station, picnic tables, water, and toilets. The trailhead is on the south side of Channel Dr., opposite the east end of the parking area.

Your route, the Cobblestone Trail, starts in a wooded area. Douglas-fir, coast live oak, black oak, California bay, and bigleaf maple are some of the native trees that grace this park. Alternately moderate and level, the route rises through rocky terrain, which may become muddy during wet weather. Stands of tall manzanita, some of them top heavy and bent toward the ground, line the trail.

After traversing an open, grassy field, the route bends sharply left and is crossed by a trail that has been closed for restoration. At a junction, the Frog Pond Trail goes

**Turkeys**
This park is one of the best places in the North Bay to see wild turkeys—look in damp ravines or along the edges of clearings for large flocks of these dark, iridescent birds, which are slightly smaller than their domestic cousins.

straight, but your route, the Cobblestone Trail, curves left. Gaining elevation on a gentle grade, you enjoy a pleasant stroll through oak groves and across open fields, one holding the remains of an old orchard.

*Santa Rosa/Petaluma*

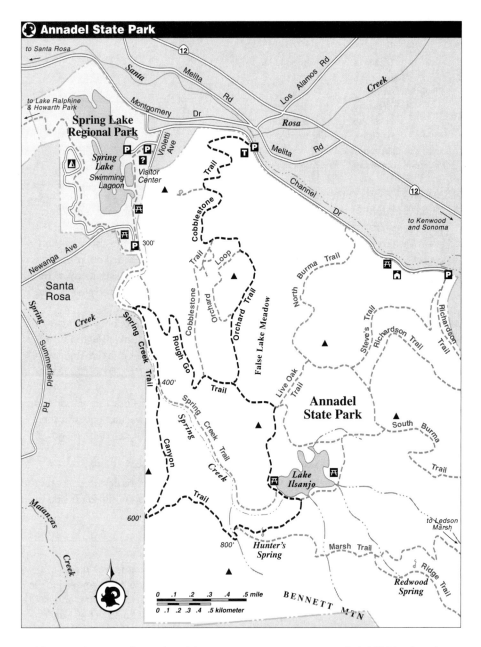

Annadel State Park

Now passing a trail on the right, you enter forest. At a junction with a dirt road —closed on your left but open on your right as the continuation of the Cobblestone Trail—you go straight, now on the Orchard Trail. After passing an unsigned trail, right, you make a long tra-verse across a wooded hillside that drops left, then climb to an open area.

Passing the remains of a several cobble-stone quarries, right, you soon reach a fork marked by a trail post, where you stay left, still on the Orchard Trail. Ahead, in the dis-tance to the southeast, rises Bennett

Mountain, at 1887 feet the highest point in Annadel State Park, its slopes dappled in fall with colorful foliage. Around 2 miles, you come to a T-junction with the Rough Go Trail, where you turn left.

Climbing on a gentle grade, the Rough Go Trail soon meets the Live Oak Trail, left, and then bends right, finding a level course. At last nearing Lake Ilsanjo, named for the former property owners, Ilsa and Joe Coney, you bear right at a fork, and then pass a trail, left. The area ahead is used as a spillway for the lake during periods of high water. If the spillway is flooded, you can detour around and over it by means of a trail, right, and a bridge about 100 feet to your right.

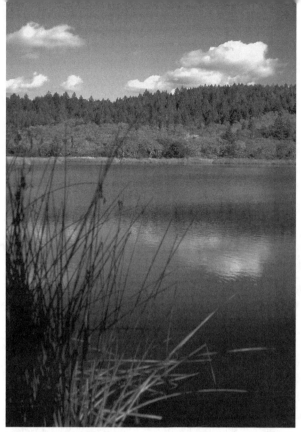

Lake Ilsanjo, named for former property owners Ilsa and Joe Coney, reflects clouds and sky.

About 25 feet ahead, your route becomes paved, and 100 feet or so farther it arrives at a T-junction with a dirt road. Turning left, you walk about 200 feet to a picnic table in the shade of a large oak, where a short path leads down to the lake, a lovely body of water. Just past the picnic table is a concrete dam on Spring Creek, which forms the lake.

Bearing left across the 100-yard-long dam, you pass the Spring Creek Trail, right, a wonderful route but closed during the rainy season. On the far side of the dam, your route, a dirt road, swings left and begins a gentle climb. Topping a low rise, the road descends to a junction, where you turn right on the Canyon Trail, also a dirt road. The road climbs southwest through a dense, fern-floored forest, passing Hunter's Spring, a favorite haunt of wild turkeys.

Soon you reach a junction, which has a picnic table to the left and a rest bench to the right. The dirt road heading left is the

Marsh Trail, part of the Bay Area Ridge Trail. You continue straight on the Canyon Trail, here also part of the Bay Area Ridge Trail. The road drops to cross a watercourse, which drains through a culvert under the road, then comes into an open area. You continue to descend over very rocky ground on a gentle grade, passing a trail, left, that goes through a locked gate.

Leaving open grassland, you enter forest and soon cross a bridge over Spring Creek.

**Hawks**

The great expanse of open fields here favors aerial hunters such as red-tailed and red-shouldered hawks. Hard to distinguish from one another against a bright sky, they are best told apart by their calls: a single whistled "keer" for the red-tailed hawk, and a repeated crying "keer, keer, keer" for the red-shouldered.

Just across the creek, at about 5 miles, the Canyon Trail ends at a T-junction with the Spring Creek Trail. To your right the Spring Creek Trail is a single track, and to your left it is a dirt road, part of the Bay Area Ridge Trail. Turning left, you enjoy a level walk beside the creek, and soon pass a gravel road heading left to a flood-control dam and levee.

Just before the road veers left to cross a wooden bridge, you turn sharply right on the Rough Go Trail. Climb to near the crest of a ridge, where you encounter a large, circular maze built of small rocks, perched on the edge of a steep hillside. Veering left here, a bit more climbing brings you to the Cobblestone Trail, left. Continuing straight, you wind uphill to close the loop at the Orchard Trail. From here, at about 7 miles, turn left and retrace your route along the Orchard and Cobblestone trails to the parking area.

# **TRIP 2** Sugarloaf Ridge State Park: Bald Mountain

| | |
|---:|:---|
| **Distance** | 6.7 miles, Semi-loop |
| **Hiking Time** | 4 to 5 hours |
| **Elevation Gain/Loss** | ±1900 feet |
| **Difficulty** | Difficult |
| **Best Times** | Spring and fall |
| **Agency** | CSP |
| **Recommended Map** | *Sugarloaf Ridge State Park* (CSP) |

**HIGHLIGHTS**  This semi-loop route, using the Lower Bald Mountain, Bald Mountain, Vista, Headwaters, Red Mountain, and Gray Pine trails, is a challenge, but well worth the effort. A superb array of trees, shrubs, and wildflowers, along with some of the best views in the Bay Area, are the rewards for tackling the rigorous climb to the summit of Bald Mountain.

**DIRECTIONS**  From Highway 12 just north of Kenwood, take Adobe Canyon Road and go northeast 3.4 miles to the entrance kiosk. If the entrance kiosk is not staffed, pay fee at the self-registration station here. Continue 0.1 mile to a dirt parking area, left.

**FACILITIES/TRAILHEAD**  The park has both family and group campsites. A visitor center, phone, and water are just southeast of the entrance kiosk. Picnic tables and a toilet are near the trailhead, which is on the northeast corner of the parking area.

The Lower Bald Mountain Trail, a single track, heads northeast from the parking area through a wet area into open grassland and finds a gentle uphill course. High on your left are rolling hills and forested ridges, but your goal, Bald Mountain (2729'), remains hidden behind them. In places, the trail enters groves of coast live oak, California bay, and madrone, where you will also find shrubs such as manzanita, coffeeberry, toyon, and poison oak. At a junction with the Meadow Trail, you veer left and soon begin a moderate uphill climb via a series of switchbacks in a densely wooded area.

**Sugarloaf Flora**

In spring, the fields beside the trailhead are dotted with wildflowers, including blue-eyed grass, yarrow, bluedicks, lupine, vetch, and blow wives. As you move ahead, you'll go through a densely wooded area. Then, as you emerge from this forest into chaparral, the change in vegetation is dramatic and fascinating for lovers of native plants—here, in addition to manzanita, you may find chamise, buckbrush, spiny redberry, bush monkeyflower, and leather oak, the latter an indicator of serpentine soil.

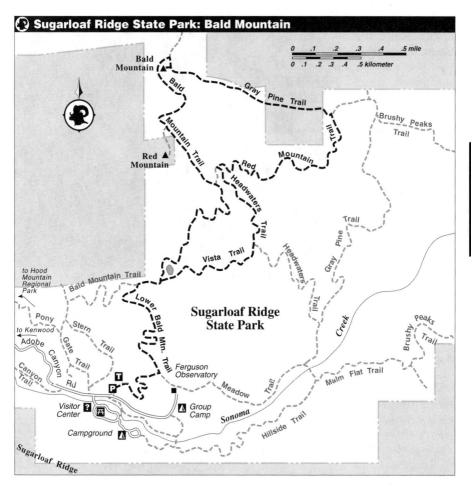

**Sugarloaf Ridge State Park: Bald Mountain**

Your trail merges with the Bald Mountain Trail, a paved road that is part of the Bay Area Ridge Trail. Bearing right on the paved road, which is attractively lined with silver lupine, you follow it steadily uphill on a

### A Peak Experience

According to *California Place Names*, more than 100 peaks in California are named Bald, but it is certainly confusing to have two so close together. Only Black and Red are more popular mountain names, and this park has one of the latter, too. Peaks visible from trailside vantage points include Mt. Diablo and Mt. Tamalpais.

moderate grade. Where the road angles sharply left, you turn onto the Vista Trail, a single track leading right and downhill. A small pond in a marshy area welcomes you to a lovely but fragile area. In the distance to the southeast rises another Bald Mountain, its open slopes planted with vineyards.

Now in a shady corridor of oak, toyon, and manzanita, you enjoy a level walk, soon reaching several small streams crossed by wooden planks. This wet area supports bigleaf maple trees, ferns, and wildflowers. The trail dips to cross a seasonal creek and then climbs on a moderate grade across an open, grassy hillside.

The route turns left and then descends steeply over loose, rocky ground to a junction, at about 2 miles, with the Headwaters Trail. Here you turn left and make a short, steep descent to a fern-filled area. Reaching Sonoma Creek but staying on its west side, the trail bends left and rises on a moderate grade. After struggling uphill over rough ground, the route finally reaches a T-junction with the Red Mountain Trail, a single track.

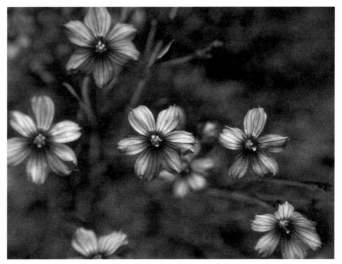

Blue-eyed grass is a member of the iris family found in grasslands.

Here you turn right and descend to a crossing of Sonoma Creek near its upper reaches. Finding a rolling course, the trail takes you back into dense forest. Now you descend steeply to a creek and cross it on a wooden bridge. Once across, the trail switchbacks right and climbs on a moderate grade, crossing a steep hillside and soon resorting to more switchbacks to surmount a steep grade. Suddenly you are atop a man-

**Summit Views**

The views from Bald Mountain on a clear day are extraordinary, ranging from the Sierra Nevada to Point Reyes, and from Snow Mountain, north of Clear Lake, to San Francisco. Two display panels — one facing north, the other south — help you identify landmarks in addition to the ones already noted. From here, Mt. Hood (the Sonoma County one) is due west, and Mt. St. Helena, at the corner of Napa, Sonoma, and Lake counties is slightly west of north. Sonoma Mountain, the backbone of Jack London State Historic Park, is southwest, and the Napa Valley is east.

zanita barren — the sandy, rocky soil here is perfect for these hardy, pioneering plants.

From this barren, you have a 360-degree view that, at last, reveals the summit of this park's Bald Mountain, slightly north of west, along with the other Bay Area summits already seen. The trail passes just south of the barren's high point, then curves counterclockwise around it. The sight of gray pines is welcome, because it means you are approaching the Gray Pine Trail, the last leg on the way to Bald Mountain.

You join the Gray Pine Trail, a dirt road, at a T-junction. Turn left and continue uphill on a moderate grade. After several steep pitches, you leave the Gray Pine Trail where it bends right, and continue west over windswept open ground a few hundred feet to the summit of Bald Mountain, at about 4 miles.

When it is time to head down, retrace your steps to the Gray Pine Trail, turn left onto it, and follow it steeply downhill for several hundred feet to a T-junction with the Bald Mountain Trail, a dirt road. Here you turn left, climb briefly, and then traverse the west side of Bald Mountain. With Red Mountain ahead, you drop steeply to a T-junction with a paved road. Here you turn left and continue downhill on pavement. Use caution while descending the road, because it is also used by service vehicles.

Passing a picnic table, right, the route levels and begins a gentle climb, in places going by exposed bands of red rock that perhaps gave the mountain its name. Where the Red Mountain Trail departs left, you continue straight, passing through a zone of chaparral. Soon the road begins a curvy course downhill, crossing a creek that flows through a culvert. When you reach the Vista Trail, continue downhill on the Bald Mountain Trail. Turn left on the Lower Bald Mountain trail and retrace your route to the parking area.

# TRIP3 Sugarloaf Ridge State Park: Meadow Loop

|  |  |
|---|---|
| **Distance** | 2.6 miles, Loop |
| **Hiking Time** | 1 to 2 hours |
| **Elevation Gain/Loss** | ±300 feet |
| **Difficulty** | Moderate |
| **Trail Use** | Good for kids |
| **Best Times** | Spring and fall |
| **Agency** | CSP |
| **Recommended Map** | *Sugarloaf Ridge State Park* (CSP) |

**HIGHLIGHTS** Using the Creekside Nature, Hillside, and Meadow trails, this lovely loop explores a forested hillside south of Sonoma Creek at the foot of Sugarloaf Ridge, and then circles back through meadows full of spring wildflowers, just north of the creek. Along the way, you pass the Robert Ferguson Observatory, which offers public astronomy programs; for information call (707) 833-6979 or visit www.rfo.org.

**DIRECTIONS** From Highway 12 just north of Kenwood, take Adobe Canyon Road and go northeast 3.4 miles to the entrance kiosk. If the entrance kiosk is not staffed, pay fee at the self-registration station here. Continue 0.1 mile to a dirt parking area, left.

**FACILITIES/TRAILHEAD** The park has both family and group campsites. A visitor center, phone, and water are just southeast of the entrance kiosk. Picnic tables and a toilet are near the trailhead, which is on the northeast corner of the parking area.

Just right of a picnic area is the trailhead for the park's self-guiding Creekside Nature Trail. Following this single-track trail into a forest of Douglas-fir, coast live oak, and California bay, you have a wooden fence on your right, guarding the steep drop to Sonoma Creek. After several hundred feet you reach a fork. Here you bear left and soon reach a clearing and the park's campfire center, where evening programs are held. At a four-way junction with a cement path, turn right and cross Sonoma Creek on a large wooden bridge. About 50 feet ahead, you come to a T-junction with a paved road, where you turn left.

Now in the park's campground, you follow the road southeast, passing a junction with another paved road to a turnaround. Between camp sites 25 and 26, the Creekside Nature Trail continues as a dirt-and-gravel path, heading southeast. The trail crosses an open area dotted in spring with wildflowers. Reaching Rattlesnake Creek, a seasonal stream, you cross it and then begin a moderate climb.

At a T-junction, you turn right on the Hillside Trail, climbing on a gentle and then moderate grade. Passing a picnic table and then two water tanks, the trail changes to a dirt-and-gravel road and soon begins to descend via sweeping S-bends. Your descent

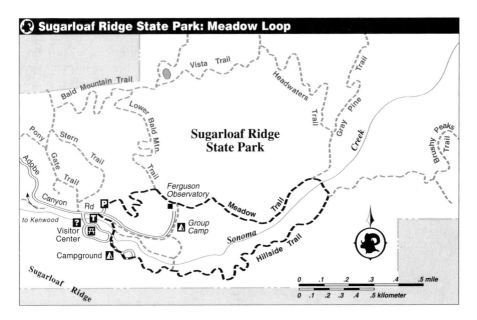

## Sugarloaf Ridge State Park: Meadow Loop

### Birds and Flowers of Note

Wildflowers beside the trail include California poppies, blue-eyed grass, mule ears, yarrow, lupine, and bluedicks.

The marshy areas in the park provide nesting habitat for red-winged blackbirds, and your passing may be noted, even disputed, by these territorial birds.

is interrupted by several brief uphill pitches, but soon you reach a meadow graced with oaks and wildflowers, and arrive at a junction with the Brushy Peaks Trail, right.

Your road continues straight from here with a new name, the Meadow Trail. After several hundred feet, as the road makes a left-hand bend, you pass the Gray Pine Trail, right. A wood bridge takes you across beautiful Sonoma Creek, where a picnic table invites you to sit and be serenaded by birdsong in the shade of bigleaf maple and white alder. Now emerging from the trees, your route crosses open ground where deer may be grazing in the tall grass.

A large meadow, left, holds Sonoma Creek, and behind it rises Sugarloaf Ridge, its steep sides densely clad with trees and chaparral. After crossing a seasonal tribu-

tary of Sonoma Creek, which flows under the road through a culvert, you pass a gate and then reach a paved parking area for the the Ferguson Observatory.

Across the parking area to the west are picnic tables and a toilet. Between them and the observatory is the continuation of your route, the Meadow Trail, here a rocky dirt track climbing on a moderate grade. Soon your reach a fork marked by a trail post, where you stay on the Meadow Trail by veering left. Now the route wanders through wildflower meadows and wooded groves. A gentle descent through a wet area returns you to the parking area.

### Robert Ferguson Observatory

The observatory was named for the late Bob Ferguson, a Petaluma astronomer dedicated to involving young people in astronomy. It is operated by the Valley of the Moon Observatory Association, and houses both a 40-inch and a 20-inch telescope, along with smaller telescopes. The observatory is open to the public for observation, classes in telescope making, and group meetings. More information is available at www.rfo.org.

# *TRIP4* Jack London State Historic Park

| | |
|---|---|
| **Distance** | 2.9 miles, Semi-loop; with out-and-back option on the Mountain Trail, 8 miles |
| **Hiking Time** | 2 to 3 hours; with out-and-back option, 4 to 5 hours |
| **Elevation Gain/Loss** | ±450 feet; with out-and-back option ±1300 feet |
| **Difficulty** | Moderate; with out-and-back option, difficult |
| **Trail Use** | Good for kids, Mountain biking allowed[1] |
| **Best Times** | All year |
| **Agency** | CSP |
| **Recommended Map** | *Jack London State Historic Park* (CSP) |
| **Notes** | [1]Bicycles are not allowed on single-track trails, and must instead use the Lake Service Road to reach the Mountain Trail |

**HIGHLIGHTS** Jack London's ranch, a beautiful redwood forest, and a vista point with superb views are the attractions of this semi-loop trip that uses the Lake, Upper Lake, and Mountain trails. You can extend the trip with an out-and-back option, via the Mountain Trail and then the short Mountain Spur, to just below the 2463-foot summit of Sonoma Mountain. (This adds 5.1 miles to the described route.) After your hike, be sure to visit the park's fine visitor center and museum, open daily 10 A.M. to 5 P.M., devoted to the work of its namesake author. From the museum, which is next to a parking area just east of the entrance kiosk, you can walk to London's grave site and the remains of his elaborate mansion, called Wolf House, which was destroyed by fire in 1913, a month before the Londons were scheduled to move in.

**DIRECTIONS** From Highway 12 just north of Sonoma Valley Regional Park, take Arnold Dr. southwest to Glen Ellen. At 0.9 mile, Arnold Dr. crosses a bridge over Calabazas Creek and begins to turn left. Here you bear right onto London Ranch Road, which is heavily used by bicyclists. Go 1.3 miles to the park's entrance kiosk; turn right just past the kiosk into a large paved parking area. If the entrance kiosk is not staffed, pay fee at the self-registration station in the parking area.

**FACILITIES/TRAILHEAD** A visitor center and museum with displays, books, and helpful staff is located next to a separate parking area, just east of the entrance kiosk. Picnic tables, water, and a toilet are near the parking area. The trailhead is on the parking area's southwest side, just behind the self-registration station. Equestrians must use a trailhead located a few hundred feet northwest of the hiking trailhead.

Follow a paved path, which soon changes to a dirt-and-gravel road leading through a shady picnic area. Passing three stone barns, left, you come to a T-junction with another dirt-and-gravel road, part of the Bay Area Ridge Trail. Turn right and pass London's cottage, left, which the author purchased in 1911 and where he died in 1916. The cottage is open to visitors on weekends from 12 to 4 P.M.

Rising dramatically behind London's vineyard is Sonoma Mountain, a long ridge capped by a 2463-foot summit, which is on

### The Pig Palace
The vineyard to the southwest was kept by London's heirs when they sold the rest of the property to the state in 1978. You may see signs for the Pig Palace—an elaborate stone piggery designed by London as a home for prize breeding pigs and built in 1915.

private land just west of the park boundary. About 75 feet from the T-junction, you bear right at a fork onto a dirt road, signed LAKE

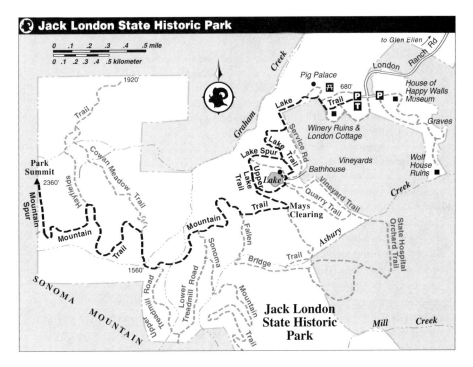

Jack London State Historic Park

and PIG PALACE. Several hundred feet ahead, the trail from the equestrian trailhead, labeled Lake Trail on the park map, joins from the right.

You continue straight, now on the Lake Trail, and in 100 feet pass a hiking-only trail to the Pig Palace. Follow the road as it curves left and soon pass another trail, right, to the Pig Palace. As the road bends sharply left around a corner of the vineyard, you pass a closed trail, right. Before reaching a gate across the road, turn right on the hiking-only Lake Trail. (Bicycles and horses must stay on the road.)

Soon you enter a magical redwood forest and climb moderately past a closed trail to meet a trail signed UPPER LAKE TRAIL, but listed on the park map as the Lake Spur. Turn right and climb to a T-junction, at about 1 mile. Here you turn right, now without doubt on the Upper Lake Trail. After a couple of hundred feet, your route turns sharply left, and now you enjoy a level walk among towering redwoods. (Also found in this park are stands of Douglas-fir, black

**London's Lake**
Created by a stone dam built in 1915, London's Lake was designed as an irrigation reservoir, but soon became a swimming hole where London and his wife, Charmian, entertained their guests. The Londons' bathhouse, which you can visit later, is made of redwood and sits back from the shore on the lake's northeast corner.

oak, blue oak, coast live oak, California bay, madrone, and bigleaf maple.)

Just after an abandoned road joins sharply from the right, you reach a junction with the Mountain Trail, a wide dirt road. Turn right and climb out of the redwood realm to a big grassy meadow called Mays Clearing, which in spring is full of blue-eyed grass, California buttercup, vetch, and false lupine. A rest bench just ahead beckons you to pause and enjoy the stunning view, which extends southeast to Mt. Diablo.

From here, you can extend the trip by following the Mountain Trail, a dirt road, and then the Mountain Spur, a short trail, to the park boundary, about 1 mile northeast of the summit of 2463-foot Sonoma Mountain. To return from Mays Clearing, retrace your route to the junction of the Upper Lake and Mountain trails. At this junction, the Mountain Trail makes an almost 180-degree bend to the right, and you follow it downhill on a gentle and then moderate grade.

As you approach the lake, you pass a path leading left to a stone dam, and then the Quarry Trail, right. Just ahead is a T-junction with a dirt road, drawn incorrectly on the park map. The road heading right is labeled Vineyard Road on the map, and

here you turn left and walk toward the lake, with the stone dam in front of you. Your route then turns right and runs parallel to the dam. Once on the far side of the dam, you can see London's bathhouse and a picnic area with tables, left.

Now you are on the Lake Service Road, but only briefly. Where the road begins to descend, leave it and bear left, coming in about 50 feet to the Lake Trail, a wide dirt path for hiking only. As you follow it downhill, you pass a faint trail, left, to the bathhouse, shown on the map as the Upper Lake Trail. Your trail soon narrows and then closes the loop at the Upper Lake Trail (Lake Spur on map). From here, continue straight on the Lake Trail and retrace your route to the parking area.

## TRIP5 Sonoma Valley Regional Park

| | |
|---|---|
| **Distance** | 2.6 miles, Loop |
| **Hiking Time** | 1 to 2 hours |
| **Difficulty** | Easy |
| **Trail Use** | Leashed dogs, Good for kids |
| **Best Times** | All year |
| **Agency** | SCRPD |
| **Recommended Map** | *None* |

**HIGHLIGHTS**  This small park is big on rewards: a fine picnic area shaded by oaks, a surprisingly varied loop trail that runs through a streamside corridor and then climbs a forested ridge to a high point with great views, and a 1-acre dog-exercise enclosure. For a full-day outing, combine a hike here with a visit to any of the nearby state parks: Jack London, Sugarloaf Ridge, or Annadel.

**DIRECTIONS**  From Highway 12 northbound in Sonoma, use the junction of Broadway and Napa St., on the south side of the Plaza, as the 0.0-mile point. Follow Highway 12 west and then northwest for a total of 6.6 miles to the park entrance, left.

From Highway 12 southbound, south of Kenwood, use the junction with Arnold Dr. as the 0.0-mile point. Continue 0.4 mile to the park entrance, right, and go 0.2 mile to a paved parking area with a self-registration station, then follow the directions above.

**FACILITIES/TRAILHEAD**  There are picnic tables, water, and a toilet near the trailhead, which is on the south end of the parking area, at a metal gate.

A paved multi-use path leaves the parking area and wanders through a large, open field graced here and there with a few venerable native oaks and some planted trees. After about 150 feet, you pass a gravel

road leading uphill to two large water tanks. The path curves to a junction with a dirt-and-gravel road, left, that you will use on the return part of this loop. You continue on the paved path, which descends gently

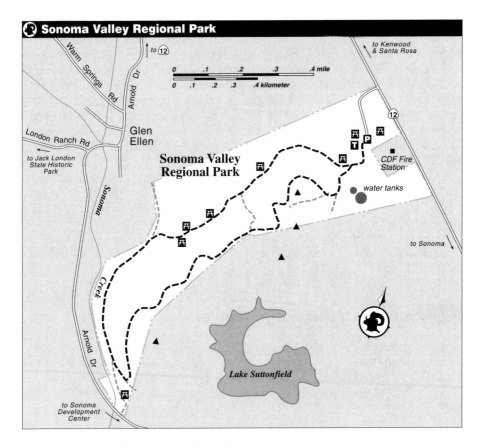

Sonoma Valley Regional Park

to Kenwood & Santa Rosa

to ⑫

Warm Springs Rd

Arnold Dr

London Ranch Rd

Glen Ellen

to Jack London State Historic Park

**Sonoma Valley Regional Park**

Sonoma Creek

Arnold Dr

Creek

CDF Fire Station

water tanks

to Sonoma

Lake Suttonfield

to Sonoma Development Center

past several oak-shaded picnic tables and then finds a mostly level course.

Entering a savanna of mostly blue oak, you follow a seasonal creek that crisscrosses under the trail through culverts. Soon a hiking-only trail departs left, and then an unsigned single track rises right. Several more trails take off left and uphill: ignore them all. Soon a dirt path joins from the right, and then your path bends left. Sonoma Mountain, a high, forested ridge that forms the backbone of Jack London State Historic Park, rises to the southwest.

At a junction where the paved path continues straight, you turn left onto a single-track trail that heads uphill. After about 75 feet you come to a fork, marked by a trail post, where you bear left onto a rocky track that climbs across a steep hillside. Curving right, the trail approaches the crest of a hill,

**The Trees of Sonoma County**

Joining the blue oak in this park are black oak, valley oak, California buckeye, California bay, and manzanita. Oregon ash, a tree that turns brilliant yellow in fall, grows from the creek bed. You'll also find madrone, which invites comparison with its smaller cousin, manzanita. Madrone has orange bark and large, shiny green leaves, whereas manzanita has burgundy bark and small, pointed leaves that range from gray to dark green.

Many of the oaks and other trees and shrubs in this park are draped with beautiful strands of lace lichen, which resembles the Spanish moss of the Southern U.S.

the top of which is on private land, behind a barbed-wire fence. A path, right, goes through a gap in the fence, but you continue straight, soon dropping steeply over rough ground.

Now a level traverse across a steep hillside brings you to a junction, where a trail goes downhill and left. Soon the hiking-only trail you passed earlier joins from the left, and now your route runs along the top of a ridge and then crosses to its left side. Ignore the trails going right at the next two junctions, and instead follow your trail as it bends sharply left, then jogs back to the right. With the two water tanks near the parking area in view, you come to a four-way junction, where you turn left.

Early spring is a good time to spot birds at Sonoma Valley Regional Park.

Now out in the open, the trail passes near the top of a hill, where a short path leads to a rest bench and a vantage point with fine views. Past this spur, the main trail widens as it descends steeply over a bed of loose rock and gravel. Reaching a T-junction with a dirt road, you turn left. Then, after about 75 feet, you merge with a dirt-and-gravel road and bear left. Ahead is the paved path you used at the start of this loop. Bear right on it and retrace your route to the parking area.

## TRIP 6 Shiloh Ranch Regional Park

| | |
|---|---|
| **Distance** | 3.8 miles, Loop |
| **Hiking Time** | 2 to 3 hours |
| **Elevation Gain/Loss** | ±750 feet |
| **Difficulty** | Moderate |
| **Trail Use** | Mountain biking allowed |
| **Best Times** | Spring and fall |
| **Agency** | SCRPD |
| **Recommended Map** | *None* |

**HIGHLIGHTS** This loop, using the Big Leaf, Ridge, Pond, and Creekside trails, explores a forested enclave north of Santa Rosa on the east side of Highway 101. For a longer outing, combine a visit here with one to nearby Foothill Regional Park, on the east side of Highway 101, about 3 miles northwest of here.

**DIRECTIONS** From Highway 101 in Windsor, take the Shiloh Road exit and go east 1.5 miles to Faught Road. Turn right and go 0.1 mile to the park entrance, left, and a paved parking area with a self-registration station.

**FACILITIES/TRAILHEAD** There are restrooms, picnic tables, phone, and water near the trailhead, which is on the north end of the parking area.

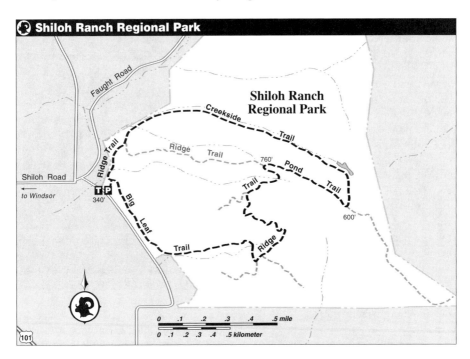

Shiloh Ranch Regional Park

Heading north on the Big Leaf Trail, a rocky dirt road, you soon pass the Ridge Trail, left, which you will use on the return part of this loop. The road curves sharply right and follows a shady course under the arching limbs of coast live oaks, valley oaks, and madrones. Beside the road are common shrubs such as manzanita, toyon, coyote brush, poison oak, and bush monkeyflower. After several hundred feet, you pass an alternate trail from the parking area, right, and soon a horse trail from the parking area merges on your right.

A vineyard slopes uphill from Faught Road and borders the trail. As the road bends left and begins a moderate climb, you encounter tall Douglas-firs and bigleaf maples, the latter combining with the vineyard's grape and nearby poison oak to create a dazzling display of fall foliage. A ravine, right, holds a seasonal creek, and the road swings right to cross it. Soon the vegetation thins and you are in a savanna of mostly blue oak, where a power-line tower and a rest bench mark a junction and the end of the Big Leaf Trail.

Now you bear left on the Ridge Trail and continue a moderate climb that soon eases. The next junction is with the Mark West Creek Trail, right. Here you continue straight on a narrow crest running generally north to a T-junction. Turning right, still on the Ridge Trail, you descend a dirt road on a gentle grade. A deep canyon is left, and your route angles down into it, switchbacks left, and climbs out.

At about 2 miles, turn right on the Pond Trail, a dirt road, and climb gently, with views of Mt. St. Helena northeast through the trees. Now the road loses elevation, gently at first, then on a moderate grade. Where the road begins to bend left, you turn sharply left onto the Creekside Trail, a single track marked with a trail post. Now you head north toward a lovely pond ringed with willows and cattails. Several rest benches invite you to contemplate this small artificial oasis in the midst of mostly open, rolling hills.

Passing the earthen dam at the northwest end of the pond, you continue straight, following a northwest course that soon puts you back in a dense forest. Ferns and mosses give this place a rain-forest feel. The trail threads its way between two steep-sided hills, with a narrow ravine downhill and right. Now the trail descends into the ravine, where two creek beds, which may be dry, merge. Your route drops briefly into their joined bed and then climbs out.

With the ravine still on your right, you climb on a moderate grade to a T-junction with the Ridge Trail, a dirt road. Turning right and walking downhill, you soon pass a

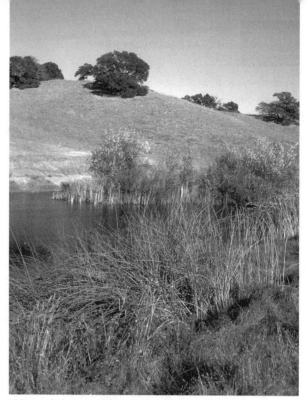

Visit a secluded pond on the aptly named Pond Trail.

junction with an overgrown dirt road, right. Here your road curves left and comes to a seasonal creek, which you cross. Now you meet the Big Leaf Trail to close the loop. Turn right and retrace your route to the parking area.

## TRIP 7 Armstrong Redwoods State Reserve/Austin Creek State Recreation Area

| | |
|---|---|
| **Distance** | 5.6 miles, Loop |
| **Hiking Time** | 4 to 5 hours |
| **Elevation Gain/Loss** | ±1750 feet |
| **Difficulty** | Difficult |
| **Best Times** | All year |
| **Agency** | CSP |
| **Recommended Map** | *Armstrong Redwood State Reserve/Austin Creek State Recreation Area* (CSP) |

**HIGHLIGHTS** This athletic loop, using the East Ridge, Pool Ridge, Discovery, and Pioneer trails, explores the high ground east of Fife Creek in Armstrong Redwoods State Reserve, and then continues north into the Austin Creek State Recreation Area. Groves of old-growth coast redwoods are the prime attraction in the reserve, but the recreation area boasts fine forests of Douglas-fir, oak, and California bay, along with sweeping vistas from the route's high point. The last 0.5 mile of the loop takes you past the Colonel Armstrong and Parson Jones trees, both more than 300 feet high.

**DIRECTIONS**  From Highway 116 in Guerneville, 0.1 mile west of the bridge across the Russian River, go north on Armstrong Woods Road 2.3 miles to the visitor-center parking area, right.

**FACILITIES/TRAILHEAD**  Family campsites are available near Bullfrog Pond, via a steep, narrow 2.5-mile road (campsites are first come, first served; no vehicles over 20 feet; no trailers or other towed vehicles). Beside the parking area are a visitor center with interpretive displays, books, maps, and helpful staff, as well as a ranger station, restrooms, picnic tables, phone, and water. The trailhead is about 75 feet south of the visitor center.

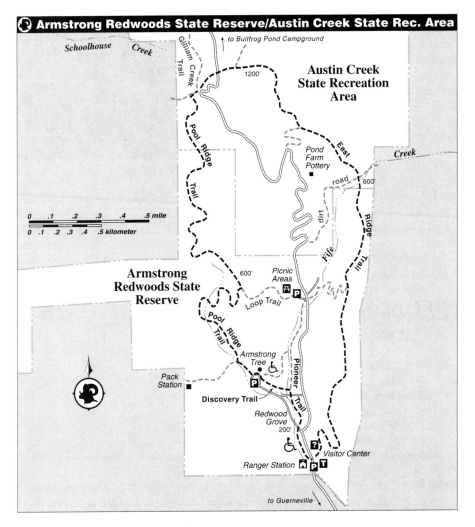

The East Ridge Trail, your route, starts as a paved path just south of the visitor center. The trail soon changes to dirt and finds a moderate course via well-graded switchbacks up the steep east wall of the canyon holding Fife Creek, the reserve's main watercourse. Most of the reserve's towering coast redwoods are found along Fife Creek, but there are many on this hillside too, mixed with Douglas-fir, California bay, tanbark oak, evergreen huckleberry, hazelnut, and bigleaf maple.

After some relentless climbing, the trail gains the crest of a ridge and turns north, following it uphill. Now on a rolling course with some steep sections, you stay right at a fork, then rejoin the left-hand branch after about 150 feet. Staying left at the next fork, you reach a junction, about 50 feet ahead. (To shorten the route, turn left here, descend the trail, then follow paved roads and the Pioneer Trail south to the parking area.)

The forest at the ridgetop is less dense than in the canyon, making way for species such as coast live oak, madrone, black oak, and Oregon oak. The warmer, drier microclimate here encourages shrubs such as manzanita, toyon, coffeeberry, and coyote brush.

You continue straight on the East Ridge Trail, with the crest of a ridge uphill and right, and a steep drop to your left. Dropping into a ravine that holds a tributary of Fife Creek, the trail turns left to cross a bridge, and then comes to a four-way junction with a dirt road, just west of the tributary. You have just left Armstrong Redwoods State Reserve and are now in Austin Creek State Recreation Area. Across the road is the continuation of the East Ridge Trail, which rises on a moderate grade, curves left, and then traverses a large clearing at about 2 miles.

At a junction with a dirt road, left, you continue straight, passing Pond Farm. About 60 feet beyond where a road joins from the left, you reach a fork. Here the dirt road bends left, but your route, the East Ridge Trail, a single track, veers right and uphill. Now in a forest of Douglas-fir, climbing past the ranger's residence, you join a dirt road that curves right, and then begin a steep climb that eases to moderate. Passing an overgrown dirt road, left, your route swings left to cross a seasonal creek,

---

**Pond Farm**

Pond Farm was the site of an artists colony active from 1949 to 1952. Marguerite Wildenhain (1889–1981), a famous Bauhaus-trained ceramicist who left Europe and emigrated to the U.S. to escape Nazi persecution, helped found the farm. She led countless seminars and workshops, and made her home here until her death.

---

and then resumes its relentless climb on a rocky, eroded track.

Crossing a shallow ravine, left, the trail, now a single track, works its way steeply uphill. Leaving the forest, you make a rising traverse across an open slope, where a fine view extends south across the Russian River all the way to Mt. Tamalpais. Spurred on by this scenic reward, you soon reach a flat spot and a grove of trees, left, that makes a perfect picnic spot. Here your trail meets a dirt road, across which are several trails into an area signed as closed.

From this junction, take a moment to climb a short distance to a vantage point for views that stretch from Jackson Mountain, topped with communication towers, to Sonoma Mountain, and, on a clear day, to Mt. Diablo. Then descend the dirt road southwest to paved Armstrong Woods Road, which you cross. You continue downhill, aided by a few wooden steps, until you reach a small parking area adjacent to a dirt road and the trailhead for the Gilliam Creek Trail.

---

**Camping Options**

Four remote backcountry camps — Manning Flat (two camps), Tom King, and Gilliam Creek — are located near East Austin Creek in a far corner of the recreation area, a few hundred feet above sea level. To reach them, hikers use the Gilliam Creek Trail, just ahead, or the Austin Creek Trail, and descend about 1000 feet to the camps.

To find your route, the Pool Ridge Trail, bear right on the dirt road and follow it west a few hundred feet to a junction, where you turn left. The single-track Pool Ridge Trail heads south and descends on a moderate grade over loose dirt and gravel, crossing an open, grassy hillside graced by a large valley oak. Finding level ground, the trail hugs a hillside that drops left, and then pursues a rolling course which takes you across several ravines and back into Armstrong Redwoods State Reserve.

A few downhill switchbacks bring you to a sunny area of chaparral—chamise, scrub oak, toyon, coffeeberry, and bush monkeyflower—and then back into a dense forest. After a moderate descent, the route

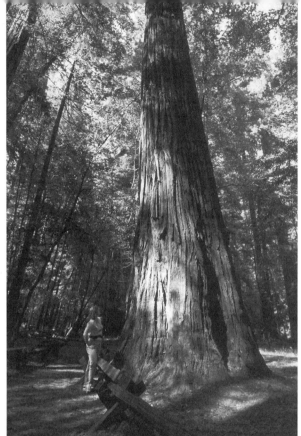

The Pioneer Trail leads to some of the Bay Area's biggest coast redwoods.

levels and reaches a junction not shown on the park map, at about 4 miles. A trail, signed here as the Loop Trail, rises to the right, but you continue straight on the Pool Ridge Trail, now a wide path of loose dirt, in places badly eroded. At the next junction, marked by a trail post, you pass a trail signed PICNIC AREA, and follow the Pool Ridge Trail, signed ARMSTRONG TREE, as it curves right.

You descend via switchbacks into a deep canyon that holds a tributary of Fife Creek. After several crossings of the watercourse, which may be dry, you enjoy a mostly level and then a downhill walk among massive redwoods. Reaching a dirt-and-gravel road that leads to a pack station, right, you turn left and soon come to a paved road, part of a loop. To the right are restrooms and the Depression-era Redwood Forest Theater, once used for artistic performances but now a place of quiet contemplation. You

turn left and walk through the parking area for the Discovery Trail, a route especially designed for the visually impaired, but one that can be enjoyed by all park visitors.

Leaving the parking area, you begin a level walk on a dirt hiking path. On the right is a nylon rope, stretched between posts, to serve as a guide for blind or visually impaired visitors, and there are markers along the way in English and Braille describing features of the reserve and its magnificent trees. After about 100 feet, you come to the Colonel Armstrong Tree, 308 feet high, 14.6 feet in diameter, and, at more than 1400 years old, said to be the reserve's most ancient tree.

Just past the Armstrong Tree is a fork marked by a trail post, where you bear right. Most members of the redwood-forest community can be found here, including tanbark oak, hazelnut, wild rose, and redwood sorrel. Reaching a paved road, you bear left and cross Fife Creek, which flows under the

---

**A Giant Exhibit**

A display created from the cross-section of a redwood that began its life in 948 AD shows some important dates in world history: 1215, the signing of the Magna Carta; 1492, the landing of Columbus in the New World; 1776, the Declaration of Independence; 1906, the San Francisco earthquake. Sadly, the last date, 1978, is the year the tree was felled by vandals.

---

road. Once on the east side of the creek, turn right, cross the road, and join the Pioneer Trail heading south.

A few feet beyond the display of historical dates is a another paved road. Left is the Parson Jones Tree, at more than 310 feet high said to be the preserve's tallest. It is 13.8 feet in diameter and more than 1300 years old. Crossing the paved road, you rejoin the Pioneer Trail and soon reach Armstrong Woods Road, with the reserve's entrance kiosk to your right. After crossing the road, turn right and in a few paces reach the visitor center and the parking area.

## TRIP 8 Sonoma Coast State Beach: Bodega Head Loop

| | |
|---|---|
| **Distance** | 1 mile, Loop |
| **Hiking Time** | 1 hour or less |
| **Difficulty** | Easy |
| **Trail Use** | Good for kids |
| **Best Times** | All year |
| **Agency** | CSP |
| **Recommended Map** | *Sonoma Coast State Beach* (CSP) |

**HIGHLIGHTS**  The jutting promontory of Bodega Head is a fine place to come face to face with the elemental forces — sun, sea, and sky — that preside over California's coast, and the easy loop trail that circles the head presents you with fine vistas almost every step of the way. This hike can easily be combined with others on the Sonoma coast to make a full-day outing.

**DIRECTIONS**  From Highway 1 just north of the town of Bodega Bay, turn west onto East Shore Road, signed here for Bodega Head and Westside Park Marinas. Go 0.3 mile to a stop sign at Bay Flat Road and turn right. Continue straight — first on Bay Flat Road, then on West Shore and Westside roads — for a total of 3.7 miles to a large dirt-and-gravel parking area at the end of the road.

**Facilities/Trailhead**  There are toilets at the trailhead, which is on the southeast side of the parking area.

You set off on a level, single-track trail heading almost due east, passing two trails, one left, the other right. Directly below are Campbell Cove and the two rock jetties that form the entrance channel to Bodega Harbor. Just across the channel is a sandy finger of land called Doran Beach, a popular county park. Bodega Head itself is the tip of a large, mostly treeless peninsula jutting south from the Sonoma coast mainland.

The hilly terrain around you is covered with grasses and scrub vegetation such as coyote brush, blackberry vines, and yellow bush lupine. This can be a beautiful, sunny paradise or a bleak, windswept barren — the only constant here is the mournful note of the channel marker

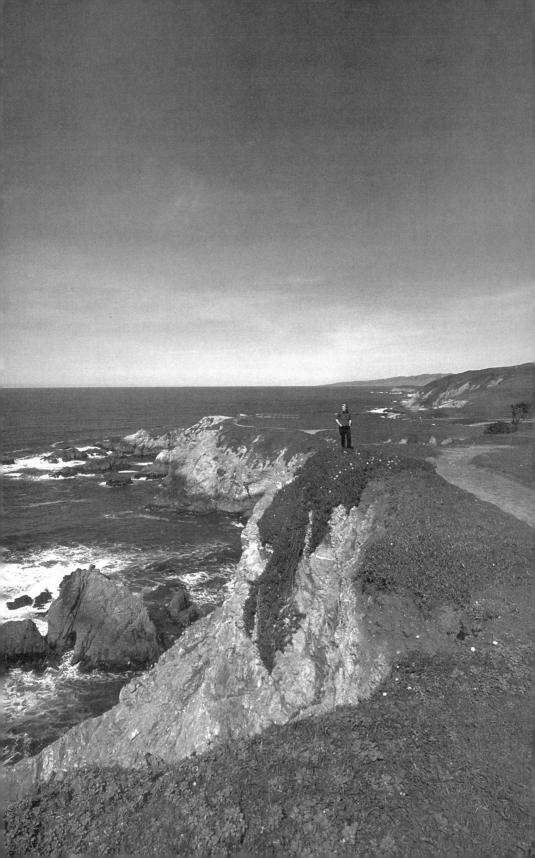

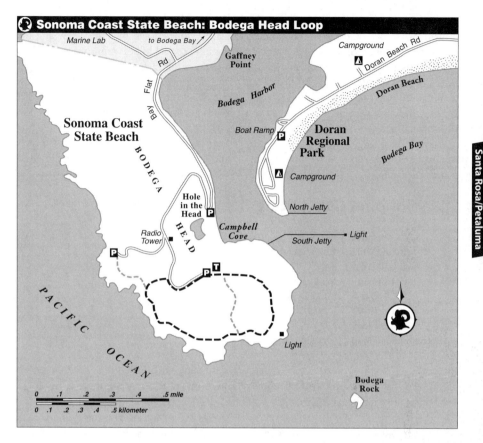

**Sonoma Coast State Beach: Bodega Head Loop**

warning boaters of the narrow harbor entrance.

After passing another trail heading left, your route begins its clockwise curve around Bodega Head, and soon, if the day is clear, you can make out Tomales Point and the entrance to Tomales Bay to the south-east, Point Reyes to the south, and even the Farallon Islands. Bodega Bay is the enor-mous semicircle of water between Bodega Head and Tomales Bay. A trail plunges left down a steep ravine, but your route contin-ues to bend right. Just offshore to the south-east is a big rock used as a roost by sea birds and as a haul-out for seals, whose barking you may hear.

A large nautical marker of red and white squares topped by a light is uphill and right. Below and left, waves crash against the

**Watch Your Step!**

The southeast face of Bodega Head is a sheer cliff, so use caution as you approach it. Avoid mishaps by stopping whenever you admire the view and, as you hike, by paying attention to where you place your feet.

head's rocky foundations. As the trail turns west and rises on a gentle grade, you are confronted with the wide Pacific Ocean, magnificent no matter what the weather or the season.

As your trail crests a rise, you pass a trail, right, and then swing left and downhill. Daubs of color are added to the scene by the yellow-and-red flowers of seaside paint-brush, and the magenta blooms of iceplant,

The 1-mile loop trail around Bodega Head offers fine views of the Pacific Ocean.

a succulent that carpets California's coastal dunes and sandy roadside embankments. Just offshore, lines of brown pelicans or cormorants may be cruising low over the waves. Where a trail heads downhill and left to a promontory, your route bends right, hugging the cliffs, with no fence to keep you from the abyss.

Jagged, knife-edged ridges jut proudly toward the ocean and slice down to the water's edge. Enjoying a level walk, you begin to get views to the northeast, across Bodega Harbor to the town of Bodega Bay and the Sonoma coastal hills. Passing another trail to a promontory, left, your route swings right and descends, soon passing within about 6 feet of a dirt road, right. Cross over to the dirt road and follow it downhill for about 100 yards to a low metal gate and a wooden fence. Step over the gate, bear right across a dirt-and-gravel turnout, and then get on the paved road that leads uphill to the parking area.

## TRIP 9 Sonoma Coast State Beach: Kortum Trail

| | |
|---|---|
| **Distance** | 3.7 miles, Out-and-back |
| **Hiking Time** | 2 to 3 hours |
| **Elevation Gain/Loss** | ±400 |
| **Difficulty** | Moderate |
| **Trail Use** | Good for kids |
| **Best Times** | All year |
| **Agency** | CSP |
| **Recommended Map** | *Sonoma Coast State Beach* (CSP) |

**HIGHLIGHTS**  This out-and-back trip on part of the Kortum Trail parallels the Pacific Ocean on a coastal prairie just west of Highway 1. For most of the way the route is within sight of the crags and cliffs that rise from the water's edge. For a more ambitious outing, try starting at Wright's Beach, about 1.5 miles south; in that case the round-trip distance would be 7.6 miles. The Kortum Trail is often done as a car-shuttle trip — the entire route from Wright's Beach to Goat Rock is 3.8 miles. This hike can easily be combined with others on the Sonoma coast to make a full-day outing.

**DIRECTIONS**  From Highway 1 northbound just north of the town of Bodega Bay, use the junction of Highway 1 and East Shore Road, the turnoff to Bodega Head, as the 0.0-mile mark. Go north 7.1 miles to the entrance to Shell Beach. Turn left and go 0.1 mile to the parking area.

From Highway 1 southbound just south of Jenner, use the junction of Highway 1 and Highway 116 as the 0.0-mile mark, and go south 1.9 miles to the entrance to Shell Beach, right. Turn right and go 0.1 mile to the parking area.

**FACILITIES/TRAILHEAD**  There are restrooms near the trailhead, which is on the northwest corner of the parking area.

Leaving the parking area, you head northwest on a single track through coastal scrub — mostly coyote brush — and across the open, flat coastal prairie. This wide and grassy expanse stretches from Highway 1 to the rocky cliffs that border the Pacific. The scenic cove of Shell Beach is downhill and left. A gully with willow thickets is also left, and you pass a trail heading in that direction that goes to a vantage point at the edge of the seaside cliffs.

Ahead, as you proceed, you can see two large rocks, one in the ocean, a roost for sea birds, and the other on dry land. At some time in the not-too-distant past, both were underwater, but geological forces uplifted

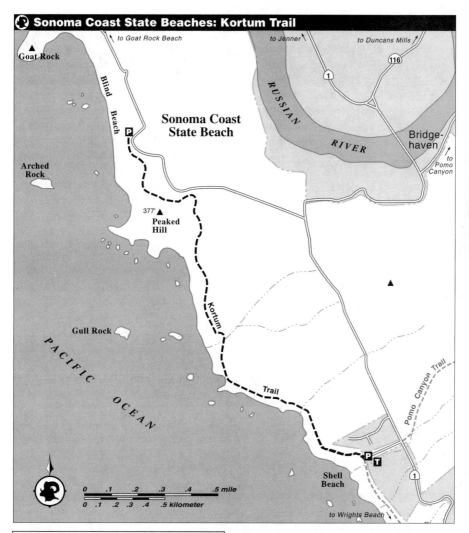

**Sonoma Coast State Beaches: Kortum Trail**

to Goat Rock Beach · to Jenner · to Duncans Mills

Goat Rock

Blind Beach

**Sonoma Coast State Beach**

Arched Rock

377' Peaked Hill

Gull Rock

Kortum Trail

PACIFIC OCEAN

RUSSIAN RIVER

Bridge-haven

to Pomo Canyon

Pomo Canyon Trail

Shell Beach

0 .1 .2 .3 .4 .5 mile
0 .1 .2 .3 .4 .5 kilometer

to Wrights Beach

## The Kortum Trail

This trail, which stretches nearly 4 miles from Wright's Beach to Goat Rock, honors Bill Kortum, a dairy veterinarian and coastal-preservation advocate who helped defeat a proposed nuclear power plant at Bodega Bay. Kortum, who served in the 1970s as a Sonoma County supervisor, was also active in the fight to preserve public access to lands acquired by the Sea Ranch development, and this effort led to passage of the Coastal Act of 1972 and the creation of the Coastal Commission and the Coastal Conservancy.

the marine terrace you are standing on and put the rocks in their present alignment. The San Andreas fault, chief architect of California's coastline, is just offshore here.

Beyond the two rocks rises Peaked Hill, and beyond it are the Sonoma coastal mountains north of the Russian River, which empties into the ocean near the town of Jenner. A path, left, leads to a promontory, and if you turn and look southeast, you can see the hulking form of Bodega Head in the distance. Now a trail veers left, but your route goes right and through a gap in a barbed-wire fence. Just beyond the

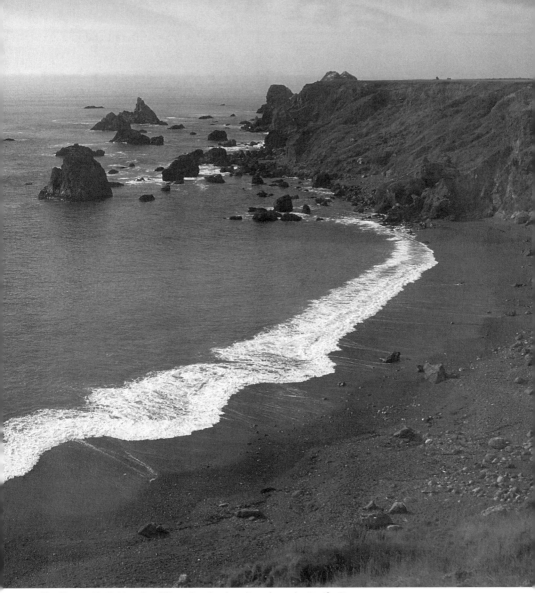

The Kortum Trail skirts the cliffs and rocky shoreline along the Pacific Ocean.

fence, a trail branches right, but you continue straight, stepping across a narrow fissure in the ground.

The trail forks again, and you stay right. Many paths lead toward the ocean, and soon your route does too, coming to the edge of a cliff above a lovely cove with a sandy beach. Now you are joined by a trail coming sharply from the right, and soon you descend into a verdant gully which may be wet. The next gully has a bridge over it. After crossing it the route turns left, and then comes to a fork, marked by a trail post, where you bear right.

In the open fields around you may find sparrows and western meadowlarks, and the off-shore rocks may hold pelicans, cormorants, and common murres.

Just beyond where a trail joins sharply from the left, you pass through a gap in a

**Rock Pillars**

Pillars of rock, at one time sea stacks in the ocean, jut upward from the coastal prairie. Some of these pillars were used during World War II as bombing-practice targets. One, called Sunshine Rocks, is today used for practice by local climbers because it offers a bomb-proof belay spot.

barbed-wire fence. Immediately you come to a narrow trail heading left, but you continue straight on the wider path. Now the trail drops into a shallow, wildly overgrown ravine, which holds a bridged creek. As the trail rises from the ravine bottom, you pass a trail, left, but your route continues uphill over wooden steps and bends right. At about 1 mile, the trail dips into and out of another shallow ravine, and then swings right, toward a jumble of rock pillars.

At an unmarked fork, you stay right, passing the rock pillars. Just past the pillars, a path heads right, but you continue straight, now climbing on a moderate grade. The trail markers here are round wood posts with the tops cut at a 45-degree angle. Fine views, which get better with each step, extend southeast along the coastline toward Bodega Head, and beyond to Point Reyes. A trail leads left toward Peaked Hill, the high point on a ridge you will soon surmount. Ignoring that trail, you continue

straight up the ridge, pass through a gap in a barbed-wire fence, and then turn left.

Now you have a paved road uphill and right, and a short trail branches to it. You stay on the main trail, which runs parallel to the road, and head for a saddle between Peaked Hill and a lesser summit. When you reach the saddle, where a trail heads left, an entirely new vista is waiting for your enjoyment, this one sweeping northwest along the Sonoma coast, north of the Russian River.

Now descending from the saddle on a moderate grade, you have a beautiful view ahead to Goat Rock, a flat-topped giant joined to the mainland by a narrow strip of sand. Beyond it are the mouth of the Russian River and the town of Jenner. To your left is Arched Rock, a wave-eroded outpost. Be careful not to look and walk at the same time, as the trail is rocky and needs your complete attention.

Soon the route levels and traverses a grassy hillside, coming to a barbed-wire fence with a gap, and then the paved road you approached a few minutes ago. Walking along its shoulder, you reach the parking area for Blind Beach, which is just southeast of Goat Rock. You can reach the beach via a dirt-and-gravel road. On the northeast side of the parking area are restrooms. When you are ready to return, retrace your route to the parking area at Shell Beach.

Santa Rosa/Petaluma

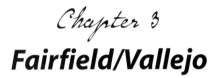

*Chapter 3*

# Fairfield/Vallejo

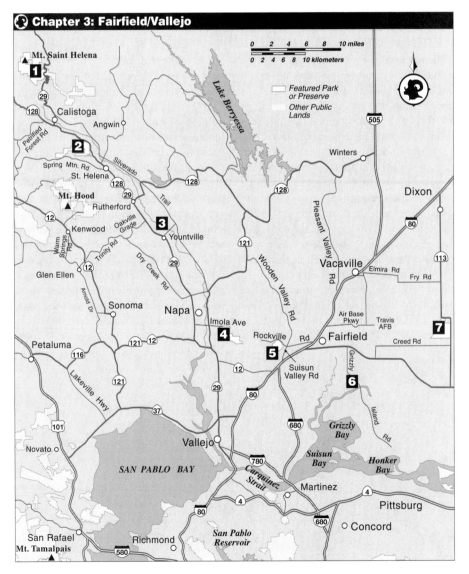

Mt. Saint Helena

1

29

128

Calistoga

Angwin

Petrified Forest Rd

Lake Berryessa

0   2   4   6   8   10 miles
0  2  4  6  8  10 kilometers

☐ Featured Park or Preserve
☐ Other Public Lands

505

Winters

2

Spring Mtn. Rd
St. Helena

Silverado

128

128

128

Dixon

80

Mt. Hood

Rutherford

Trail

12

Oakville Grade

3

Yountville

Kenwood

Warm Springs Rd

Trinity Rd

Dry Creek Rd

29

121

113

Pleasant Valley Rd

Vacaville

Elmira Rd    Fry Rd

Glen Ellen

12

Arnold Dr

Sonoma

Napa

Imola Ave

Wooden Valley Rd

Air Base Pkwy    Travis AFB

7

Petaluma

116

121   12

4

Rockville    Rd    Fairfield

Creed Rd

Lakeville Hwy

121

12

29

Suisun Valley Rd

5

Grizzly

6

Island Rd

101

37

680

Grizzly Bay

Novato

Vallejo

80

780

Suisun Bay

Honker Bay

SAN PABLO BAY

Carquinez Strait

Martinez

4

Pittsburg

80

4

680

Concord

San Rafael
Mt. Tamalpais

Richmond

San Pablo Reservoir

580

# TRIP 1 Robert Louis Stevenson State Park: Mt. St. Helena

| | |
|---|---|
| **Distance** | 10.6 miles, Out-and-back |
| **Hiking Time** | 4 to 6 hours |
| **Elevation Gain/Loss** | ±2100 feet |
| **Difficulty** | Difficult |
| **Trail Use** | Mountain biking allowed[1] |
| **Best Times** | Spring and fall |
| **Agency** | CSP |
| **Recommended Map** | *Bothe-Napa Valley State Park & Robert Louis Stevenson State Park* (CSP) |
| **Notes** | [1]Using alternate trailhead, about 0.2 mile ahead on the left side of Highway 29, at a gated fire road |

**HIGHLIGHTS** This out-and-back route, a "must-do" for lovers of high places, takes you to the 4339-foot North Peak of Mt. St. Helena, the tallest summit in the North Bay. Using an 0.8-mile single-track trail and a 4.5-mile section of the Mt. St. Helena Trail, a dirt road, the route is exposed for much of its length to sun, wind, and weather. The difficult rating comes from distance and elevation gain, not steepness. Pick a cool day with unlimited visibility, and you will reap all the magnificent scenic rewards this hike has to offer.

**DIRECTIONS** From the intersection of Highways 128 and 29 in Calistoga (at Lincoln Ave.), go northwest 8.7 miles on Highway 29 to a small parking area on the left side of the road at the highway's summit. If this area is full, park in the large area just across the highway. The trailhead for bicycles is about 0.2 mile ahead on the left side of Highway 29, at a gated fire road. Parking for this trailhead is on the right side of the highway, just past the fire road.

**FACILITIES/TRAILHEAD** There are picnic tables beside the parking area. The trailhead is on the west side of Highway 29, next to the small parking area. If you need to cross Highway 29, do so carefully!

Ascend a set of wooden steps to the trail, here a wide dirt track, and pass a sign with information about the park's namesake, the author of *The Silverado Squatters*, *Treasure Island*, and other books. The trail rises gently in a dense forest of Douglas-fir, tanbark oak, California bay, madrone, and bigleaf maple. Mixed in with the taller trees are coffeeberry, hazelnut, poison oak, and California nutmeg, an evergreen with spine-tipped needles.

Following the switchbacks uphill over rocky ground, you soon reach a more open, sunny area, where chaparral shrubs prevail. Back in dense forest, you soon pass a stone marker indicating the site of the Stevensons' honeymoon cabin, nothing of which remains. Just past the marker, the route makes a sharp right-hand switchback, and you climb a gently angled slab of rock.

At a junction with the Mt. St. Helena Trail, a dirt road, you turn left, now with a good view of the rocky abutments and ramparts on the mountain's southeast flank. In a very rocky area, the road bends right and passes a trail post.

Both gray and knobcone pines, each having needles in bundles of three, are

### The Toll House

From the mid-1800s to 1900, the rugged hills of Napa County were studded with mines that produced cinnabar, an ore of mercury, as well as silver and gold. A toll road to Calistoga, the railhead, ran nearby, and as you begin your climb you may see what remains of the old toll house — its concrete foundation.

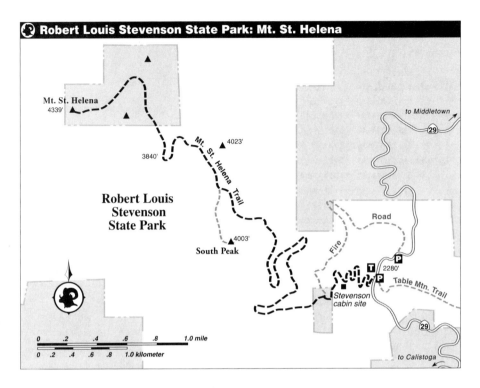

## Robert Louis Stevenson State Park: Mt. St. Helena

found on the mountain. Gray pines have large cones, and needles nearly a foot long, whereas knobcone pines have smaller, egg-shaped cones, and needles from 3 to 7 inches long. Knobcone pines are adapted to fire: heat opens the cones and releases their seeds.

At a clearing beneath a dramatic, eroded cliff, the road makes an almost 180-degree bend to the right. From this point on, the feeling of isolation becomes more and more intense as you follow the well-graded road upward at a steepness that alternates between easy and moderate.

Around 2 miles, at a wide clearing crossed by power lines, you make a 180-degree turn to the left. Another sharp turn, this one right, aims you almost due north and soon brings you to very eroded ground. On your right, outcrops of rock fractured into columns may remind you of Devils Postpile in the Sierra. Now on a moderate grade, you have sweeping views east and northeast toward the series of ridges and summits that form the

> **Volcanic Activity**
>
> Although it is made of volcanic rock, Mt. St. Helena itself is not a volcano. But nearby volcanoes, quiet for several million years and no longer recognizable because of erosion and fault movement, once spewed layers of ash that can still be seen in road cuts along Highway 29.

border between Napa and Yolo counties; beyond lies the Central Valley.

You pass the road to South Peak (4003'), left, at around 3.5 miles. Continuing straight, past mostly scrub vegetation, you have a fine view of the Napa Valley, framed by a V-notch formed by two intervening ridges. Reaching a clearing, you pass a road, left, that heads toward several communication towers. Your route swings left and finds a level course, with North Peak in view at last. Soon a turnaround marks the spot where the well-graded road ends and a short, steep, rocky track to North Peak begins.

**Moniker Mystery**

How Mt. St. Helena got its name is uncertain. According to *California Place Names,* the first recorded climb took place in 1841 by a Russian, J. G. Woznesenski. A replica of the plaque left on the summit by the 1841 Russian party is on the southwest side of the communication facilities. It is even said that Princess Helena de Gagarin, a niece of the Czar, climbed the mountain and bestowed upon it the name of her patron saint. Perhaps a more likely derivation is the name of a Russian ship, the *Saint Helena,* whose crew may have spotted the peak from off the Northern California coast.

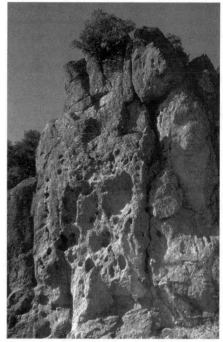

Eroded rock formations rise steeply beside Mt. St. Helena Trail.

Passing several communication facilities, you arrive at last on the summit of North Peak—in the Bay Area, only Copernicus Peak on Mt. Hamilton is higher, by a mere 34 feet. The 360-degree views, on a clear day, are stunning, taking in all the familiar North Bay summits, plus Lassen Peak and even Mt. Shasta, 192 miles away. After you have finished enjoying this spectacular vantage point, retrace your route to the parking area.

# *TRIP 2* Bothe–Napa Valley State Park

| | |
|---:|:---|
| **Distance** | 4.5 miles, Semi-loop |
| **Hiking Time** | 2 to 3 hours |
| **Elevation Gain/Loss** | ±950 feet |
| **Difficulty** | Moderate |
| **Best Times** | Spring and fall |
| **Agency** | CSP |
| **Recommended Map** | *Bothe–Napa Valley State Park & Robert Louis Stevenson State Park* (CSP) |

**HIGHLIGHTS** This semi-loop, using the Ritchey Canyon, Redwood, Coyote Peak, and South Fork trails, explores the lush riparian habitat along Ritchey Creek and the wonderful upland forest and chaparral surrounding Coyote Peak. Spring and fall are the best times to visit. During the rainy season, it may be impossible to ford Ritchey Creek—as required on the return part of this route—and a detour using the Ritchey Canyon Trail and the Ritchey Creek Campground road may be required. However, *except* during the rainy season, the first parts of the Redwood and the Ritchey Canyon trails are heavily used by equestrians, mostly riders from the nearby horse concession, and may be carpeted with horse dung.

**DIRECTIONS** From Highway 29 northbound in St. Helena, go 5 miles from the first St. Helena stoplight (at Pope St.) to the park entrance, left. After 0.1 mile you reach the entrance kiosk. If the entrance kiosk is not staffed, pay fee at the self-registration station in the parking area just ahead and right. Continue another 0.3 mile to the parking area for the Ritchey Creek trails, right.

From Highways 29 or 128 southbound in Calistoga, go 3.5 miles from their merger (Lincoln Ave.) to the park entrance, right. Then follow directions above.

**FACILITIES/TRAILHEAD** The park has a campground with 50 sites that can be reserved; call (800) 444-7275. A visitor center near the entrance kiosk, open most weekends, has books and maps. A phone and a swimming pool are near the parking area; there is a water fountain on the trail within the first 0.5 mile. The trailhead is on the west end of the parking area.

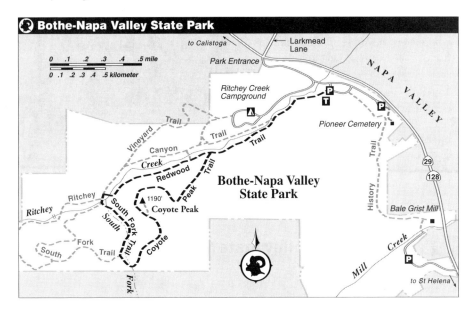

Heading west on the Ritchey Canyon Trail, you soon cross a paved road and then pass a junction with a trail, right. You merge with a dirt-and-gravel road coming from the left. At about the 0.5-mile point, the Ritchey Canyon Trail branches right, but your route, the Redwood Trail, continues straight and begins to climb on a moderate and then gentle grade. Soon you reach a junction with the Coyote Peak Trail, where you turn left and begin a winding uphill course on a moderate grade that changes in places to steep.

Dropping slightly to cross a small seasonal stream, the route curves right and climbs. Bending left, the trail, now rocky and eroded, emerges from the trees and traverses an area of chaparral. Still gaining elevation, in some places steeply, you reenter a dense forest. The trail here is a narrow track gouged out of a steep hillside falling away to your right. Magnificent manzanitas —tall, bulky, and twisted—grow in company with chaparral pea and yerba santa.

Around 2 miles, the route forks: the trail to the forested summit of Coyote Peak (1170') goes left, and the Coyote Peak Trail goes right. Turning right and descending over loose dirt and rock, you cross a divide and then begin to climb. Soon veering right,

**Trees & Trout**

The wooded area bordering Ritchey Creek is home to a wonderful variety of trees, including California bay, coast redwood, Douglas-fir, madrone, valley oak, and bigleaf maple. The creek itself holds a run of steelhead trout, federally listed as a threatened species.

the shrub-lined trail affords you here and there a view back toward Coyote Peak. Now you follow a rolling downhill course and cross a tributary of Ritchey Creek. Where the Coyote Peak Trail ends, you continue straight on the South Fork Trail, descending steeply in places.

Stepping across the tributary, you continue your descent to a bridge. Once across, you turn right, and in about 100 feet reach a junction with the Spring Trail, a dirt road. Here you turn right and follow the road as it crosses Ritchey Creek, which flows beneath it through a culvert. About 75 feet farther, you reach a junction offering a confusing array of trails. From here, your route, the Redwood Trail, a single track, veers sharply

right and heads back toward Ritchey Creek. Once beside it, you soon come to a spot where you can cross the creek on rocks.

If you are able to cross Ritchey Creek, follow it downstream. The trail soon makes a steeply rising traverse across a hillside that drops left. After leveling and then descending, you are back beside the bubbling creek, enjoying a walk through groves of redwoods. After passing a trail, left, that leads across the creek to the Ritchey Canyon Trail, you soon reach the junction with the Coyote Peak Trail. From here, retrace your route to the parking area.

**High Water**

During periods of high water, crossing Ritchey Creek may be impossible. If it is, return to the Spring Trail and turn right. Follow the dirt road, now called the Ritchey Canyon Trail, as it bends right and runs northeast, parallel to Ritchey Creek. When you reach Ritchey Creek Campground, follow the paved campground road to the park entrance road and turn right, returning to the parking area.

## TRIP3 Napa River Ecological Reserve

| | |
|---|---|
| **Distance** | 1.3 miles, Semi-loop |
| **Hiking Time** | 1 hour or less |
| **Difficulty** | Easy |
| **Trail Use** | Leashed dogs, Good for kids |
| **Best Times** | Late spring through fall |
| **Agency** | CDF&G |
| **Recommended Map** | *Trail Guide Napa River Ecological Reserve* (Napa – Solano Audubon Society) |

**HIGHLIGHTS** This semi-loop explores a small reserve wedged between the Napa River and Conn Creek near the Napa Valley town of Yountville. Traversing some of the last remaining old-growth riparian habitat in the Napa Valley, the trail brings you into a realm of oaks, birds, butterflies, and wildflowers. **Boldface** numbers in the route description refer to numbered markers along the trail, which are keyed to a trail guide published by the Napa – Solano Audubon Society. Access to the Nature Trail is impossible during the rainy season, because a footbridge over the Napa River, the trail's sole access, is removed. To find out if the bridge is in place, call the California Dept. of Fish and Game, (707) 944-5500.

**DIRECTIONS**  From Highway 29 in Yountville, take the Madison St. exit and go northeast 0.25 mile to Yount St. Turn left onto Yount St., and then immediately right onto Yountville Cross Road. Go 0.9 mile to the reserve's parking area, left.

**FACILITIES/TRAILHEAD**  There is a toilet at the trailhead, which is on the northwest side of the parking area.

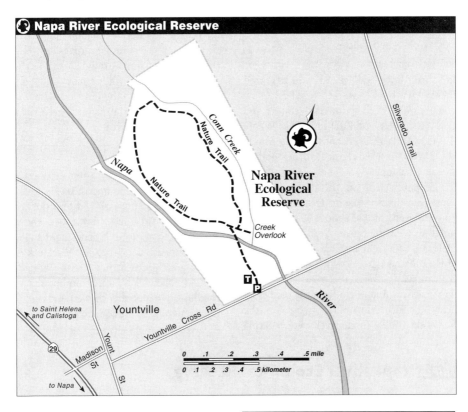

The trail heads northwest across an open, weedy field, with a vineyard on the left and a dirt-and-stone levee, right. About 100 yards from the trailhead, you climb over the levee, which has a trail running along its top, and descend toward the Napa River. Large valley oaks, one of the reserve's prime attractions, offer shade here. Once on the gravelly riverbed itself, you lose the trail, and the signs here are not much help.

About 75 feet past the top of levee, you arrive at a clearing; here the next trail post, partially hidden by brush, directs you left. Walk about 125 feet upstream and then turn right. About 100 feet ahead is a wooden bridge, which gets removed during the rainy

**The Birds & the Beasts**

According to the Napa–Solano Audubon Society, 146 different species of birds have been observed on the reserve, including 67 nesting species (the rest pass through, either on migration or local wanderings), such as wood ducks, woodpeckers, swallows, and owls. Migration brings an influx of songbirds, and in spring, butterflies and wildflowers add color to the landscape. Mammals that live here include deer, raccoons, skunks, squirrels, opossums, and minks, although most of these are active at night, when the reserve is closed.

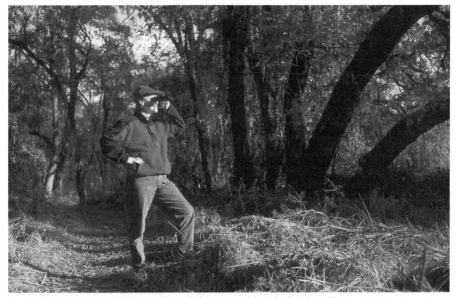

The self-guiding Nature Trail loops through this preserve beside the Napa River.

season. Once across the river, you veer left on a dirt trail and climb to a junction. Here you turn right and follow a short spur trail that leads to marker **1**, overlooking Conn Creek, named in honor of John Conn, an early Napa Valley settler. The land this reserve occupies was once called the Yountville Camp Grounds, and large religious camp meetings were held here from 1851 until 1879.

Now back at the junction, go right on a dirt trail for about 15 feet to the start of the Nature Trail loop. A nearby box is supposed to contain trail brochures but may be empty. Bearing right at the fork, you soon come to marker **2**, indicating poison oak. The level trail meanders through lush woodland on a wedge of high ground between the Napa River and Conn Creek.

One of the factors that make this reserve a great birding area is the presence of different habitats close together. For some reason, birding is often most successful on the border between habitats, such as the edge of a marsh, creek, or meadow. Here, a large meadow, left, may offer good viewing.

Marker **3** describes lace lichen, which is actually two life forms, an alga and a fun-

gus, growing in a symbiotic relationship. Lichen is sensitive to air quality, so it is heartening to see so much of it here. Marker **4** refers to dead trees, called snags, used by acorn woodpeckers to store acorns for the winter.

Dropping to cross a gully, the route returns to shade, arriving at marker **5**, a good place to listen for birds. As the trail bends left, you come upon a rest bench and marker **6**. The nearby town of Yountville

---

**Napa River Flora**

In addition to valley oak and bay, trees found on the reserve include coast live oak, Oregon ash, bigleaf maple, white alder, and Fremont cottonwood. Among trees, shrubs, and grasses, some nonnative species can pose a threat to natives, but others are harmless. Among the most unwelcome here are eucalyptus, French broom, English plantain, and Italian thistle. The few fruit trees you may see in the reserve, although not native, provide food for birds and deer, and are not considered harmful.

was named for George C. Yount, a North Carolinian who came to California in 1831. Five years later, Yount was granted a rancho, called Rancho Caymus, in the Napa Valley, the present site of the town of Yountville. The name of the rancho lives on as a vineyard in Rutherford that produces some of the Napa Valley's finest wine.

At marker **7**, be sure to stop and admire a large, ropy vine of California wild grape, perhaps more than 100 years old. Also here are two kinds of blackberry—California, a native, and Himalayan, an import from Europe. Now veering left again, you find marker **8** and a bed of periwinkle, another visitor from Europe, a spreading ground

cover with blue flowers that may bloom year-round.

An overlook at marker **9** gives you a chance to view the Napa River. Here, at a wide spot, the rushing current during high water has undercut the far bank. When enough ground has been lost, trees will topple into the river, providing quiet pools for fish, among them migratory steelhead trout, federally listed as a threatened species. The trail now bends right and reaches the south end of the meadow, where marker **10** indicates two shrubs, wild rose and snowberry. When you reach the junction at the start of the Nature Trail loop, bear right and retrace your route to the parking area.

# TRIP 4 Skyline Wilderness Park

| | |
|---|---|
| **Distance** | 6 miles, Loop |
| **Hiking Time** | ±1200 feet |
| **Elevation Gain/Loss** | 3 to 4 hours |
| **Difficulty** | Moderate |
| **Trail Use** | Mountain biking allowed |
| **Best Times** | Spring and fall |
| **Agency** | SPCA |
| **Recommended Map** | *Skyline Wilderness Park* (SPCA) |

**HIGHLIGHTS**  Wildflowers and scenic vistas are the attractions of this unique park, run by the Skyline Park Citizens Association. True to its name, the Skyline Trail, combined here with the Buckeye Trail to form a loop, clings to high ground for most of its length, as befits a segment of the Bay Area Ridge Trail. The Skyline Trail comes down only near Lake Marie, your destination. Park maintenance is a volunteer effort, so some trails may be in better shape than others — long pants are advised. The park welcomes equestrians and bicyclists as well as hikers. Bicyclists must wear helmets; the park is closed Thanksgiving and Christmas.

**DIRECTIONS**  From Highway 29 in Napa, take the Imola Ave./Lake Berryessa/Highway 121 North exit and go east 2.9 miles on Imola Ave. to the park entrance, right. After paying a fee at the entrance kiosk and getting a map, bear right and go about 200 feet to a paved parking area.

**FACILITIES/TRAILHEAD**  A campground adjacent to the parking area hosts RVs year-round, and tent camping during spring and summer. Also in the park are picnic and barbecue areas, a disc-golf course, an activity center, a cookhouse, a social center for meetings and indoor parties, and an equestrian arena. Picnic tables, restrooms, and water are beside the parking area. The trailhead is on the southwest corner of the parking area.

This park, on land formerly used by Napa State Hospital, was created by concerned

citizens who were unwilling to see the State of California sell state land to private

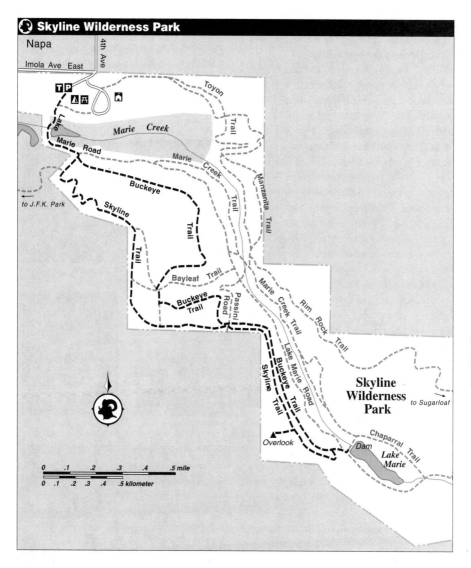

developers. With the help of various conservation groups, a unique deal was struck: the state leased the land to Napa County, which in turn leased it to the Skyline Park Citizens Association. The park, which opened in 1980, depends on user fees and volunteer efforts to keep it open.

You walk south from the parking area, past the Martha Walker Native Habitat Garden, right. After about 400 feet, you come to a T-junction with a rough paved road, where you turn right. Passing the

**The Walker Garden**
Martha Walker, who died at age 78 in 1983, was a botanist who taught at the community college, hosted a radio program, and wrote a column in the *Napa Valley Register*. Her namesake garden, designed to attract birds, is worth a visit. It contains both native and nonnative plants, bird feeders, a bird path, and a duck pond.

garden's entrance, right, you continue another 400 feet and, at the next T-junction, turn left onto Lake Marie Road.

After about 100 feet, the dirt road merges with a paved road, where you veer left. Before reaching the Napa State Hospital gate, you turn right onto a dirt road, passing Lake Louise, left, and Lake Camille, right. After approximately 200 feet, the road bends left and reaches a junction. Here you turn right on the Skyline Trail, a dirt-and-gravel road that is part of the Bay Area Ridge Trail, and climb moderately amid stands of coast live oak, California bay, blue oak, and California buckeye.

After a few hundred feet, you pass the Buckeye Trail, your return route, left. Ahead is the Lower Skyline Trail, also left. About 50 feet farther, you turn left on the Skyline Trail. The steep, rocky trail makes a series of rising switchbacks, rewarding you with a fine view northwest toward the City of Napa and the lower Napa Valley.

A rising traverse eventually puts you atop a ridge and brings you to a junction with the Bayleaf Trail, left. Veering slightly right, you begin to descend on a moderate grade, in places stepping down over large rocks. At a junction marked by a trail post, you stay on the Skyline Trail by going straight. After reaching a low point, the trail rises gently to a junction with a connector to the Buckeye Trail, left. Again you continue straight, and soon begin a winding, moderate ascent through a brushy area.

After leveling briefly, at about 2 miles the trail plunges through forest to Passini Road. Cross Passini Road and continue climbing on the Skyline Trail. At an unsigned fork, you bear right. After about 15 feet the trail forks again, but this time you bear left. After a rolling course, you pass a short trail, right, leading to an overlook, right. The view southwest from this overlook is terrific, taking in the marshlands around the mouth of the Napa River, the northern end of San Pablo Bay, and, on a clear day, other Bay Area landmarks.

> **Wildflowers!**
> In spring, the park's grassy hillsides are dotted with California poppies, Ithuriel's spears, blue-eyed grass, bluedicks, yellow Mariposa lilies, Chinese houses, and lupine.

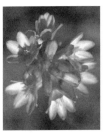

bluedicks

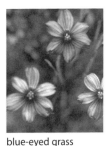

blue-eyed grass

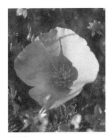

California poppy

Ithuriel's spear

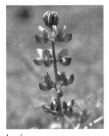

lupine

yellow Mariposa lily

Now the Skyline Trail descends on a moderate grade to meet your return route, the Buckeye Trail, left. You continue straight on the Skyline Trail, soon passing the first of three access paths to Lake Marie. When you reach the second, veer left and descend to the lake, built in 1908 to provide water for the state hospital farm. A nearby rest bench invites you to stay awhile. When you are ready to set off again, retrace your route to the junction of the Skyline and Buckeye trails.

You continue straight, now on the Buckeye Trail, a single track. Maintaining a mostly level grade, the route soon takes you out of deep forest and across hillsides of California sagebrush, coffeeberry, toyon, and bush monkeyflower. Back in the woods, at an unsigned fork, you stay right and descend to Passini Road. Turn right, and in about 40 feet pick up the continuation of the Buckeye Trail, left.

Passing a connector to the Skyline Trail, left, you bear right and walk through a gap in a rock wall. This wall and the park's many other rock walls were probably built by 19th century settlers and ranchers. In about 200 feet, you pass another connector to the Skyline Trail, left, and in 150 feet or so, reach a four-way junction, where you go straight. Continuing straight on the Buckeye Trail, the route rises to cross a rock rib, then descends through a lovely forest. Eventually you return to the Skyline Trail, where you turn right and then left on Lake Marie Road to retrace your route to the parking area.

# TRIP5 Rockville Hills Regional Park

|  |  |
|---|---|
| **Distance** | 4.6 miles, Loop |
| **Hiking Time** | 2 to 3 hours |
| **Elevation Gain/Loss** | ±600 feet |
| **Difficulty** | Moderate |
| **Trail Use** | Mountain biking allowed, Leashed Dogs |
| **Best Times** | Spring and fall |
| **Agency** | FCSD |
| **Recommended Map** | *Rockville Hills Regional Park* (FCSD) |

**HIGHLIGHTS**  Nine miles of trails through this 610-acre open space beckon visitors to enjoy blue oak savannas, grasslands decorated with colorful spring wildflowers, and several lakes for picnicking. Using the Rockville, Fire, Green Valley, Black Oak, Middle Mystic, Mystic, Arch, and Quarry trails, this lovely loop ranges through the park's varied habitat, including a "rock garden" of volcanic and sedimentary cliffs that rise above Upper Lake.

There is a fee to use the park; call (707) 428-7714 for more information.

**DIRECTIONS**  From I-80 eastbound west of Fairfield, take the Suisun Valley Road exit and go north 1.5 miles to Rockville Road. Turn left and go 0.7 mile to the park entrance, left.

From I-80 westbound in Fairfield, take the West Texas St./Rockville Road exit, go 0.3 mile, and bear right on Rockville Road. Continue another 3.7 miles to the park entrance, left.

**FACILITIES/TRAILHEAD**  There are no facilities at the trailhead, which is on the west corner of the parking area.

Passing the Quarry Trail, right, you go straight on the Rockville Trail, part of the Bay Area Ridge Trail. Climbing moderately on an eroded dirt road, you pass several unofficial trails and wander through a blue oak savanna before arriving at a paved road and a five-way junction. Here you cross the road and angle right on the Fire Trail, passing Lower Lake, left. Following a dirt road, you continue straight to a T-junction at Upper Lake.

Here you turn left and walk south on the dam that forms the lake. Curving right around the lake, you come to a four-way

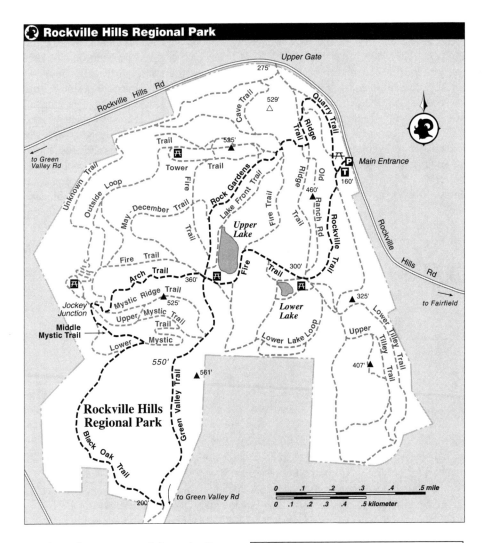

## Rockville Hills Regional Park

junction, where you turn left on the Green Valley Trail, also part of the Bay Area Ridge Trail. Immediately the route forks, but you stay left, on a dirt road. Climbing on a moderate grade, you crest a ridge with views southeast to Suisun Bay and Mt. Diablo. The Mystic Ridge and Upper Mystic trails depart right, but you continue straight, passing through a gap in a barbed-wire fence.

Now on a wide, dirt path, you climb moderately through a wooded area to a T-junction that is not shown on the park map. Here you turn right and stay atop the ridge. The hills on the western skyline form the boundary

### Springtime Bonuses

Spring is a good time to look and listen for birds. Oak titmouse, white-breasted nuthatch, western bluebird, and acorn woodpecker have all been spotted here. Also plentiful in spring are colorful grassland wildflowers, among them lupine, linanthus, California poppies, Chinese houses, owl's-clover, goldfields, and bluedicks.

between Solano and Napa counties. Behind you, at the head of Cook Canyon, rise the

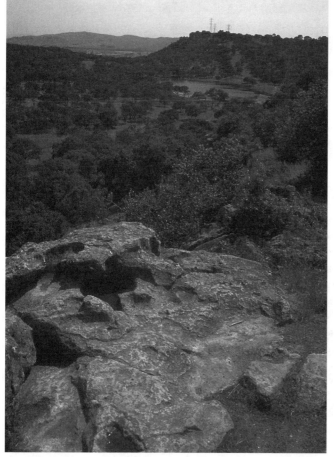

The Rock Gardens are outcrops of volcanic rock to the north and west of Upper Lake.

left at the next fork on the Arch Trail.

A venerable, moss-shrouded blue oak beside the trail looks like it may come to life and start waving its outstretched limbs at any moment. Follow the Arch Trail to where it merges with the Green Valley Trail, closing the loop. Now go straight, heading north on a dirt road with Upper Lake on your right. Where the Fire Trail veers left, you continue straight, soon climbing toward the Rock Gardens. Soon the May– December Trail veers left, but you angle right and head northwest through a rocky area where trails wander left and right (warning: the park map is no help here).

Twin Sisters. Losing elevation in the shade of coast live oaks, you bear left at a fork with an unofficial trail and cross under some power lines. On rocky ground, you near a fence, left, marking the park boundary.

At an unsigned junction, you turn right on the Black Oak Trail, a single track. Curving right and climbing on a gentle grade, you pass stands of blue, valley, and, finally, black oak. At about 2 miles, you go through a gap in a barbed-wire fence and pass the Lower Mystic Trail, left. Then, about 100 yards ahead, you turn sharply left on the Middle Mystic Trail. At a T-junction, called Jockey Junction on the park map, turn right. At a fork about 75 feet ahead, bear right on the Mystic Ridge Trail, then

Descending to a saddle, you turn right on a wide dirt path and follow it to a T-junction with the Fire Trail, where you turn left. After a moderate climb over open ground, you pass the Cave Trail, left, and then meet a paved road. Turn left, descend on a gentle grade, and then angle right on the Quarry Trail, which descends through stands of manzanita, toyon, and oak. Now near Rockville Road, you come to a fork, where you bear right and continue downhill.

Crossing a rocky area, you pass a quarry site and a vernal pool. The trail wanders through a picnic area and then meets the Rockville Trail beside the trailhead. Turn left here and return to the parking area.

# TRIP 6 Rush Ranch

| | |
|---:|:---|
| **Distance** | 2.2 miles, Loop |
| **Hiking Time** | 1 to 2 hours |
| **Difficulty** | Easy |
| **Trail Use** | Good for kids |
| **Best Times** | Fall through spring |
| **Agency** | SLT |
| **Recommended Map** | *Rush Ranch Marsh Trail Guide* (Rush Ranch Educational Council) |

**HIGHLIGHTS** Acquired in 1988 by the Solano County Farmlands and Open Space Foundation (now Solano Land Trust), this ranch has more than 2000 acres of significant habitat, including a more than 5-mile-long boundary between wetlands and upland grasslands. There are a dozen rare or endangered species here, including the clapper rail, the salt marsh harvest mouse, and the Delta smelt. An easy loop along the self-guiding Marsh Trail lets you sample some of this protected open space.

**Boldface** numbers in the route description refer to numbered markers along the trail, which are keyed to the *Rush Ranch Marsh Trail Guide* pamphlet, available at the visitor center, or online at www.rushranch.org.

**DIRECTIONS** From I-80 in Fairfield, take the exit for Highway 12, also signed for Rio Vista and Suisun City. At 4.2 miles, turn right on Grizzly Island Road and go 2.4 miles to the ranch entrance, right. Go 0.2 mile to a large gravel parking area, left.

**FACILITIES/TRAILHEAD** There are picnic tables and toilets near the parking area. A visitor center with displays, brochures, and other information is a few hundred feet southwest of the parking area, just past the livestock corrals. Other ranch buildings and displays of farming equipment are nearby. The trailhead is just left of the visitor center, a small white building.

You head west through a grove of eucalyptus, marker **1**, a nonnative species from Australia planted extensively in the Bay Area. Although unsuited for lumber, the trees provide windbreaks and habitat for some birds and small mammals. Marker **2**, just ahead, is for the transition zone between the coastal plain and the Central Valley. Joined on the left by a dirt road, you veer right and enjoy a level walk.

Once through a gap in a barbed-wire fence, you climb on a gentle grade to a junction, where a short trail goes right to an overlook atop a hill with 360-degree views that reach from Mt. Diablo and Suisun Marsh northward to the Vaca Mountains. Circling clockwise around the hill, marker **3**, you come to marker **4**, for the boundary, or ecotone, between grasslands and salt marsh. Passing a reconstructed Native American tule house and a road, left, you enter a managed wetland, marker **5**. Beginning in the late 1800s, this area was managed for farming and waterfowl through the regulation of water by tide gates.

Now on a rough path atop a levee, you pass marker **6**, where otters sometimes cross from the managed marsh, right, to the salt marsh, left. Other mammals found here include skunks, raccoons, and opossums. The blackberry vines, marker **7**, are not marsh plants, so their seeds were probably deposited here by birds or the wind. Marker **8** is for one of the many tide gates that regulate water flow seasonally into and out of the marsh. Cattails and tules, marker **9**, are common marsh plants. Across Suisun

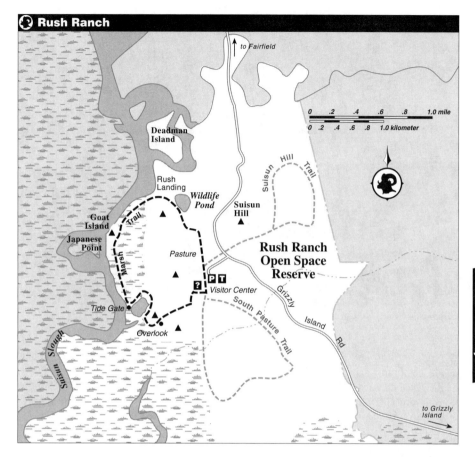

**Rush Ranch**

to Fairfield

0   .2   .4   .6   .8   1.0 mile
0  .2  .4  .6  .8  1.0 kilometer

Deadman
Island

Rush
Landing

*Wildlife
Pond*

Suisun   Hill   Trail

Suisun
Hill

Goat
Island

Japanese
Point

*Pasture*

**Rush Ranch
Open Space
Reserve**

Marsh Trail

Trail

Tide Gate

P  T

? ⓘ  Visitor Center

Grizzly

South Pasture Trail

Island

Overlook

Suisun Slough

Island  Rd

to Grizzly
Island

Fairfield/Vallejo

Slough, marker **10**, is more of Rush Ranch and the buildings of a private hunting club.

Common reed, also called phragmites, marker **11**, is a tall plant found in fresh or brackish water. Marker **12** indicates Goat Island and a viewpoint on the bluff above. Marker **13** is for the rocks, or riprap, that reinforce the levee. Climbing over a barbed-wire fence via a stile, you come to marker **14**, indicating the outflow tide gate you just passed. Turning left, you follow a faint dirt road through grassland, marker **15**. Slightly higher elevation makes it harder for marsh water to flood this area, and this creates a habitat that is different from the one you just left.

With the Potrero Hills ahead, you pass a rest bench and climb gently to marker **16**.

---

**The Birds & the Flowers**

More than 120 species of birds have been recorded at Rush Ranch, with the best birding being in winter. In addition to ducks, geese, and shorebirds, the ranch is home to many common songbirds, including the red-winged blackbird, northern mockingbird, western mead-owlark, marsh wren, and mourning dove. Grassland flowers here include California poppies, blue-eyed grass, California buttercup, lupine, and butter-and-eggs. Growing in the marsh are pickleweed, salt-grass, jaumea, brass buttons, and fat hen.

---

From here, you can see Rush Landing, a cove where boats from San Francisco and Sacramento used to land. A path from marker

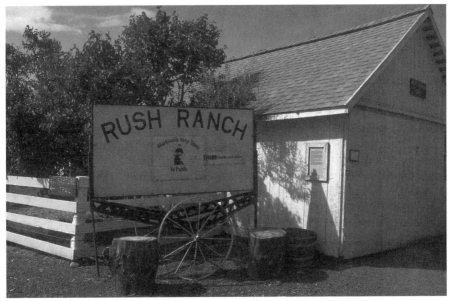

Farm buildings and displays of old farming equipment greet visitors to Rush Ranch.

**17** heads north toward Hill Slough. The trail bends right and passes a wildlife pond, marker **18**, fed by a spring and also by runoff from Suisun Hill. Nonnative Harding grass, marker **19**, was planted here in the 1940s as forage for cattle. This grassland habitat, marker **20**, provides habitat for rodents, which are prey for raptors and owls. Marker **21**, near the parking area, is for a small horse stable, one of several ranch buildings.

## TRIP 7 Jepson Prairie Preserve

| | |
|---|---|
| **Distance** | 0.7 miles, Loop |
| **Hiking Time** | 1 hour or less |
| **Difficulty** | Easy |
| **Trail Use** | Good for kids |
| **Best Times** | Spring |
| **Agency** | SLT/UCNRS |
| **Recommended Map** | *None* |

**HIGHLIGHTS** This easy, self-guiding loop takes you through what preserve authorities describe as "the best remaining, unspoiled stand of native bunchgrass prairie in the Central Valley." Along the way, you'll learn why the Nature Conservancy thought this seemingly empty stretch of ground, actually teeming with life, was important enough to buy and protect. If you visit in spring, you'll be rewarded with colorful displays of wildflowers. On weekends from mid-March through Mother's Day, there are guided tours of the preserve at 11 A.M. For more information, call Solano Land Trust (707) 432-0150 or visit www.solanolandtrust.org. **Boldface** numbers in the route description refer to numbered markers along the trail, which are keyed to the *Jepson Prairie Self Guided Nature Trail* brochure. Parts of this brochure are summarized in the description, below.

**DIRECTIONS** From the intersection of Highway 12 and Highway 113, east of Fairfield, take Highway 113 north, then west, 8.2 miles to Cook Lane. Turn left and go 0.7 mile to a parking area, left.

**FACILITIES/TRAILHEAD** There are picnic tables and a toilet beside the parking area. The trailhead is on the west side of Cook Lane, across from the parking area.

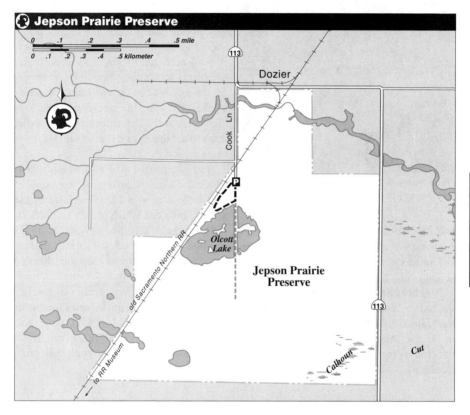

## Jepson Prairie Preserve

From the trailhead, you follow a path through the grass to marker **1**. Jepson Prairie contains a variety of habitats, including sloughs, playas, vernal pools, swales, and grassland. With Olcott Lake, a large playa lake, or undrained basin, ahead, you soon reach marker **2**. Unlike in nearby farmlands, early settlers found the sand and clay soils here were unsuited for agriculture, and this helped spare the area from development.

Marker **3** is for the adaptation of local plants and animals to the Bay Area's Mediterranean climate—dry in summer, wet in winter. The bumps in the landscape seen from marker **4** are called "mima-mounds," and explanations for them range from temperature changes, to wind erosion, to burrowing animals, to earthquakes. You pass through a swale, a water-trapping depression underlain by clay, to marker **5**.

Now the path approaches a tall power line tower used as a perch by birds. The annoying sounds come from a nearby go-cart course. Most nonnative plants, marker **6**, can't grow in swales or vernal pools, yet they are widespread on the higher ground of the preserve. Most of these, such as wild oats and thistles, came from Europe back when California was a colony of Spain and then Mexico. Fencing, grazing, planting,

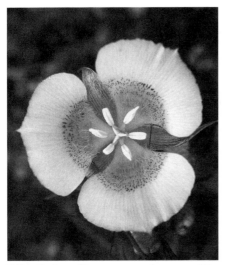

Yellow Mariposa lilies are among the many wild-flowers found at the Jepson Prairie Preserve.

thought to have used fire to keep land open and stimulate preferred species, and modern land managers often do the same. Mt. Diablo, about 30 miles south, is visible from marker **10**.

As the waters of rain-filled Olcott Lake, marker **11**, recede, a variety of colorful wildflowers flourish and bloom around its shore. These include meadowfoam, popcorn flower, goldfields, and downingia. Grassland wildflowers here include brodiaeas, white hyacinths, and Mariposa lilies. Marker **12** is for the rare plants and animals, such as the Delta green ground beetle, that caused the Nature Conservancy to purchase Jepson Prairie in 1980.

You go straight at a four-way junction beside the lake. The linkage between upland and wetland, marker **13**, is illustrated by the tiger salamander, which breeds and is born in Olcott Lake, but lives most of its life in grassland. Several species of shrimp, marker **14**, live in the lake, and the cysts they lay survive the dry summer. Among the birds that rest and feed here during migration, marker **15**, are geese, ducks, and shorebirds. Herons and egrets circle the lakeshore, and raptors patrol the skies. When you reach Cook Lane, turn left and go about 100 yards to the parking area.

and development, signs of which are evident from marker **7**, all took their toll on California's most fragile habitats, such as vernal pools, grasslands, and marsh lands.

You bear right at a fork to marker **8**, for the Native Americans who used this area to hunt, fish, and gather seeds and building materials. Purple needle grass, a native bunchgrass that benefits from fire, is near marker **9**. The Native Americans are

# Chapter 4
## Concord/Walnut Creek

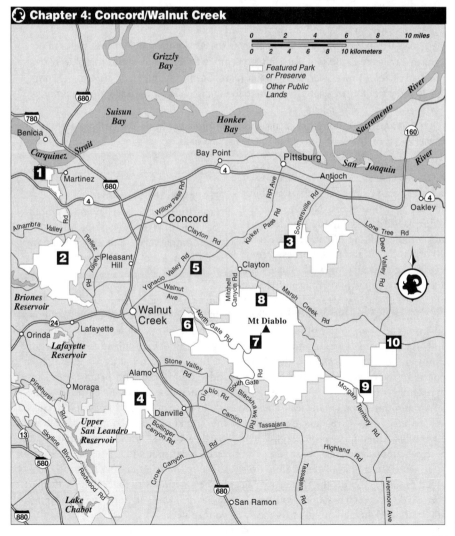

Featured Park
or Preserve

Other Public
Lands

0   2   4   6   8   10 miles
0   2   4   6   8   10 kilometers

Grizzly
Bay

Suisun
Bay

Honker
Bay

Sacramento River

Carquinez Strait

Benicia

Bay Point

Pittsburg

San Joaquin River

160

Martinez

Antioch

Oakley

Alhambra Valley Rd

Willow Pass Rd

Concord

Clayton Rd

Kirker Pass Rd

Somersville Rd

Lone Tree Rd

Deer Valley Rd

Pleasant
Hill

Reliez Valley Rd

Ygnacio Valley Rd

Clayton

Briones
Reservoir

Walnut
Ave

Mitchell Canyon Rd

Marsh Creek Rd

Walnut
Creek

North Gate Rd

Mt Diablo

Lafayette

Lafayette
Reservoir

Orinda

Stone Valley Rd

Alamo

South Gate Rd

Morgan Territory Rd

Pinehurst Rd

Moraga

Diablo Rd

Blackhawk Rd

Camino Tassajara

Danville

Upper
San Leandro
Reservoir

Bollinger Canyon Rd

Highland Rd

Skyline Blvd

Redwood Rd

Crow Canyon Rd

Tassajara Rd

Livermore Ave

Lake
Chabot

San Ramon

**1** **2** **3** **4** **5** **6** **7** **8** **9** **10**

780 680 4 24 13 580 880

117

# TRIP 1 Carquinez Strait Regional Shoreline

| | |
|---:|:---|
| **Distance** | 2.8 miles, Semi-loop |
| **Hiking Time** | 1 to 2 hours |
| **Elevation Gain/Loss** | ±1100 feet |
| **Difficulty** | Moderate |
| **Trail Use** | Mountain biking allowed |
| **Best Times** | Fall through spring |
| **Agency** | EBRPD |
| **Recommended Map** | *Carquinez Strait Regional Shoreline* (EBRPD) |

**HIGHLIGHTS**  Circling a high ridge overlooking Carquinez Strait, this route has some steep sections, but your efforts are rewarded by terrific views of the strait, Suisun Bay, the west delta, Mt. Diablo, and the hills of Napa and Solano counties. Using the California Riding and Hiking Trail, and the Franklin Ridge Loop Trail, your route explores open grassland, oak savanna, and shady, tree-lined ravines.

**DIRECTIONS**  From Highway 4 in Martinez, take the Alhambra Ave./Martinez exit and go north 2 miles to Escobar St. Turn left, go 0.1 mile to Talbart St. and turn right. Follow Talbart St. for 0.1 mile, veer left onto Carquinez Scenic Dr. and go 0.3 mile to the John A. Nejedly staging area, left. The lower parking area has some shade; the upper area has spaces for horse trailers.

**FACILITIES/TRAILHEAD**  There are picnic tables and toilets beside the parking area. The trailhead is on the west end of the upper parking area.

**G**o through a gate and walk across a large, grassy field, coming after about 200 feet to a trail post. Now follow the California Riding and Hiking Trail, a single-track trail, walking through stands of California bay, California buckeye, coast live oak, and eucalyptus, with a creek on your left. The California Riding and Hiking Trail is part of the Bay Area Ridge Trail. The trail widens and begins a moderate climb and crosses an open, grassy hillside. A steep climb leads to a T-junction atop a ridge. Turn right on the Franklin Ridge Loop Trail, a dirt road, and follow it north, enjoying magnificent views.

As you round a bend in the trail, you can see Carquinez Strait, the narrow passage between Suisun and San Pablo bays. When you reach an unsigned fork, bear left, passing a rest bench. Now descending over eroded ground, drop off the ridge via a big S-bend. As you reach a saddle, you pass a path leading right and uphill to an oak-

> **Don't Miss the View**
> From the ridge, Suisun Bay with its moth-ball fleet of WW II Navy ships, Mt. Diablo, the Central Valley, and even the snow-capped peaks of the Sierra are visible.

adorned summit. Here your route bends left and continues to descend. At the next junction, an unsigned fork, bear right through an oak woodland to a T-junction.

Turn left, continuing on the Franklin Ridge Loop Trail, and begin a gentle and then moderate climb. At a four-way junction, you turn left and walk uphill, still on the Franklin Ridge Loop Trail. You head northeast and, after a moderate climb, reach a flat spot and a T-junction. To close the loop, turn left and walk about 250 feet to the junction with the trail from the parking area. Here you turn right and retrace your route.

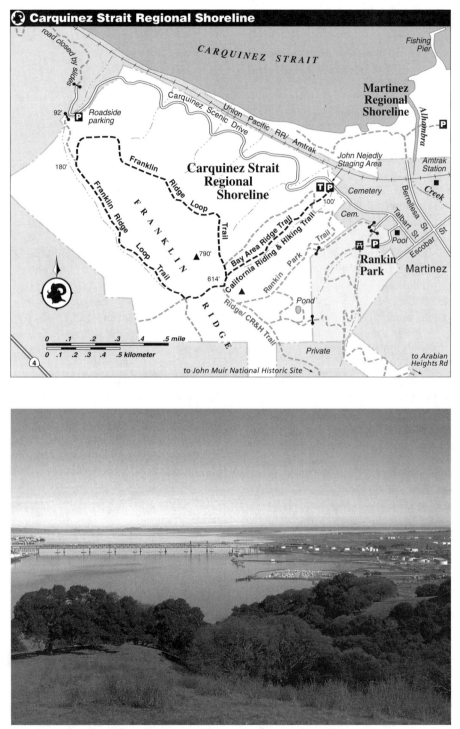

The Franklin Ridge Loop Trail offers great views of Carquinez Strait and beyond.

# TRIP 2 Briones Regional Park

| | |
|---:|:---|
| **Distance** | 4.8 miles, Loop |
| **Hiking Time** | 3 to 4 hours |
| **Elevation Gain/Loss** | ±1050 feet |
| **Difficulty** | Moderate |
| **Trail Use** | Mountain biking allowed, Leashed dogs |
| **Best Times** | Fall through spring |
| **Agency** | EBRPD |
| **Recommended Map** | *Briones Regional Park* (EBRPD) |

**HIGHLIGHTS** This loop, which includes all or parts of the Diablo View, Spengler, Pine Tree, and Orchard trails, and part of Old Briones Road Trail, gives you a chance to explore the East Bay's largest developed regional park, an area of deep, wooded canyons, forested slopes, oak savannas, and open, grassy ridges. The varied habitat attracts a large variety of birds, from chickadees to golden eagles. The plant life along this route is equally diverse, with a wide range of trees, shrubs, and wildflowers.

**DIRECTIONS** From Highway 4 in Martinez, take the Alhambra Ave. exit and go 0.5 mile south on Alhambra Ave. to Alhambra Valley Road. Turn right and go 1.25 miles to Reliez Valley Road. Turn left and go 0.5 mile to the Alhambra Creek Valley entrance, marked by a sign. Turn right and follow the entrance road 0.8 mile to the parking area.

**FACILITIES/TRAILHEAD** Water (may not be available because of contamination) and a toilet are near the trailhead, which is on the southeast corner of the parking area.

Pass through a gate next to an information board and turn immediately left onto the Diablo View Trail, a dirt road. Soon you pass the Tavan Trail, left, and now the slope changes from gentle to moderate as you ascend via well-graded S-bends toward the top of a ridge, where a fine view of Mt. Diablo awaits. At a fork marked by a trail post, stay on the Diablo View Trail as it bends left and makes a gentle climb along a ridgetop.

Turning right at a T-junction, you follow a rolling course to a clearing. Soon you come to a four-way intersection and the end of the Diablo View Trail. Here you turn right on the Spengler Trail, an eroded dirt road, and descend moderately. After passing through a gate, you continue to descend over easy and then moderate ground to Alhambra Creek. Just past the creek is a junction, where you stay on the

### Trees and Birds of Briones

Trees and shrubs in this park include coast live oak, valley oak, blue oak, California bay, California buckeye, blue elderberry, coffeeberry, and hillside gooseberry. The park also attracts a variety of songbirds, including chestnut-backed chickadees, woodpeckers, warblers, dark-eyed juncos, western bluebirds, sparrows, western meadowlarks, and horned larks. Birds of prey, such as red-tailed hawks, red-shouldered hawks, and vultures are common, and even golden eagles have been spotted here.

Spengler Trail as it bears left, then swings sharply right and climbs. Around 2 miles, the route emerges from forest and leads past one of the two Maricich Lagoons to a

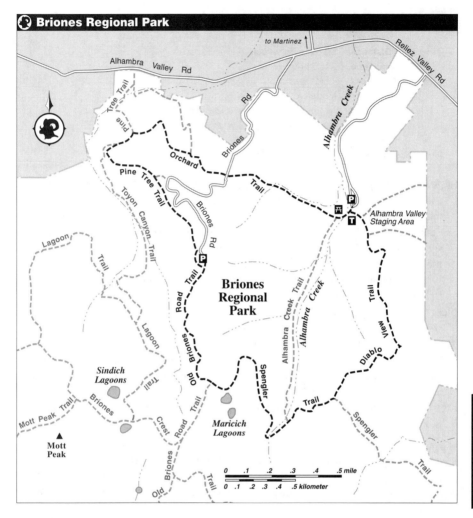

## Briones Regional Park

Alhambra Valley Rd

to Martinez

Reliez Valley Rd

Pine Tree Trail

Orchard

Briones Rd

Pine Tree Trail

Alhambra Creek

Briones Trail

Toyon Canyon Trail

Briones Rd

Alhambra Valley Staging Area

Lagoon Trail

**Briones Regional Park**

Alhambra Creek Trail

Alhambra Creek

View Trail

Old Briones Road Trail

Lagoon Trail

Diablo

*Sindich Lagoons*

Spengler

Trail

Spengler

Briones

Mott Peak Trail

Crest Briones Road Trail

*Maricich Lagoons*

▲ Mott Peak

Old Briones Trail

| 0 | .1 | .2 | .3 | .4 | .5 mile |
| 0 | .1 | .2 | .3 | .4 | .5 kilometer |

T-junction with Old Briones Road Trail. Here you turn right and walk downhill, past a gate and a junction with an unsigned path, left. You follow Old Briones Road Trail downhill to a parking area, right, at the end of Briones Road, with an information board, a gate, and water. Before the gate, find a single-track trail that skirts the left side of a wooden fence beside paved Briones Road. Follow this trail for about 200 feet, pass through a gap in the fence, then turn left and walk along the fence until you reach a gate. Go through the gate and climb through an area of chaparral.

Now descending, you bear left on the Pine Tree Trail, a dirt road. Where the Toyon Trail heads sharply left, you continue straight, passing an unsigned path, right, and coming to a fenced pond. At the southeast corner of the pond, you join the Orchard Trail, a dirt road that bends right. Stay on the Orchard Trail past the Rancho Briones Equestrian Facility and then cross Briones Road. With Mt. Diablo ahead in the distance, descend on a moderate grade, then wander beside a tributary of Alhambra Creek. At a T-junction with the Alhambra Creek Trail, go left to the parking area.

# TRIP3 Black Diamond Mines Regional Preserve

| | |
|---|---|
| **Distance** | 5.5 miles, Semi-loop |
| **Hiking Time** | 3 to 5 hours |
| **Elevation Gain/Loss** | ±1450 feet |
| **Difficulty** | Moderate |
| **Trail Use** | Mountain biking allowed, Leashed dogs |
| **Best Times** | Fall through spring |
| **Agency** | EBRPD |
| **Recommended Map** | *Black Diamond Mines Regional Preserve* (EBRPD) |

**HIGHLIGHTS** This hike, in one of the East Bay's most remote, beautiful, and historic parks, uses the Nortonville and Black Diamond trails to visit part of California's largest coal-mining area, which was active from the 1860s until the early 1900s. On the edge of the Central Valley, the preserve is best enjoyed during cool weather. In late winter and spring, wildflowers abound, and during this time, before the trees and shrubs leaf out, the preserve's numerous birds are easiest to spot.

**Boldface** numbers in the route description refer to numbered markers along the trail, which are keyed to the EBRPD map and its accompanying text.

**DIRECTIONS** From Highway 4 in Antioch, take the Somersville Road exit and go south, staying in the left lane as you approach and pass Buchanan Road. At 1.5 miles, follow Somersville Road as it continues straight, while the main road, now called James Donlon Blvd., bends sharply left. At 2.6 miles from Highway 4, you reach the entrance kiosk, park office, and emergency phone; continue another 0.9 mile to a large parking area, right, with an overflow area, left.

**FACILITIES/TRAILHEAD** There are picnic tables, water, and a toilet near the trailhead, which is on the south end of the parking area.

You head south on Somersville Road, passing the Stewartville Trail, left, and then join the Nortonville Trail. When you reach a fork, bear right, continuing gently uphill toward Rose Hill Cemetery. Along the way, you pass the Manhattan Canyon Trail, left. Now climbing on a moderate grade, you reach a junction with a short trail to the Rose Hill Cemetery, certainly worth a visit.

Now the route climbs on a moderate grade toward Nortonville Pass, a notch in the western skyline. Just before reaching the pass, you meet the Black Diamond Trail, left, which you will use later on your return. Descending from the pass into the valley where Nortonville once was, you soon reach a T-junction and the end of the Nortonville Trail. Here you turn left on the Black Diamond Trail and climb to a junction with paved Black Diamond Way.

> **Rose Hill Cemetery**
>
> Most of the graves here are from the mid- to late 1800s, when this was California's largest coal-mining area. Five mining towns were active, all nearby—Nortonville, Somersville, Stewartville, West Hartley, and Judsonville.

Continue straight on the now-paved Black Diamond Trail, climbing on a gentle grade past a pond, left. The road makes several S-bends and reaches a clearing. At about 2 miles, a short trail goes left to Jim's Place, **4**, and the Coal Canyon Trail. Continuing uphill, you reach a junction with the Cumberland Trail, right, which leads to two mining sites, **5** and **6**. The Black Diamond Trail climbs on a moderate grade through a blue-oak savanna. Gaining elevation, you

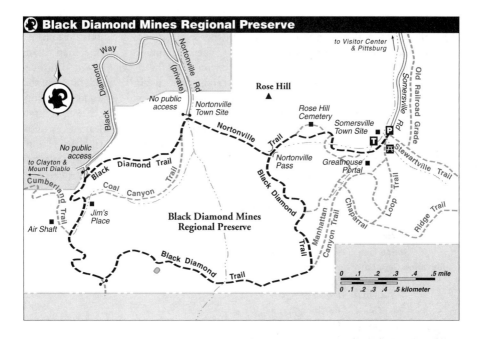

## Black Diamond Mines Regional Preserve

Way

Nortonville Rd (private)

to Visitor Center & Pittsburg

Somersville Rd

Old Railroad Grade

No public access

Nortonville Town Site

**Rose Hill** ▲

Rose Hill Cemetery

Somersville Town Site

Nortonville Trail

Stewartville Trail

No public access

to Clayton & Mount Diablo

Black Diamond Trail

Trail

Nortonville Pass

Greathouse Portal

Black Diamond

Cumberland Trail

Coal Canyon

Loop Trail

Chaparral

Ridge Trail

Air Shaft

Jim's Place

**Black Diamond Mines Regional Preserve**

Manhattan Canyon Trail

Black Diamond Trail

Black Diamond Trail

0  .1  .2  .3  .4  .5 mile
0  .1 .2 .3 .4  .5 kilometer

### Flora & Bird Life

This preserve is characterized by rolling hills, grassland, and blue-oak savanna. Other native trees include coast live oak, gray pine, Coulter pine (this is the northernmost location of this species, which is found only in California and northern Mexico), and California buckeye. There are also prominent stands of nonnative trees, including tree-of-heaven and black locust, which flowers fragrantly in the spring. The preserve has several types of manzanita, including the highly restricted Mt. Diablo variety, known by its stemless, clasping gray-green leaves and white flowers tinged with pink.

Many birds are found here, from huge turkey vultures to tiny hummingbirds, and from aerialists like the American kestrel to ground dwellers such as the golden-crowned sparrow.

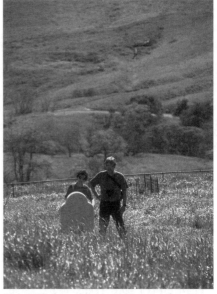

Rose Hill Cemetery holds the remains of coal miners who came searching for "Black Diamonds."

get views of Mt. St. Helena, the hills of Oakland and Berkeley, Mt. Tamalpais, and, perhaps, the Sierra.

You follow an open ridgetop to a junction with a wide dirt road, left—the continuation of the Black Diamond Trail. You descend east to a fenced pond, then roller-

Concord/Walnut Creek

coaster through a wooded area. Across a deep valley, left, are the exposed rock cliffs of the Domengine Formation, 52-million-year-old marine sandstone that contains the coal for which this area became known.

Now the route enters a dry, rocky area, then swings north past a pond and reenters forest. Around 4 miles, you pass the steep Manhattan Canyon Trail, right, and then wander through an area of chaparral—

chamise, bush monkeyflower, black sage, pitcher sage, yerba santa, and manzanita.

Where a connector to the Manhattan Canyon Trail heads right, you continue straight and begin a moderate climb. Passing through a cattle gate and reentering oak woodland, the route makes several changes of direction before leaving the trees and descending to Nortonville Pass. From here, turn right on the Nortonville Trail and retrace your route to the parking area.

# TRIP4 Las Trampas Wilderness

| | |
|---|---|
| **Distance** | 6.1 miles, Loop |
| **Hiking Time** | 4 to 6 hours |
| **Elevation Gain/Loss** | ±2150 feet |
| **Difficulty** | Difficult |
| **Trail Use** | Leashed dogs |
| **Best Times** | Fall through spring |
| **Agency** | EBRPD |
| **Recommended Map** | *Las Trampas Regional Wilderness* (EBRPD) |

**HIGHLIGHTS**  This rugged loop joins all or parts of the Chamise, Las Trampas Ridge, Corduroy Hills, Madrone, Virgil Williams, Del Amigo, Sulphur Springs, Trapline, and Mahogany trails, leading you through an remarkable variety of terrain, from sun-baked chaparral to shady forest. Some of the best views in the East Bay of Mt. Diablo are to be found on this loop, which passes through a stunted forest of scrub oak and other interesting plant communities. Bring plenty of water and start early; the parking area gate may be locked at 5 P.M.

**DIRECTIONS**  From I-680 in San Ramon, take the Crow Canyon Road/San Ramon exit and go west 1.1 miles on Crow Canyon Road to Bollinger Canyon Road. Turn right and go 4.5 miles to the end of the road, past the first Las Trampas Wilderness entrance, and turn left into the parking area.

From I-580 eastbound in Castro Valley, take the Center St./Crow Canyon Road exit, go left over the freeway, then right on Castro Valley Blvd., which soon becomes E. Castro Valley Blvd., 0.7 mile to Crow Canyon Road. Turn left and go 7.5 miles to Bollinger Canyon Road, then follow the directions above.

From I-580 westbound in Castro Valley, take the Castro Valley exit, turn left onto E. Castro Valley Blvd. and go 0.1 mile to Crow Canyon Road. Turn right and follow the directions above.

**FACILITIES/TRAILHEAD**  There are picnic tables, a toilet, and water (may not be available year-round) beside the parking area. The trailhead is on the northeast side of Bollinger Canyon Road, about 0.1 mile southeast from the parking area.

Go through a gate and follow the single-track Chamise Trail as it climbs past a junction with the Bollinger Canyon Trail via switchbacks.

As the trail bends left, you pass a junction with the Mahogany Trail, part of your return route. To the northeast is Las Trampas Ridge, a rugged, chaparral-covered

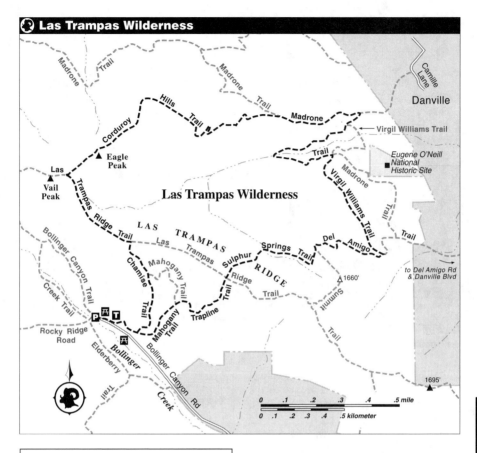

## Las Trampas Wilderness

(map labels:)
Madrone Trail · Hills Trail · Corduroy · Madrone Trail · Madrone Trail · Danville · Camille Lane · Virgil Williams Trail · Eagle Peak · Trail · Eugene O'Neill National Historic Site · Las Vail Peak · Las Trampas Ridge Trail · Las Trampas Wilderness · Virgil Williams Trail · Trail · Bollinger Canyon Trail · LAS TRAMPAS · Las Trampas Ridge Trail · Springs Trail · Del Amigo · Trail · Chamise Trail · Mahogany Trail · Sulphur Springs Trail · RIDGE · 1660' · to Del Amigo Rd & Danville Blvd · Creek Trail · Ridge Trail · Summit Trail · Rocky Ridge Road · Mahogany Trail · Trapline · Trail · Elderberry Trail · Bollinger Creek · Bollinger Canyon Rd · 1695'

0  .1  .2  .3  .4  .5 mile
0  .1  .2  .3  .4  .5 kilometer

### Chamise

Chamise is a hardy, widespread shrub, which grows here with two other chaparral plants, buckbrush and black sage. Looking like a small evergreen tree, chamise sports white flowers in late spring.

barrier you will soon cross. The Chamise Trail ends at a T-junction, and you bear left on the Las Trampas Ridge Trail, enjoying views of Mt. Diablo, northeast, and Rocky Ridge, sporting a lone communication tower, southwest. Passing through a fence, you descend a steep, narrow track, muddy at times, past stands of scrub oak.

Now the trail follows a rolling course on the edge of a steep canyon, right. Soon you reach a fence, right, and a junction with the Corduroy Hills Trail, at about 1 mile. Here your route, a single track, turns right and descends steeply to an open, grassy hillside. After crossing a divide, you scramble uphill over rocky ground and boulders to a cliff just west of Eagle Peak, a convenient rest stop with fine views. On level ground, you reach a trail junction where the Corduroy Hills Trail continues left, and a spur trail to Eagle Peak heads right. The Corduroy Hills, true to their name, are characterized by deeply convoluted canyons and ridges.

After turning left and descending some steps, you traverse the north side of Eagle Peak on a trail carved in a steep cliff. Soon you begin to descend steeply, then less so, along the crest of a ridge. After leveling and then climbing, the route drops to a T-junction with a wide dirt road. Turn left and

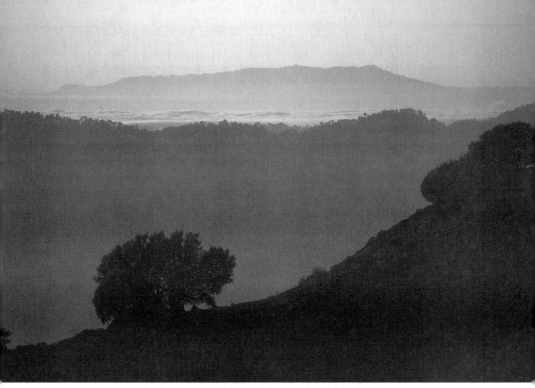
Las Trampas Wilderness lies between Mt. Diablo and the Berkeley/Oakland Hills.

continue to descend, soon joining a road coming from the right-hand branch of the T. Where the Corduroy Hills Trail ends, you merge with the Madrone Trail.

At about 3 miles, the road makes an almost 180-degree bend right, and soon you reach a dense forest with a creek on your left. The road bends left, crosses the creek, and climbs to a four-way junction. Here you turn right on the Virgil Williams Trail, a single track that climbs through dense forest on moderate and occasionally steep grades.

At a T-junction with the Del Amigo Trail, a dirt road, you turn right and attack the steepest part of the route. Where the grade finally eases, the route enters a lovely clearing, bends sharply left, and reaches a junction. You turn right on the Sulphur Springs Trail, a dirt road, and descend into a shady, creek-filled canyon. At about 5 miles, you turn left, cross the creek, and then climb moderately, now on a single track.

At a four-way junction, you go straight on the Trapline Trail, and after about 100 feet reach a saddle on the crest of Las

**Tao House**

Nearby Tao House, one-time home of playwright Eugene O'Neill (1888–1953), is a National Historic Site, owned and operated by the National Park Service. It was in Tao House, where he lived from 1937 to 1944, that O'Neill wrote *The Iceman Cometh* and *A Long Day's Journey Into Night*, two of his best-known dramas. Arrangements to visit Tao House can be made by calling (925) 838-0249.

Trampas Ridge. Through a gap in a barbed-wire fence, you follow the rocky path downhill through a corridor of chaparral, then through forest. You join the Mahogany Trail, a single track joining from the right, and continue to descend beside a creek in a steep ravine, right. You reach a bridge over the creek and, once across, begin to climb. At a junction with the Chamise Trail, you continue straight and retrace your route to the parking area.

# TRIP5 Lime Ridge Open Space

| | |
|---|---|
| **Distance** | 3.3 miles |
| **Hiking Time** | 2 to 3 hours |
| **Elevation Gain/Loss** | ±850 feet |
| **Difficulty** | Moderate |
| **Trail Use** | Mountain biking allowed[1] |
| **Best Times** | Fall through spring |
| **Agency** | WCOSTD |
| **Recommended Map** | *Lime Ridge Open Space* (WCOSTD) |
| **Notes** | [1]Bicycles are not allowed on the Lime Ridge Trail, and must instead stay on dirt roads to complete the trip. |

**HIGHLIGHTS** This athletic loop, a perfect cool-weather outing, uses the Ohlone, Manzanita, Lime Ridge, and Paraiso trails to explore the rugged, chaparral-clad hills northwest of Mt. Diablo on the border of Concord and Walnut Creek.

**DIRECTIONS** From I-680 in Walnut Creek, or Highway 24 eastbound (just before the merge with I-680), take the Ygnacio Valley Road exit and go northeast 3.5 miles to Oak Grove Road. Turn right and go 0.4 mile to Valley Vista Road. Turn left and go 0.8 mile to a parking area, right.

**FACILITIES/TRAILHEAD** There are no facilities at the trailhead, which is on the east end of the parking area.

Y ou go through a gate and walk uphill to an information board and the Ohlone Trail. Bearing left, you climb moderately on a dirt road to a junction, where the Paraiso Trail, which you will use later, joins from the right. Turning left, you soon go through a gate into the Walnut Creek Open Space Lime Ridge Preserve, which is closed to dogs.

Descending through a narrow ravine, you come to a T-junction, where you turn right on the Manzanita Trail. Climbing steeply, you follow a rocky dirt road that soon provides great views in exchange for the effort. After passing the Buckeye Trail, left, you reach a saddle where a number of

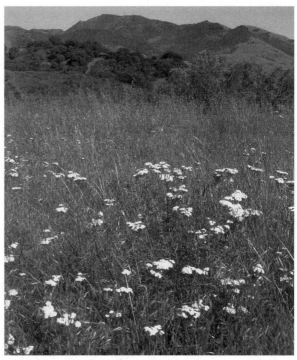

Lime Ridge Open Space: meadow with yarrow frames view of Mt. Diablo.

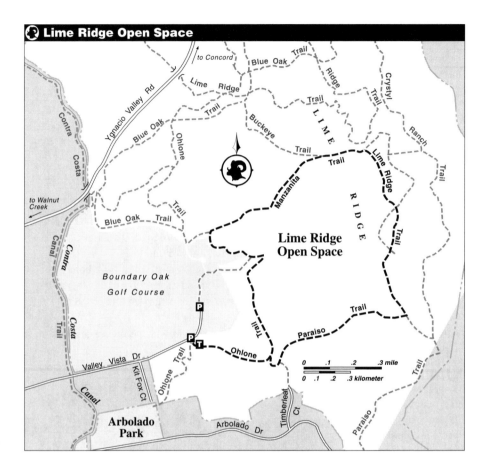

**Lime Ridge Open Space**

Boundary Oak
Golf Course

**Lime Ridge
Open Space**

L I M E

R I D G E

to Concord

Blue Oak  Trail

Lime  Ridge

Ridge

Crystyl

Trail

 Trail

Ohlone

Buckeye

Trail

Ranch

Ygnacio Valley Rd

Blue Oak

Trail

Manzanita

Lime  Ridge

Trail

Contra  Costa

to Walnut
Creek

Blue Oak   Trail

Trail

Trail

Canal

Contra

Trail

Costa
Trail

P

P T

Trail

Paraiso

Ohlone

Ohlone  Trail

Valley  Vista  Dr

Kit Fox Ct

Canal

0    .1    .2    .3 mile
0  .1  .2    .3 kilometer

Trail

Paraiso

**Arbolado
Park**

Arbolado  Dr

Timberleaf

Ct

---

**Lime Ridge Flora**

Coast live oaks, blue oaks, and California buckeyes line the route, which also passes hillsides of chaparral, mostly chamise, toyon, California sagebrush, yerba santa, manzanita, and black sage.

---

trails meet. Turning right, you follow the Lime Ridge Trail, a dirt road, through a corridor of chaparral. At an unsigned fork, bear left and descend a set of steps, then follow a single-track trail to the base of a power-line tower.

With the tower on your right, follow the trail alongside, and then atop, a ridge. A rolling course soon brings you to a junction with a dirt road, where you angle right. After 100 feet or so, you rejoin the Lime Ridge Trail by veering left. The trail soon merges with the dirt road you just left, and now you have an open, ridgetop climb. Topping a rise, you descend to a saddle and a junction with the Paraiso Trail, where you turn right.

Descending a dirt road on a gentle grade, you pass stands of chaparral pea, which produce beautiful magenta flowers in late spring and early summer. After meeting the Timberleaf Court Trail, left, your road curves right and closes the loop by joining the Ohlone Trail. Here you turn left and retrace your route to the parking area.

# TRIP 6 Diablo Foothills Regional Park

|                      |                                             |
|----------------------|---------------------------------------------|
| **Distance**         | 6.1 miles, Loop                             |
| **Hiking Time**      | 3 to 4 hours                                |
| **Elevation Gain/Loss** | ±1300 feet                               |
| **Difficulty**       | Difficult                                   |
| **Trail Use**        | Mountain biking allowed, Leashed dogs       |
| **Best Times**       | Spring and fall                             |
| **Agency**           | EBRPD, City of Walnut Creek                 |
| **Recommended Map**  | *Diablo Foothills Regional Park* (EBRPD)    |

**HIGHLIGHTS** If you enjoy a challenging route, take this roller-coaster ride through the foothills just west of Mt. Diablo State Park. Using the Castle Rock, Shell Ridge Loop, Briones-to-Mt. Diablo Regional, Twin Ponds, Hanging Valley, and Stage Road trails, you'll make two connected loops through the park, with a short jaunt into neighboring Shell Ridge Open Space, enjoying oak savannas, wildflower-dotted hillsides, and a variety of birds.

**DIRECTIONS** From I-680 in Walnut Creek, or Highway 24 eastbound (just before the merge with I-680), take the Ygnacio Valley Road exit and go northeast 2.3 miles to Walnut Ave. Turn right, go 1.6 miles to Oak Grove Road, and turn right. At 0.1 mile, Oak Grove Road changes to Castle Rock Road, and you continue straight. At 1.7 miles you come to the trailhead parking area.

**FACILITIES/TRAILHEAD** There are no facilities at the trailhead, which is on the north end of the parking area, on the west side of the road.

You climb on a single-track trail, past a gate that prevents access by bicycles and horses during wet weather. Meeting the Castle Rock Trail, a dirt road, you turn sharply right, then stay left at a fork. The road climbs on a gentle and then moderate grade. At the next junction you also stay left, passing through a blue oak savanna. Gaining a ridgetop, you wind uphill through chaparral—chamise, black sage, toyon, California sagebrush—with a view, left, of impressive sandstone cliffs.

Climbing very steeply over rough ground, you meet the Shell Ridge Loop Trail at a T-junction. Turning left, you roller-coaster along an exposed ridgetop to a junction, where you stay right. Now descending on a moderate and then steep grade past a trail, left, you drop into a wooded valley and a junction with a connector to the Briones-to-Mt. Diablo Regional Trail. Turn right and walk through

**Borges Ranch**

Borges Ranch, the former home of Walnut Creek pioneers Frank and Mary Borges, today is a base of activities for Shell Ridge Open Space. Livestock lives at the ranch, which offers displays on ranching life, and also serves as a ranger station and residence. For information about educational programs and group use, call (925) 944-5766 or visit www.ci.walnut-creek.ca.us/openspace/osborges.htm.

a canyon, passing the Buckeye Ravine Trail, left. When you meet the Briones-to-Mt. Diablo Regional Trail, a dirt road, turn right and go through a gate into Shell Ridge Open Space.

Where a dirt road veers right at about 2 miles, you continue straight past the Borges

Concord/Walnut Creek

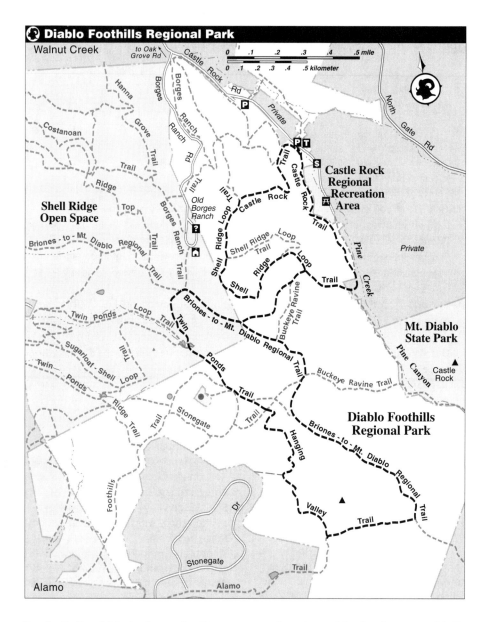

## Diablo Foothills Regional Park

Ranch Trail, which leads to the Borges Ranch. Bearing left, you come to a fork, where you again stay left, now on the Twin Ponds Trail, a dirt road that goes between two ponds. Beyond the ponds is a junction, where you continue straight and soon return to the regional park. Climbing moderately past a water tank and a paved road, you veer right at a fork and come to a four-way junction with the Stonegate Trail, spelled STONE GATE on some signs. (To shorten the route, turn left on the Stonegate Trail, go about 0.2 mile to a junction with the Briones-to-Mt. Diablo Regional Trail, and follow the description below.)

Go straight now on the Hanging Valley Trail, following a rolling course until the trail climbs steeply over a rise. The view from

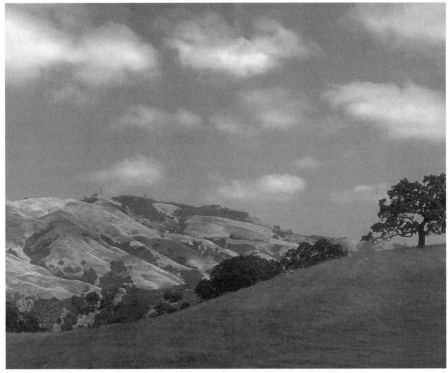

Diablo Foothills Regional Park; oak-topped hill frames view of Mt. Diablo's west side.

here of a housing development reinforces the importance of protecting open space. Stay on the Hanging Valley Trail as it turns left at a junction with the Alamo Trail. Climbing on a moderate grade, with Mt. Diablo dominating the skyline, you reach a T-junction with the Briones-to-Mt. Diablo Regional

**Spring Bonuses**

Spring brings birds in abundance to the Mt. Diablo area; among the ones you may find here are western scrub-jays, barn swallows, northern orioles, western bluebirds, northern mockingbirds, red-winged blackbirds, and flycatchers.

Raptors, including a pair of peregrine falcons, have been known to nest in the park.

Wildflowers to look for on display include California poppies, paintbrush, Ithuriel's spears, asters, bellardia, Mariposa lilies, and clarkias.

Trail, a dirt road. Turn left and continue climbing.

Beyond a saddle, the road descends past a pond at about 4 miles, and then curves right and meets the Stonegate Trail, left. You veer right, then left at a junction with the Buckeye Ravine Trail. Still on the Briones-to-Mt. Diablo Trail, you come over a rise and then descend past a second Buckeye Ravine Trail to the junction that closes this loop. Here you turn right and retrace your route to the Shell Ridge Loop Trail. Turn right at the T-junction and follow a level course through a steep-walled canyon.

Soon the Shell Ridge Trail ends, and you turn left on the Stage Road Trail, a dusty dirt road. After about 0.1 mile, you branch left on the Castle Rock Trail, which skirts Castle Rock Regional Recreation Area. When you reach the short trail to the parking area, turn right and retrace your route.

# TRIP 7 Mt. Diablo State Park: Grand Loop

| | |
|---|---|
| **Distance** | 6.5 miles, Loop |
| **Hiking Time** | 3 to 5 hours |
| **Elevation Gain/Loss** | ±2200 feet |
| **Difficulty** | Difficult |
| **Trail Use** | Mountain biking allowed[1] |
| **Best Times** | Fall through spring |
| **Agency** | CSP |
| **Recommended Map** | *Trail Map of Mt. Diablo State Park and Adjacent Parklands* (CSP) |
| **Notes** | [1]Bicycles are not allowed on the Summit and Juniper trails, and must instead use Summit Road to descend from Devils Elbow to the parking area |

**HIGHLIGHTS**  A complete circle around Mt. Diablo, the East Bay's tallest peak, plus a trip to the summit, make this one of the region's premier hikes, and a great way to learn more about the trees, shrubs, and wildflowers that struggle for survival on the rugged mountain's upper reaches. This strenuous route uses Deer Flat, Meridian Ridge, and Prospectors Gap roads, and the North Peak, Summit, and Juniper trails.

**DIRECTIONS**  From I-680 in Danville, take the Diablo Road/Danville exit and follow Diablo Road 3 miles east to Mt. Diablo Scenic Blvd. Turn left onto Mt. Diablo Scenic Blvd. — which soon becomes South Gate Road — and go 3.7 miles to the South Gate entrance station. Continue on South Gate Road another 3.2 miles to Park Headquarters and a junction with North Gate and Summit roads. Turn right onto Summit Road and go 2.3 miles to a paved parking area at a sharp bend in the road, at the entrance to the Juniper Campground.

**FACILITIES/TRAILHEAD**  There are picnic tables, water, and a toilet near the trailhead, which is on the north end of the parking area.

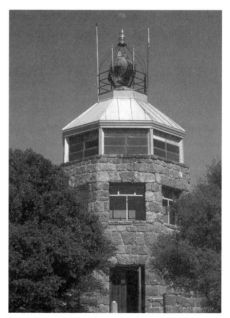

Follow either of two paved roads downhill into the Juniper Campground. From the point where they join, continue walking northwest on a gated dirt road, signed as Deer Flat Road/Mitchell Canyon Fire Road but called Deer Flat Road on the Mt. Diablo State Park trail map.

Passing Burma Road, left, you follow the road as it descends via well-graded S-bends, giving you a look at Mt. Diablo's 3849-foot summit. Deer Flat, which you soon reach, is one of the prettiest spots on Mt. Diablo, especially in fall, when bigleaf maple, California wild grape, and poison oak add touches of color to the scene.

Deer Flat Road ends here, and you turn right on Meridian Ridge Road. Soon the route turns north and skirts Bald Ridge as it begins to climb. With the grade now steep, you pass Deer Flat Creek Trail, left. At about 2 miles you reach Murchio Gap, an impor-

Tower atop Mt. Diablo's 3849-foot summit.

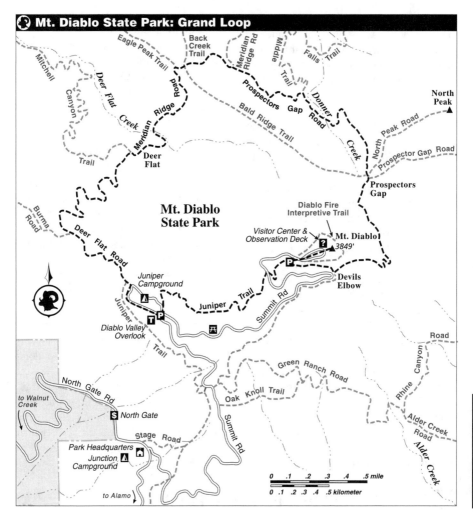

## Mt. Diablo State Park: Grand Loop

Eagle Peak Trail

Back Creek Trail

Meridian Ridge Rd

Middle Trail

Falls Trail

Mitchell Canyon

Deer Flat Creek

Meridian Ridge Road

Prospectors Gap Road

Bald Ridge Trail

Donner Road

Donner Creek

North Peak Road

North Peak ▲

Prospector Gap Road

Prospectors Gap

Deer Flat

Meridian Trail

Mt. Diablo State Park

Diablo Fire Interpretive Trail

Visitor Center & Observation Deck

Mt. Diablo ▲3849'

Burma Road

Deer Flat Road

Juniper Campground

Juniper Trail

Summit Rd

Devils Elbow

Diablo Valley Overlook

Trail

Rhine Canyon

Road

North Gate Rd

to Walnut Creek

**S** North Gate

Green Ranch Road

Oak Knoll Trail

Alder Creek Road

Alder Creek

Stage Road

Summit Rd

Park Headquarters

Junction Campground

to Alamo

0  .1  .2  .3  .4  .5 mile

0  .1  .2  .3  .4  .5 kilometer

tant junction with many trails. Here you angle right and follow Meridian Ridge Road east. After a gentle descent, you come to a junction, where you go straight, now on Prospectors Gap Road.

As you follow Prospectors Gap Road southeast, it holds a level course. Past the Middle Trail, left, you descend slightly to within earshot of Donner Creek. Now comes a steep climb, at first in shade but then in the open. A final pitch brings you, with relief, to Prospectors Gap. Here you turn right on the North Peak Trail, one of the few single tracks on Mt. Diablo open to

bicycles, but one that requires excellent skills.

### Devil Mountain Trees

Many of the trees and shrubs growing in the park are adapted to hot, dry conditions, including gray pine, California juniper, chamise, manzanita, toyon, and yerba santa. Gray pine, interior live oak, canyon live oak, and blue oak grow on the upper slopes of Mt. Diablo, and their shade is welcome on hot days.

The North Peak Trail, rutted and rocky in places, climbs across an open hillside and soon passes an unsigned trail, right. As you near a rocky ridge, at about 4 miles, the slope becomes more pronounced, with a severe drop-off, left. As you come into the open and switchback across the ridge, you are rewarded with a stunning 180-degree view. At Devils Elbow, a sharp bend in paved Summit Road, make a sharp right and begin climbing the Summit Trail, which rises through chaparral to the summit's lower parking area.

To reach the mountain's 3849-foot summit from the lower parking area, turn right and follow signs for the continuation of the Summit Trail, which runs between the two paved roads linking the summit's lower and upper parking areas. Take the Summit Trail uphill about 0.2 mile.

After resting and enjoying the scenery, retrace your steps to the lower parking area, then continue walking west across pavement until you find a trail post marking the Juniper Trail, a single track. From here, descend steeply, past some fenced-in communication equipment, to Summit Road. Cross carefully, turn right, and walk uphill a short distance to a trail post, left, marking the continuation of the Juniper Trail.

> **Summit Museum**
> The stone building at the summit was built by the Civilian Conservation Corps (CCC) from 1938 to 1940. It remained mostly unused until 1993, when the Mount Diablo Interpretive Association opened its visitor center there to hold information about the mountain's geology, flora, and fauna. Unfortunately, at press time the center was closed because of budget constraints, with no reopening date set. Restrooms, water, and a phone are still available, and you can climb to the observation deck for spectacular 360-degree views, enhanced by free binoculars, that sometimes include the snowcapped Sierra. To check whether the center has reopened, call (925) 837-2525.

The route loses elevation via switchbacks and then continues to descend along the crest of a broad ridge. At a saddle, you come to a junction with an unsigned trail, right, to Moses Rock Ridge. A trail post with an arrow pointing left directs you to the continuation of the Juniper Trail, which drops through groves of bay and juniper to the parking area.

## TRIP 8 Mt. Diablo State Park: Hidden Falls

|  |  |
|---|---|
| **Distance** | 6.6 miles, Loop |
| **Hiking Time** | 3 to 4 hours |
| **Elevation Gain/Loss** | ±1650 feet |
| **Difficulty** | Difficult |
| **Best Times** | Fall through spring |
| **Agency** | CSP |
| **Recommended Map** | *Trail Map of Mt. Diablo State Park and Adjacent Parklands* (MDIA) |

**HIGHLIGHTS**  This route, using the Bruce Lee, Back Creek, Meridian Point, Middle, and Falls trails, and Back Creek, Meridian Ridge, and Donner Canyon roads, samples the north side of Mt. Diablo. Cool, shady canyons, exposed rocky ridges, chaparral-covered hillsides, and oak woodlands provide a terrific assortment of trees, shrubs, wildflowers, and birds. During the rainy season, a set of hidden waterfalls is another incentive, if needed, to try this route.

**DIRECTIONS** From I-680 in Walnut Creek, or Highway 24 eastbound (just before the merge with I-680), take the Ygnacio Valley Road exit and go northeast 7.6 miles to Clayton Road. Turn right and go 2.9 miles (Clayton Road becomes Marsh Creek Road) to Regency Dr. Turn right and go 0.6 mile to a dead-end; park along the side of the street.

**FACILITIES/TRAILHEAD** There are no facilities at the trailhead, which is on the north side of Regency Dr., about 200 feet before its end.

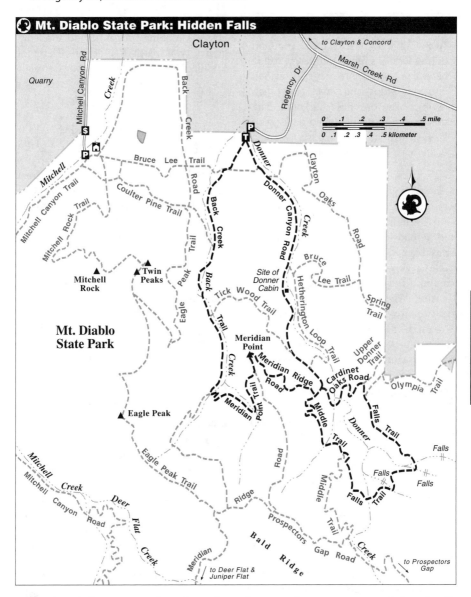

Mt. Diablo State Park: Hidden Falls

**G**o downhill on a paved road to the paved Bruce Lee Trail, named to honor a leading equestrian and trail builder, not the martial arts expert. Turn left and walk several hundred feet to the Mt. Diablo State Park boundary at Regency Gate. Past a trail to Mitchell Canyon Road, right, your road forks. You stay right and, after about 100 yards, reach a junction marked by a trail post. Here your route, the Bruce Lee Trail, heads right, and Donner Canyon Road, which you will use later, goes left.

---

**Trees to Look For**

Two of the Bay Area's three common deciduous oaks, blue and valley, reside here. Blue oak has light gray bark divided into long strips, and small, blue-green leaves. Valley oak has checkered, dark gray bark and deeply lobed dark-green leaves. Also here are coast live oak, California buckeye, and California bay.

---

In open grassland, you come to a four-way intersection. From here, the Bruce Lee Trail continues west to Mitchell Canyon, and a road joining sharply from the left heads back to Donner Canyon. Your route, Back Creek Road, angles left and contours around a ridge before dropping into Back Canyon. Where Back Creek Road turns right to cross Back Creek, you go straight, now on the Back Creek Trail, a dirt road.

Beyond a gate, the Back Creek Trail becomes a single track that climbs gently over rocky terrain, alternating between open and wooded areas and making several crossings of Back Creek. Past the Tick Wood Trail, left, a small canyon branches left from Back Canyon. About 100 yards beyond where the canyons branch, you come to a clearing and the Meridian Point Trail. Turn left, cross Back Creek on rocks, and then switchback up a steep embankment.

At the head of the side canyon, you cross a small creek and turn sharply left to climb out of the canyon. At about 2 miles, you reach a junction with Meridian Ridge Road. Turn left and descend steeply to Meridian Point, where the route bends sharply right. After descending steeply for about 0.5 mile from Meridian Point, you reach a junction, where you turn right on the Middle Trail.

A gentle climb on a single track takes you through chaparral and stands of manzanita—tall, twisted remnants of a 1977 fire and shrubby new growth. The route next climbs a series of switchbacks and then levels, taking you across an open hillside. After crossing a small creek, the route becomes rocky, eroded, and possibly wet in places. Climbing on gentle and moderate grades, you reach a junction. Here the Middle Trail turns right, but you go straight on the Falls Trail. The narrow track soon crosses an open and very steep hillside above Donner Creek (use caution).

Now the route drops via switchbacks to Donner Creek, and then begins a gentle climb on the creek's right-hand bank. A short distance upstream, Donner Creek bends left around a rocky rib, but your route follows a seasonal tributary to the right. Soon you cross the tributary, veer left, and begin climbing the opposite bank. As you work your way up the rocky rib, you come to a fork in the trail. Angle left—the right-hand fork rejoins your route in a few hundred feet.

Once around the rocky rib, the trail goes through a shady ravine on the right side of Donner Creek. You cross Donner Creek and then traverse an open hillside. After considerable effort, you are rewarded by a beautiful vista stretching north to the hills of Napa and Solano counties. And after reaching a

---

**Native Pines**

Two native pines, gray and Coulter, grow here. Gray pine, a tree well-adapted to dry conditions, has long gray-green needles in clusters of three, and big, spiny cones that fall to the ground when ripe. Coulter pine, a close relative, has darker green, bushier needles, stout branches turning up at the ends, and even larger cones (at 4 to 5 pounds, these are the heaviest of all the world's pine cones). Gray pines often have multiple trunks, but Coulter pines seldom do.

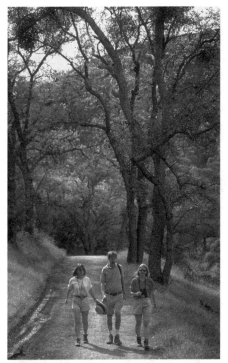

The north side of Mt. Diablo has trails that range in difficulty from easy to challenging.

flat area, there's the first waterfall, just ahead. The trail climbs, descends to a seasonal creek, and then climbs again, until you are perched on a cliff above the waterfall (again, use caution).

As the route swings east, passing through chaparral, more waterfalls pop into view, spilling across eroded, rocky cliffs. Directly under North Peak, you step across a seasonal creek and then pass a creek flowing out of Wild Oat Canyon. Now the trail bends left and then crosses several ridges, where, from around the 4-mile point, you are treated to superb views of Mt. Diablo's rugged north side. A level walk soon brings you to Cardinet Oaks Road, which you descend via S-bends to Donner Creek, which you cross.

At the junction of Cardinet Oaks, Meridian Ridge, and Donner Canyon roads, turn right and walk steeply downhill. Stay on Donner Canyon Road all the way to where the Bruce Lee Trail heads left toward Back Canyon. Closing the loop, you now retrace your route to Regency Dr.

## TRIP 9 Morgan Territory Regional Preserve

| | |
|---|---|
| **Distance** | 5.9 miles, Loop |
| **Hiking Time** | 3 to 4 hours |
| **Elevation Gain/Loss** | ±1050 feet |
| **Difficulty** | Moderate |
| **Trail Use** | Leashed dogs |
| **Best Times** | Spring and fall |
| **Agency** | EBRPD |
| **Recommended Map** | *Morgan Territory Regional Preserve* (EBRPD) |

**HIGHLIGHTS** This is one of the most remote and scenic parks in the East Bay, perched at 2000 feet on the southeastern edge of Mt. Diablo State Park, within sight of Livermore, Altamont Pass, and the Central Valley. Seclusion and wilderness make hiking here a special experience; this loop, which uses the Coyote, Stone Corral, Volvon Loop, and Volvon trails, takes full advantage of these attributes, dropping into a deep canyon, then climbing lofty Bob Walker Ridge. This is a region of extremes: hot in summer, cold in winter, and potentially windy all year.

**DIRECTIONS** From I-580 in Livermore, take the North Livermore exit and go north on North Livermore Ave., and then west on its continuation, Manning Road. At 4.4 miles from the interstate, just after a sharp bend to the west, you turn right onto Morgan

Territory Road, and go 6.3 miles to the parking area, right. (Use caution: much of Morgan Territory Road is narrow and winding.)

From I-680 in Walnut Creek, or Highway 24 eastbound (just before the merge with I-680), take the Ygnacio Valley Road exit and go northeast 7.6 miles to Clayton Road. Turn right and go 6 miles (Clayton Road becomes Marsh Creek Road) to Morgan Territory Road. Turn right and go 9.4 miles to the parking area, left. (Use caution: much of Morgan Territory Road is narrow and winding.)

**FACILITIES/TRAILHEAD**  There are picnic tables, water, and a toilet beside the parking area; there are also two toilets along the route. This trailhead is on the northeast side of the parking area.

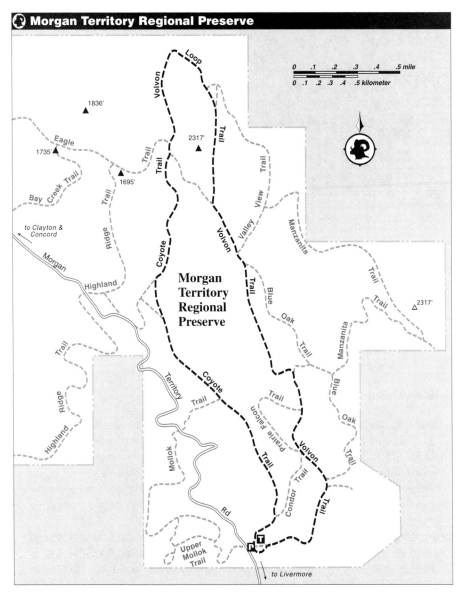

Following the Coyote Trail, left, you descend past a stock pond and a junction with the Condor Trail, and into a narrow, rocky canyon lined with black oak, California bay, and manzanita. As the descent becomes steeper, the trail makes S-bends down the hillside. In the canyon bottom, you meet a junction with the Mollok Trail, left, and then a fork, whose branches soon rejoin. Passing through the gate, you emerge from forest into grassland and leave the canyon behind.

The route stays in the middle of a large valley and soon reaches another fork. This time, follow the right-hand branch and walk uphill. Ahead is Y-junction, where you turn right on the Stone Corral Trail, a dirt road, and climb through an oak savanna. After climbing via long switchbacks, you pass the Volvon Loop Trail, right. Continue straight, past a cattle-loading pen, to the next junction. Here, at about 2.3 miles, the Eagle Trail branches left, and your route, the Volvon Loop Trail, goes right. When you reach the north end of Bob Walker Ridge, the route bends sharply right, presenting a vista that stretches east to the Central Valley and, on a clear day, the Sierra. The route stays just below the ridgecrest and passes through lovely stands of blue oak and bay. You pass the first of three connections to the Valley View Trail, left. Soon you reach a notch in the ridge and a trail, right, to the Coyote Trail. Mt. Diablo

> **Forebearers**
> The preserve is named for Jeremiah Morgan, an early settler, gold miner, and rancher. Bob Walker Ridge and the Bob Walker Regional Trail honor a photographer and environmentalist whose efforts on behalf of EBRPD from 1984 until his death in 1993 led to additional land acquisitions in Morgan Territory and on Pleasanton Ridge.

looks impressive from here, dominating the northwest skyline.

Continuing on the Volvon Trail, you pass the Valley View and Blue Oak trails, left. Tall manzanitas line the left side of the road. Where the Hummingbird Trail goes straight, you follow the Volvon Trail as it turns sharply right. Soon you pass two junctions, about 0.2 mile apart, with the Prairie Falcon Trail, right. Just beyond the second of these is a junction with the Condor Trail, also right.

When you reach a junction with the Blue Oak Trail at about 5 miles, follow the Volvon Trail as it veers right, and in about 150 feet you come to a T-junction with a dirt-and-gravel road. Turn right here and begin a gentle descent through open grassland. Stay right at a fork and follow the gently rolling road until you can see the parking area. At the next fork, veer left and descend moderately to the parking area.

## TRIP 10 Round Valley Regional Preserve

| | |
|---|---|
| **Distance** | 4.8 miles, Loop |
| **Hiking Time** | 2 to 3 hours |
| **Elevation Gain/Loss** | ±950 feet |
| **Difficulty** | Moderate |
| **Best Times** | Spring and fall |
| **Agency** | EBRPD |
| **Recommended Map** | *Round Valley Regional Preserve* (EBRPD) |

**HIGHLIGHTS** Explore this preserve, which forms an important link in the East Bay's open space chain, using the Hardy Canyon and Miwok trails. The rolling, oak-shaded hills are daubed with floral colors in spring, and the impressive expanse of Round Valley itself has few rivals in the Bay Area. This is a popular equestrian area, and the single-track Hardy Canyon Trail takes a beating.

**DIRECTIONS** From I-680 in Walnut Creek, or Highway 24 eastbound (just before the merge with I-680), take the Ygnacio Valley Road exit and go northeast 7.6 miles to Clayton Road. Turn right and go 14.8 miles (Clayton Road becomes Marsh Creek Road) to the parking area, right.

**FACILITIES/TRAILHEAD** Picnic tables, water, toilets, and an emergency phone are near the trailhead, which is on the south end of the parking area.

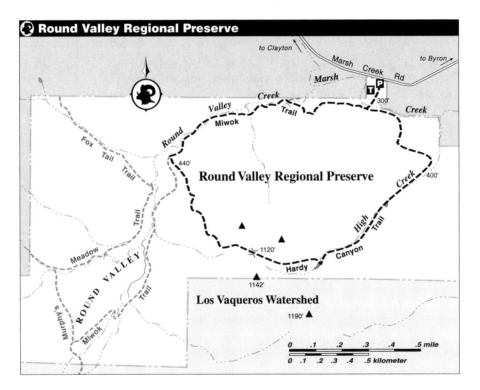

Follow a path that curves left from the trailhead to a T-junction with a dirt road. Turn right and go across a bridge over Marsh Creek. The Miwok Trail, which you will use later, is right, but you turn left on the Hardy Canyon Trail and stroll beside Marsh Creek. Staying right at a fork, you follow a rutted track through an open field and curve away from the creek. The trail rises through a blue oak savanna and then enters the canyon holding High Creek.

Emerging into a wide valley at about 2 miles, you skirt a stock pond and cross the dam that forms it. The trail, just a narrow path through the grass, angles right and climbs to a saddle just north of Peak 1142. The views here reward your efforts, and now you descend toward Round Valley, with Mt. Diablo rising in the distance. Switchbacks aid the descent, which crosses

**Round Valley Trees**
Among the trees found in this preserve are California buckeye, valley oak, blue oak, coast live oak, Fremont cottonwood, hoptree, western sycamore, and California bay.

flower-filled slopes. Dropping on a moderate grade, you curve around a ridge and meet the Miwok Trail, a dirt road, at about 3.4 miles. (You can extend the route by circling Round Valley on the Miwok and Murphy Meadow trails.)

You veer right and follow Round Valley Creek through a broad canyon. At a fork with a closed road, you stay right and climb on a gentle grade. At the next fork, unsigned, you again stay right and soon wind moderately uphill. Crossing the end of a ridge, you descend and meet the trail coming from the previous fork. Continuing straight, you follow a rolling course to the junction that closes the loop. Here you turn left and retrace your route to the parking area.

Round Valley Regional Preserve: heading west from trailhead on the Miwok Trail.

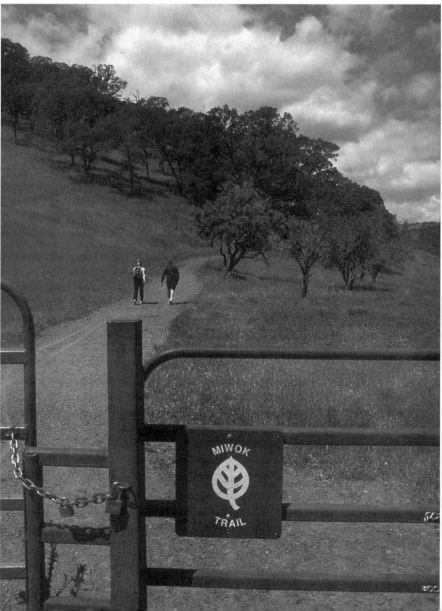

# Chapter 5
## *Berkeley/Oakland*

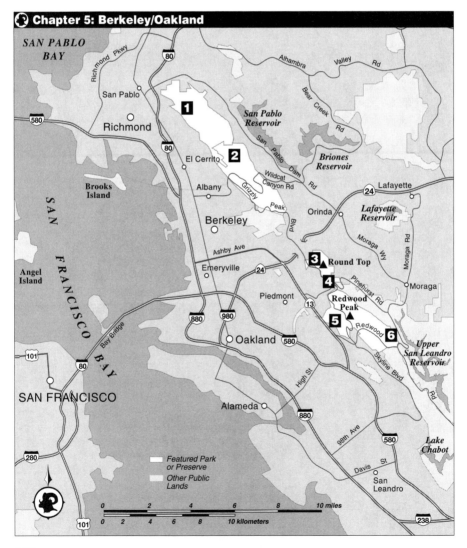

SAN PABLO BAY

Richmond Pkwy

80

Alhambra

Valley Rd

San Pablo

580

Richmond

San Pablo Reservoir

Bear Creek Rd

**1**

El Cerrito

80

**2**

Wildcat Canyon Rd

San Pablo Dam Rd

Briones Reservoir

Brooks Island

Albany

Grizzly Peak

Lafayette

24

Lafayette Reservoir

Berkeley

Orinda

SAN

Ashby Ave

Moraga Wy

Moraga Rd

Angel Island

Emeryville

24

**3** Round Top

FRANCISCO

Piedmont

13

**4**

Pinehurst Rd

Moraga

Redwood Peak

BAY

880

980

**5**

Redwood

**6**

Bay Bridge

101

Oakland

580

Skyline Blvd

Upper San Leandro Reservoir

80

High St

Rd

SAN FRANCISCO

Alameda

880

280

98th Ave

580

Lake Chabot

Davis St

San Leandro

101

■ Featured Park or Preserve

■ Other Public Lands

0    2    4    6    8    10 miles

0  2  4  6  8   10 kilometers

238

# TRIP 1 Wildcat Canyon Regional Park

| | |
|---|---|
| **Distance** | 7 miles, Semi-loop |
| **Hiking Time** | 3 to 4 hours |
| **Elevation Gain/Loss** | ±1700 feet |
| **Difficulty** | Difficult |
| **Trail Use** | Mountain biking allowed[1], Leashed dogs |
| **Best Times** | Spring and fall |
| **Agency** | EBRPD |
| **Recommended Map** | *Wildcat Regional Park* (EBRPD) |
| **Notes** | [1]Havey Canyon is closed to bicycles and horses during wet weather |

**HIGHLIGHTS**  This semi-loop takes you from the lowlands of Wildcat Creek to the high, open slopes of San Pablo Ridge, using the Wildcat Creek, Havey Canyon, San Pablo Ridge, and Belgum trails, and Nimitz Way. You are rewarded for your efforts by some of the best views in the East Bay, including a 360-degree panorama from an old Nike missile site. Exposed to sun and wind for much of the way, this hike is best done when spring wildflowers bloom or after summer's heat has abated, when the hills are golden brown. (This route is a favorite among bicyclists: walk on the right side of the trails.)

**DIRECTIONS**  From I-80 eastbound in Richmond, take the Solano Ave. exit, which puts you on Amador St. Turn left and go 0.4 mile to McBryde Ave. Turn right and follow McBryde Ave. 0.2 mile, staying in the left lane as you approach a stop sign. (Use caution at this intersection; traffic from the right does not stop.) Continue straight, now on Park Ave., for 0.1 mile to the Alvarado Staging Area, left.

From I-80 westbound in San Pablo, take the McBryde Ave. exit, turn left onto McBryde, go over the freeway and, from the intersection of McBryde and Amador, follow the directions above.

**FACILITIES/TRAILHEAD**  The Alvarado Area, northwest of the parking area, has picnic tables and water. There are toilets near the trailhead, which is on the east end of the parking area.

**F**ollow the paved remnant of Wildcat Canyon Road, closed in the early 1980s by landslides and renamed the Wildcat Creek Trail. As you make a gentle climb, you reach a junction with the Belgum Trail, left, which you will use later. Continue straight, alternating on dirt and pavement, parallel to Wildcat Creek, right. Soon the pavement ends and then you meet the Mezue Trail, left. (For a lovely glimpse of Wildcat Creek, shaded here by bay trees, turn right and walk downhill about 100 yards on a dirt path.)

The Wildcat Creek Trail follows a line of willow, white alder, and western sycamore bordering the creek, soon passing Rifle Range Road, right. Now the route climbs to

> **Wildcat Foliage**
> A mix of native and nonnative trees and shrubs, including Monterey pine, eucalyptus, California bay, blue elderberry, coffeeberry, toyon, and evergreen huckleberry, line the first part of the route. When you reach jungle-like Havey Canyon, you'll find bigleaf maple, California buckeye, and hazelnut, with an understory of western creek dogwood, snowberry, vine honeysuckle, blackberry, and ferns.

a junction with the Havey Canyon and Conlon trails, at about 2 miles. You turn left on the Havey Canyon Trail, the farthest left

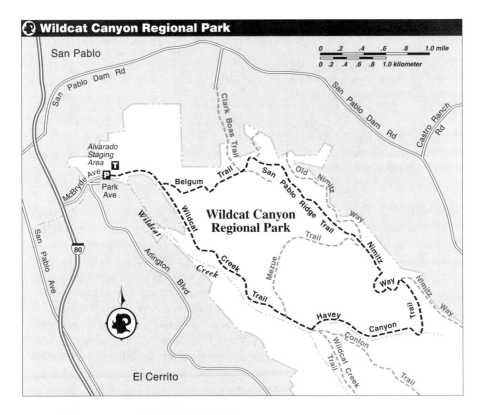

**Wildcat Canyon Regional Park**

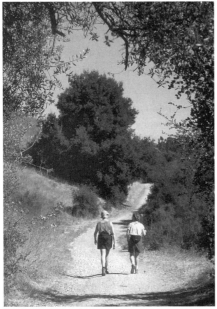

The Wildcat Canyon Trail runs between Wildcat
Canyon and Tilden regional parks.

of the trails at this junction, following a
tributary of Wildcat Creek.

As the route abruptly breaks into the
open, you have the open slopes of San
Pablo Ridge ahead, dotted with coyote
brush and stunted coast live oak. At a
T-junction with paved Nimitz Way, you
turn left. When you reach a junction with
a road heading right, at about 4 miles, take
a few minutes to make the climb to an
abandoned Nike missile site, a relic of the
Cold War, where a rest bench and
360-degree views await. The park's high
ground offers views of Mt. Tamalpais, Mt.
St. Helena, Mt. Diablo, the Santa Cruz
Mountains, San Francisco Bay, and the
Golden Gate Bridge.

Where the paved segment of Nimitz Way
ends, continue straight on a dirt road. You
come to a cattle pen and a choice of three
trails. Bear left on the Mezue Trail, then
right at a fork on the San Pablo Ridge Trail.

Now the route climbs up and over a series of high points on San Pablo Ridge, then plunges steeply northwest to a junction with the Belgum Trail, a dirt road.

Turn left, soon passing the Clark–Boas Trail, right, and then an unsigned road, left.

Now you climb to an fork, where you bear left, still following the Belgum Trail, a dirt road. The route makes a well-graded descent and closes the loop at the Wildcat Creek Trail, where you turn right and retrace your route to the parking area.

## TRIP 2 Tilden Regional Park

| | |
|---|---|
| **Distance** | 3.3 miles, Loop |
| **Hiking Time** | 1 to 2 hours |
| **Elevation Gain/Loss** | ±900 feet |
| **Difficulty** | Moderate |
| **Best Times** | All year |
| **Agency** | EBRPD |
| **Recommended Map** | *Tilden Regional Park* (EBRPD) |

**HIGHLIGHTS** This scenic loop hike takes you from the Tilden Park Environmental Education Center to the summit of Wildcat Peak via the Jewel Lake, Sylvan, Peak and Laurel Canyon trails. Terrific views of the Bay Area and a variety of plants and birds keep this route interesting throughout.

**DIRECTIONS** From I-80 in Berkeley, take the University Ave. exit and go east 2.1 miles to Oxford St. Turn left and go 0.7 mile to Rose St. Turn right and go one block to Spruce St. Turn left and follow Spruce St. 1.8 miles to an intersection with Grizzly Peak Blvd. and Wildcat Canyon Road. Cross the intersection and immediately turn left from Wildcat Canyon Dr. onto Canon Dr. There is a sign here for NATURE AREA, PONY RIDE, WILDCAT CANYON. Go downhill 0.3 mile to a junction with Central Park Dr., turn left, and go 0.1 mile to a large parking area.

From Highway 24 just east of the Caldecott Tunnel, take the Fish Ranch Road exit and go 1 mile uphill to a junction with Grizzly Peak Blvd. Turn right and go 5.4 miles to the intersection with Wildcat Canyon Road and Spruce St. mentioned above. Turn right onto Wildcat Canyon Road, then immediately left onto Canon Dr. Go downhill 0.3 mile to a junction with Central Park Dr., turn left, and go 0.1 mile to a large parking area.

**FACILITIES/TRAILHEAD** The Tilden Environmental Education Center, a short distance from the parking area, has displays, books, maps, and helpful staff. Picnic tables, restrooms, phone, and water are available. The trailhead is behind the Center, on its north side (go through the Center and out the back door to make sure you get on the correct trail).

Walk north across the lawn to the Jewel Lake Nature Trail and follow it for about 100 yards to a dirt road. Beyond the road is a junction where you turn left on the Jewel Lake and Sylvan trails, temporarily joined. At the next junction, where the trails split, you veer right on the Sylvan Trail. An easy climb brings you to Loop Road, which you cross. The continuation of the Sylvan Trail heads northwest, crosses an open hillside, then enters a eucalyptus forest.

Where the Sylvan Trail swings left, you angle right on the Peak Trail and continue climbing. Soon an unsigned trail merges from the left, but you follow the Peak Trail as it bends right and climbs to a T-junction. Turn left to visit the summit of Wildcat Peak (1250') and the Rotary Peace Monument, a

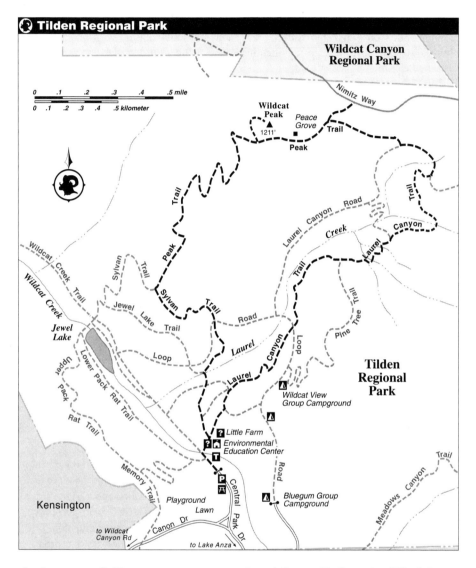

Tilden Regional Park

circular stone wall. Then retrace your route to the T-junction and continue straight on the Peak Trail as it descends past the Rotary Peace Grove, a collection of giant sequoias which, being out of their native Sierra habitat, are limited in stature.

At a junction with a connector to Nimitz Way, stay on the Peak Trail by turning sharply right. A few short switchbacks bring you to Laurel Canyon Road, where you turn left and soon reach the start of the Laurel Canyon Trail, right, at about 2 miles. (The

Laurel Canyon Trail may be difficult in wet weather. (For an alternate descent, when you reach Laurel Canyon Road, turn right, go downhill to Loop Road, turn left, and follow the directions below.)

Turn right and traverse the steep edge of Laurel Canyon. Now passing a connector to Laurel Canyon Road, right, you follow moderately graded Laurel Canyon Trail as it turns left and continues downhill. After about 100 yards, the route bends sharply right at a trail post, dips twice to cross trib-

> **Tall Tree Troubles**
> Eucalyptus is an Australian tree intro-duced to the Bay Area in the 1850s and planted extensively in the East Bay in the early 20th century as part of an ill-fated timber scheme. Although fast growing, the species of eucalyptus planted most commonly here is worthless for timber, a fact that dashed the hopes of would-be timber barons for a quick profit on their investments.

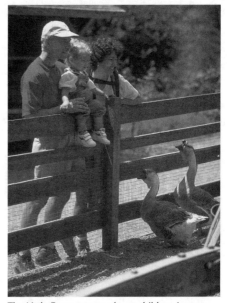

The Little Farm, sure to please children, is near the Tilden Environmental Education Center.

utaries of Laurel Creek, and then emerges from forest into a clearing.

Where the Pine Tree Trail heads left, you follow a rolling course to Loop Road, where you turn left. After about 100 feet, find the continuation of the Laurel Canyon Trail, marked by a trail post, going right. An easy descent brings you to a dirt road. Turn left and walk uphill, past an unsigned trail, which heads right. Just ahead is the fence at the corner of the Little Farm. When you reach the fence, turn right and go downhill to the visitor center.

# TRIP 3 Sibley Volcanic Regional Preserve

| | |
|---|---|
| **Distance** | 1.6 miles, Loop |
| **Hiking Time** | 1 to 2 hours |
| **Elevation Gain/Loss** | ±400 feet |
| **Difficulty** | Easy |
| **Trail Use** | Leashed dogs, Good for kids |
| **Best Times** | All year |
| **Agency** | EBRPD |
| **Recommended Map** | *Sibley Volcanic Regional Preserve* (EBRPD) |

**HIGHLIGHTS**  This delightful loop circles Round Top, an extinct volcano and one of the highest peaks in the Oakland and Berkeley hills, and also provides access to a volcanic area that will be of interest to geology buffs. The Sibley Volcanic Regional Preserve brochure and map, available free at the visitor center, has descriptions that corre-spond to numbered posts on the self-guiding Volcanic Trail.

**DIRECTIONS**  From Highway 24 just east of the Caldecott Tunnel, take the Fish Ranch Road exit and go uphill one mile to Grizzly Peak Blvd. Turn left and go 2.5 miles to Skyline Blvd. Turn left and go 0.1 mile to the preserve entrance, left.

**FACILITIES/TRAILHEAD**  A visitor center with exhibits explaining the area's volcanic past, as well as its plant and wildlife communities, is beside the parking area. There are water and toilets available. The trailhead is on the west side of the visitor center.

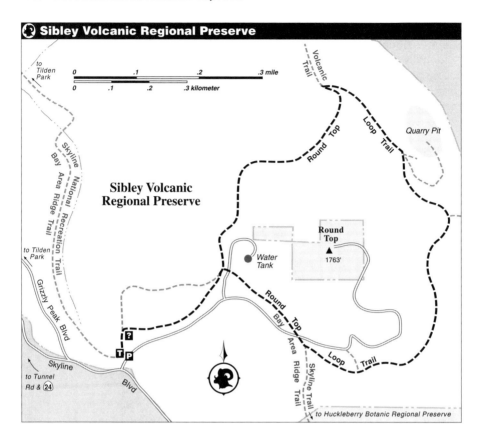

## Sibley Volcanic Regional Preserve

Just ahead of a gate, you turn right on a single-track dirt trail, signed for the Round Top Loop and Volcanic trails. Bear right and climb through stands of California bay, Monterey pine, and eucalyptus. You pass a junction, left, with a trail that leads back to the visitor center. In another 100 feet or so, you reach a four-way junction, marked by a

---

**Round Top**

Round Top (1763') was once was an active volcano, and there are three other extinct volcanoes nearby. The volcanic activity took place approximately 10 million years ago, but occasional moving and shaking along fault lines continues to this day. Quarry operations here from the 1930s to the 1960s dug into the side of Round Top, exposing the basalt lava interior of the volcano, to the delight of geologists.

---

trail post, where you turn left onto a wide dirt-and-gravel road that heads north and then northeast into the volcanic area.

A mostly level walk over rocky ground takes you around the west and north sides of Round Top to a T-junction. Here you turn right to stay on the Round Top Loop Trail. Soon you come to a viewpoint above a quarry pit, with Mt. Diablo looming on the eastern skyline. Because of its bulk and shape, Mt. Diablo could be mistaken for a volcano, but it is not, having been formed instead by a mass of rock pushing upward through sedimentary layers.

Just past the viewpoint, follow the Round Top Loop Trail as it leaves the road, heads right, and makes a rising traverse across the grassy east side of Round Top. After cresting a low ridge, you descend to a cattle gate, and now enjoy a shady stroll. Bear left at an unsigned fork, and soon you reach a junction,

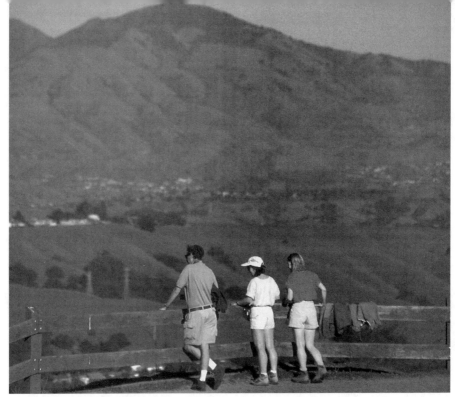

Hikers enjoy view of Mt. Diablo from quarry pit overlook on Round Top Loop Trail.

left, with the East Bay Skyline/Bay Area Ridge Trail, a route to Huckleberry Regional Preserve and Redwood Regional Park.

Go straight, and in about 125 feet, you arrive at Round Top Road. Cross the paved road and continue on the Round Top Loop Trail. Coming to a clearing, you cross a paved road leading uphill to an EBMUD water tank, and then close the loop at the four-way junction with the road to the volcanic area. Continue straight—staying left at an upcoming fork—and retrace your route to the parking area.

**A Bit of History**

The preserve, named for Robert Sibley, director and president of EBRPD from 1948 until his death in 1958, is one of the oldest East Bay regional parks. Originally called Round Top, it was dedicated in 1936, just two years after the District was formed.

## TRIP4 Huckleberry Botanic Regional Preserve

| | |
|---:|:---|
| **Distance** | 1.9 miles, Loop |
| **Hiking Time** | 1 to 2 hours |
| **Difficulty** | Easy |
| **Trail Use** | Good for kids |
| **Best Times** | All year |
| **Agency** | EBRPD |
| **Recommended Map** | *Huckleberry Botanic Regional Preserve* (EBRPD) |

**HIGHLIGHTS** This hike, an easy self-guiding loop through a 235-acre botanical treasure trove, is simply not to be missed, especially from late winter through spring, when its shrubs and flowers are in bloom. Among the highlights are two rare plants: western leatherwood and pallid, or Alameda, manzanita. **Boldface** numbers in the route description refer to numbered markers along the trail and plant descriptions in the *Huckleberry Self-Guided Nature Path* pamphlet, available at the trailhead.

**DIRECTIONS**  From Highway 24 just east of the Caldecott Tunnel, take the Fish Ranch Road exit and go uphill 1 mile to a junction with Grizzly Peak Blvd. Turn left and go 2.5 miles to a junction with Skyline Blvd. Turn left and go 0.5 mile to a parking area, left.

**FACILITIES/TRAILHEAD**  There is a toilet near the trailhead, which is on the southeast side of the parking area.

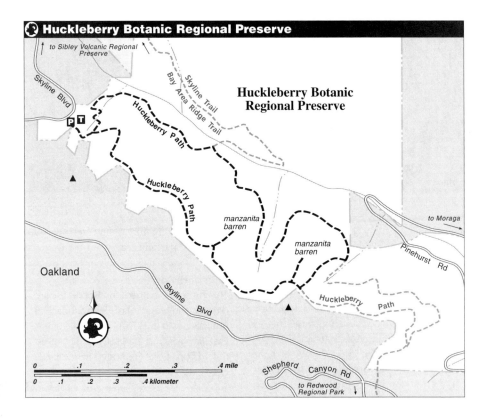

About 100 yards past the trailhead, the Huckleberry Path forks, and you descend left on a series of switchbacks through a fragrant forest of California bay and coast live oak. Soon you come to a large madrone, marker **1**, an evergreen tree with smooth, reddish bark and finely-toothed elliptical leaves. A short walk brings you to hazelnut, marker **2**, a relative of the commercial filbert. The bright green leaves of this shrub, renewed each spring, feel like pieces of soft felt. When you come to the next fork, bear right and begin to climb.

Thriving in damp areas on the forest floor is western sword fern, marker **3**. Long, pointed fronds give this fern its name and distinguish it from wood fern, marker **4**. Now the route swings left and then arrives at a grove of large bay trees, marker **5**. Here the towering bays have established dominance by depriving their would-be competitors of sunlight. Just past this grove is a junction, where you

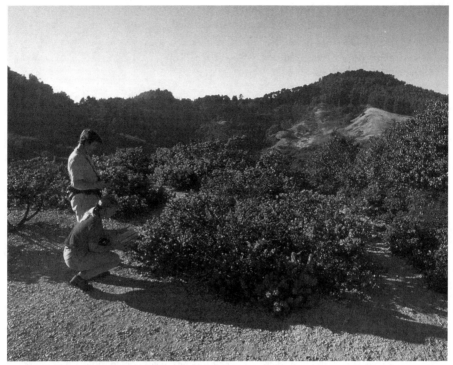

The Huckleberry Path, a self-guiding nature trail, leads to a manzanita barren.

turn right and climb via wood steps and switchbacks.

Now you reach a T-junction with the upper segment of the Huckleberry Path. Turn right, and almost immediately come to a junction, marker **6**. Here you bear right and climb to a manzanita barren—a dry, gravelly plateau in the early stage of succession from manzanita to huckleberry. Return to the main path and turn right to find Douglas iris, marker **7**, a spring bloomer. At a junction, turn right and descend through the woods.

As you begin walking on this trail, look for a short path leading right and downhill to a rare shrub called western leatherwood, marker **8**. The yellow flowers of this shrub, which gets its name from the flexibility of the wood, appear in the winter, when its branches are still bare. Climb back to the side trail, turn right, and walk to another manzanita barren, where you will find jimbrush, marker **9**, and canyon live oak, marker **10**.

Now return to the main trail, where you turn right. Walking past stands of huckleberry, marker **11**, you soon reach an area of plant succession, marker **12**. Here the manzanitas are being replaced by other, faster-growing plants, such as huckleberry and chinquapin, marker **13**. Two types of manzanita grow along this exposed stretch of trail: brittle-leaf, marker **14**, and the rare pallid, or Alameda, marker **15**.

A bit farther, you come to coast silk tassel, marker **16**. The tassel in its name refers to the flower clusters hanging in winter from male plants. The route now descends via wooden steps into dense forest, then levels in an area where you can see pinkflower currant, marker **17**. This beautiful shrub dangles its delicate flowers from bare branches in the winter. Just past marker **17** you reach a junction. Here you continue straight and retrace your route to the parking area.

# TRIP 5 Joaquin Miller Park

|  |  |
|---|---|
| **Distance** | 3.6 miles, Loop |
| **Hiking Time** | 1 to 2 hours |
| **Elevation Gain/Loss** | ±850 feet |
| **Difficulty** | Moderate |
| **Trail Use** | Mountain biking allowed[1], Leashed dogs[2] |
| **Best Times** | All year |
| **Agency** | OPR&CA |
| **Recommended Map** | *Joaquin Miller Park* (OPR&CA) |
| **Notes** | [1]Bicycles allowed on this route, but *not* allowed on the Wild Rose, Fern, and Ravine trails, or on the Palos Colorados Trail between Sinawik Cabin and Joaquin Miller Court; [2] dogs not allowed in the picnic areas |

**HIGHLIGHTS** This park, adjacent to Redwood Regional Park, offers many of its neighbor's attractions in a more intimate and less crowded setting. Using the Sunset, Cinderella, and Sequoia–Bayview trails, this loop explores forests of redwood, Monterey cypress, eucalyptus, and acacia, and offers a fine view of Oakland and San Francisco.

**DIRECTIONS** From Highway 13 northbound in Oakland, take the Joaquin Miller Road/Lincoln Ave. exit, bear right onto Joaquin Miller Road, and go 0.8 mile to Sanborn Dr., the park entrance. Turn left and go 0.1 to the ranger-station parking area, left.

From Highway 13 southbound in Oakland, take the Joaquin Miller Road/Lincoln Ave. exit, stay left, and at a stop sign turn left onto Monterey Blvd. Go several hundred feet to Lincoln Ave., turn left and cross over Highway 13. Now on Joaquin Miller Road, follow the directions above.

**FACILITIES/TRAILHEAD** A ranger station beside the parking area, with maps, brochures, and displays, is open daily from 9 A.M. to 5 P.M. Nearby are picnic tables, water, and toilets. The trailhead is in front of the ranger station.

Walk south along Sanborn Dr. in a corridor of California bay, coast live oak, madrone, and Monterey pine, toward the park entrance. Just before Joaquin Miller Road, you come to a yellow gate and turn left. Beyond the gate, go straight on a dirt-and-gravel road toward the Upper Meadow and Greenwood picnic areas. Shrubs to look for in this park include pinkflower currant, evergreen huckleberry, snowberry, hazelnut, creambush, and gooseberry.

Turn left a T-junction with the Sunset Trail, a dirt road, and follow it northwest beside Palo Seco Creek. Soon you pass the Sinawik Trail, left, and the Sunset Loop, right. Where the Palos Colorados Trail forks left, you continue straight on the Sunset Trail. With Palo Seco Creek now in a deep ravine, left, you pass the Chaparral Trail,

> **Mr. Miller**
> Joaquin Miller (1841–1913) was a colorful figure best known as a poet and an arborist. He settled in the hills above Oakland, where he planted thousands of trees and built monuments to his heroes — Moses, explorer John C. Frémont, and poets Robert and Elizabeth Barrett Browning.

unsigned, heading right and uphill. Your route narrows to a single track as it crosses a slope, which is prone to landslides.

Where the Sunset Trail swings sharply left, you turn right onto the Cinderella Trail at an unsigned junction and begin climbing steeply uphill. This section of the route may be muddy; in one place water may be flowing

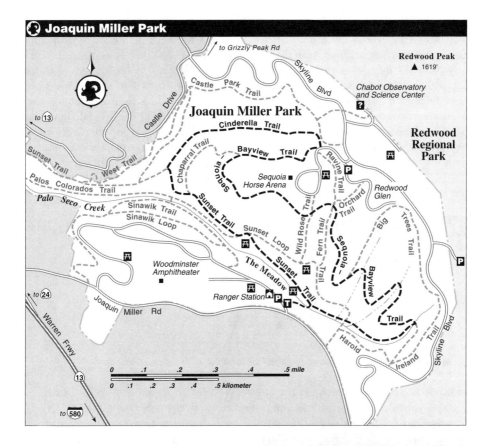

**Joaquin Miller Park**

*to Grizzly Peak Rd*

**Redwood Peak**
▲ 1619'

*Chabot Observatory and Science Center*

**Joaquin Miller Park**

Cinderella  Trail

**Redwood Regional Park**

Castle  Park  Trail

Skyline  Blvd

Castle  Drive

*to ⑬*

Bayview   Trail

Chaparral Trail

Sequoia ■
Horse Arena

Ravine Trail

Sunset  Trail

West  Trail

*Sequoia*

Palos  Colorados – Trail

Redwood
Glen

Palo  Seco  Creek

Sinawik  Trail

Wild Rose Trail

Orchard Trail

Sinawik  Loop

Sunset  Trail

Sunset  Loop

Fern  Trail

Big

Trees  Trail

Sunset

*Sequoia –*

Woodminster
Amphitheater

The  Meadow

Trail

Bayview

*to ㉔*

Ranger Station

Joaquin  Miller  Rd

Trail

Warren  Frwy

Harold

Ireland

Skyline  Blvd

Trail

⑬

0    .1    .2    .3    .4    .5 mile

0   .1   .2   .3   .4   .5 kilometer

*to ⑤⑧⓪*

across the trail from a pipe on the left. You begin a series of alternately steep and level sections to an unsigned junction just before Pine View Flat, a level clearing carpeted with wood chips.

Here you turn sharply right and follow the Sequoia–Bayview Trail, a single track, as it skirts below a parking and picnic area, with a restroom above and left. At a junction marked by a trail post, you turn right and walk about 100 feet to a T-junction. Turn right and follow the Sequoia–Bayview Trail on a level course.

Soon you pass a path, left, leading uphill to the Sequoia Arena, an equestrian facility. A bit farther, you reach a junction where your route, the Sequoia–Bayview Trail, turns left, and the Chaparral Trail goes straight. Climbing from the junction on a moderate grade, the route levels and enters

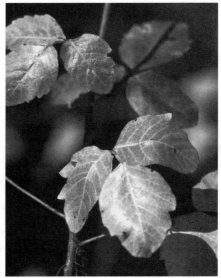

"Leaflets three, let it be," is a useful way to identify poison oak.

a magical forest — cool, quiet, and secluded — of Monterey cypress, pine, and, farther along, acacia, an import from Australia.

At about 2 miles, you pass a junction, left, with another trail to the horse arena. Now the route maintains a contour through a eucalyptus forest and then into the domain of coast redwood, a true East Bay native. Once in the redwoods, you pass junctions with the Wild Rose, Fern Ravine, and Big Trees trails. Views from clearings along the way help the trail live up to its name.

As the route finishes a right-hand bend at the head of a little canyon, you turn right on the Sunset Trail. The descent beneath towering redwoods is moderate at first, then gentle. You pass two paths heading right and uphill, the first unsigned, and the second signed as the Sunset Loop. Beyond the Greenwood picnic area, left, you close the loop at a junction beside Palo Seco Creek. Now turn left and retrace your route uphill to the parking area.

# TRIP 6 Redwood Regional Park

| | |
|---:|:---|
| **Distance** | 8.1 miles, Loop |
| **Hiking Time** | 4 to 5 hours |
| **Elevation Gain/Loss** | ±1550 feet |
| **Difficulty** | Difficult |
| **Trail Use** | Leashed dogs |
| **Best Times** | All year |
| **Agency** | EBRPD |
| **Recommended Map** | *Redwood Regional Park* (EBRPD) |

**HIGHLIGHTS** This loop, combining the Stream, West Ridge, French and Orchard trails, takes you into the heart of this unique regional park, the only one in the East Bay where coast redwoods, heavily logged in the mid-1800s, have been preserved to such an extent. The climb along the Stream Trail to Skyline Gate is easy, steepening only at the very end, and the rolling, meandering return through the redwoods via the French Trail, an alternate segment of the East Bay Skyline/Bay Area Ridge Trail, although strenuous, is not to be missed.

**DIRECTIONS** From I-580 southbound in Oakland, take the 35th Ave. exit, turn left and follow 35th Ave. east into the hills. After 0.8 mile 35th Ave. becomes Redwood Road, and at 2.4 miles it crosses Skyline Blvd., where you stay in the left lane and go straight. At 4.6 miles from I-580 you reach the park entrance; turn left and go 0.5 mile to the Canyon Meadow Staging Area.

From I-580 northbound in Oakland, take the Warren Freeway/Berkeley/Highway 13 exit and go 0.9 mile to the Carson St./Redwood Road exit. From the stop sign at the end of the exit ramp, continue straight, now on Mountain Blvd., 0.2 mile, and bear right onto Redwood Road. Go 3.2 miles to the park entrance; turn left and go 0.5 mile to the Canyon Meadow Staging Area.

From Highway 13 southbound, take the Redwood Road/Carson St. exit, turn left onto Redwood Road and follow the directions above.

There are fees for parking and dogs when the entrance kiosk is attended.

**FACILITIES/TRAILHEAD** Picnic tables, a toilet, phone, and water are near the trailhead, which is on the northwest end of the parking area. Water and toilets are also available ahead on the Stream Trail and at Skyline Gate.

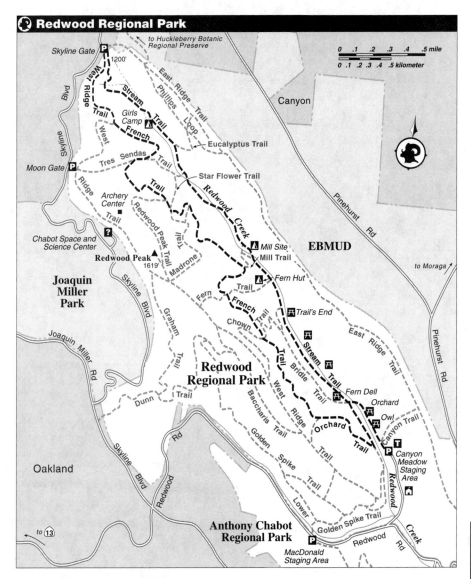

**Redwood Regional Park**

to Huckleberry Botanic
Regional Preserve

Skyline Gate

1200'

West Ridge Trail

Stream Trail

Girls Camp

French Trail

Phillips Loop

East Ridge Trail

Canyon

Eucalyptus Trail

Tres Sendas Trail

Moon Gate

West Ridge Trail

Skyline

Star Flower Trail

Archery Center

Redwood Peak Trail

Redwood Creek

Chabot Space and Science Center

Redwood Peak 1619'

Madrone Trail

Mill Site

Mill Trail

EBMUD

Pinehurst Rd

to Moraga

**Joaquin Miller Park**

Skyline Blvd

Fern Trail

French Trail

Fern Hut

Trail's End

Graham Trail

Chown Trail

Stream Trail

East Ridge Trail

Joaquin Miller Rd

**Redwood Regional Park**

West Ridge Trail

Bridle Trail

Fern Dell

Pinehurst Rd

Dunn Trail

Baccharis Trail

Orchard

Orchard Trail

Owl Canyon Trail

**Oakland**

Skyline Blvd

Redwood Rd

Golden Spike Trail

Lower Trail

Canyon Meadow Staging Area

Redwood Creek

to (13)

**Anthony Chabot Regional Park**

Golden Spike Trail

Redwood Rd

MacDonald Staging Area

0  .1  .2  .3  .4  .5 mile
0  .1  .2  .3  .4  .5 kilometer

Go northwest on the Stream Trail, a paved road, to a junction with the Canyon Trail, right. Just past this junction, the route enters a redwood grove, a taste of things to come, then emerges into the open at the Orchard picnic area. There is a play area for children here, and five more picnic areas along the Stream Trail before the pavement stops at Trail's End. The redwood twigs and needles carpeting the forest floor is called duff, and in places only western sword ferns manage to push their way through.

Beyond Trail's End, you follow the Stream Trail, now a dirt road, beside Redwood Creek, designated a Resource Protection Area along its whole length through the park. No dogs or people are allowed in the creek or on the creek banks; dogs must be on leash. You pass junctions with the Chown, Fern, and Mill trails, then cross the creek on a bridge near the Mill Site

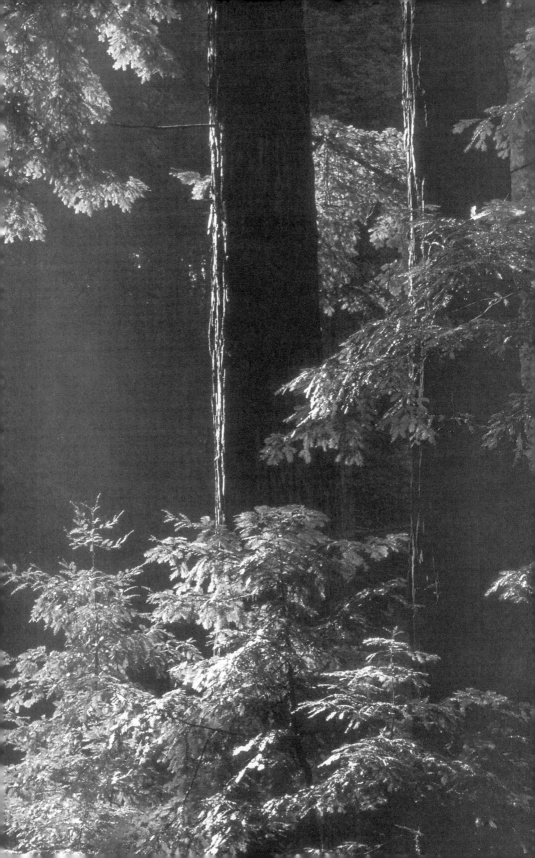

picnic area. Beyond the Mill Site, Prince Road departs right. In a large grove of redwoods you meet the Tres Sendas Trail, left. Stay on the Steam Trail as it bends right and begins a moderate climb, then levels where the Eucalyptus Trail branches right, at about 2 miles.

After crossing the creek, you reach Girls Camp, a picnic area with a stone hut, water, a restroom, and picnic tables shaded by black walnut trees. Ahead the grade steepens, and you climb via S-bends to Skyline Gate, a parking area beside Skyline Blvd. Here you turn left on the West Ridge Trail, a dirt road that is part of the East Bay Skyline/Bay Area Ridge Trail. Where the West Ridge Trail bends sharply right, about 0.6 mile from Skyline Gate, turn left on the single-track French Trail and descend through forest. The French Trail is an alternate and more scenic leg of the East Bay Skyline/Bay Area Ridge Trail.

The trail switchbacks down to a tributary of Redwood Creek and meets the Tres Sendas Trail, a wide dirt road, at about 4 miles. Continuing straight—for about the next 0.1 mile the French and Tres Sendas trails are combined—you climb moderately to the next junction and turn left to stay on the French Trail. The redwoods here, despite being second growth, grow tall, some reaching neck-craning heights.

Now the route narrows and climbs over rocky ground to a junction, right, with the Redwood Peak Trail. Continue straight, and descend moderately to a four-way junction with the Star Flower Trail, which you cross. The French Trail, now a dirt road, tops a ridge and soon reaches a junction with the Madrone Trail. Turn left and follow the French Trail, again a single track, as it makes a gradual, then steep descent.

Continue straight past junctions with the Mill and Fern trails, the latter at about 6 miles. Where the Chown Trail heads straight and climbs, you bear left and downhill. About 100 yards ahead, the continuation of the Chown Trail goes left, and

> **Away from it All**
> While not a true wilderness, given the area's history as a timber center in the mid-1800s, Redwood Regional Park, especially this section, has many wilderness attributes, including natural beauty, seclusion, and tranquillity. At the same time, it is one of the East Bay's most accessible and enjoyable parks.

here you stay right and enjoy a rolling stroll through forest. In a grove of madrone, the French Trail ends at a junction with the Orchard Trail, a wide dirt path.

Turn left and descend on a moderate grade to the Bridle Trail, a dirt road. Turn left on the Bridle Trail and go about 0.2 mile to close the loop at a junction with the Stream Trail. From here, turn right and retrace your route to the parking area.

Coast redwoods were decimated by logging, but second-growth forests remain.

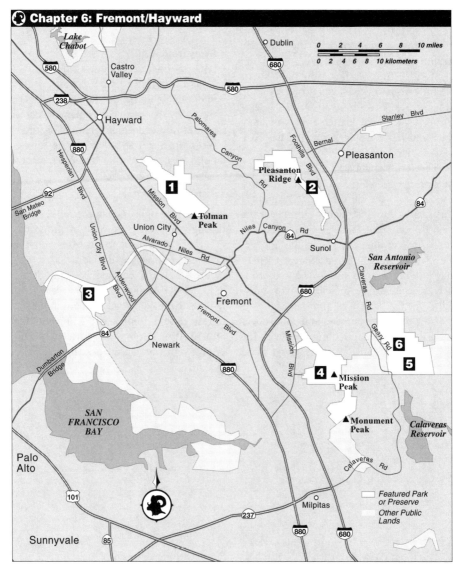

Chapter 6

# *Fremont/Hayward*

**Chapter 6: Fremont/Hayward**

Lake Chabot

580

O Dublin

680

0   2   4   6   8   10 miles

0   2   4   6   8   10 kilometers

Castro Valley

238

Stanley   Blvd

O Hayward

Palomares

Bernal

Foothills   Blvd

O Pleasanton

880

Canyon

Pleasanton Ridge ▲

**2**

Hesperian

92

San Mateo Bridge

Mission   Blvd

Blvd

84

**1**

▲ Tolman Peak

Union City   Blvd

Union City

Niles   Canyon   Rd

84

San Antonio Reservoir

Alvarado

Niles   Rd

Ardenwood   Blvd

**3**

O Sunol

Claveras   Rd

680

Fremont   Blvd

O Fremont

Geary   Rd

**6**

84

Mission   Blvd

**5**

Dumbarton Bridge

O Newark

880

**4** ▲ Mission Peak

SAN FRANCISCO BAY

▲ Monument Peak

Calaveras Reservoir

Palo Alto

Calaveras   Rd

101

Featured Park or Preserve

Other Public Lands

Sunnyvale

85

237

O Milpitas

880

680

# TRIP 1 Dry Creek Pioneer Regional Park

| | |
|---|---|
| **Distance** | 9.6 miles, Semi-loop |
| **Hiking Time** | 4 to 6 hours |
| **Elevation Gain/Loss** | ±1900 feet |
| **Difficulty** | Difficult |
| **Trail Use** | Mountain biking allowed[1], Leashed dogs |
| **Best Times** | All year |
| **Agency** | EBRPD |
| **Recommended Map** | *Garin & Dry Creek Pioneer Regional Parks* (EBRPD) |
| **Notes** | [1]Bicycles are not allowed on the South Fork or Dry Creek trails, and must instead stay on the High Ridge Loop and Tolman Peak trails to complete the trip |

**HIGHLIGHTS**  This route, combining the High Ridge Loop, Tolman Peak, South Fork, Meyers Ranch, and Dry Creek trails, explores a regional park gem — a 1563-acre oasis in the middle of one of the East Bay's most heavily industrial and residential areas. Scenery, views, and variety of habitat combine to make hiking to Tolman Peak more than just a challenging workout.

**DIRECTIONS**  From I-580 eastbound in Castro Valley, take the Hayward/Route 238 exit and follow signs for Hayward. From the first traffic light, continue straight, now on Foothill Blvd., for 1.7 miles to Mission Blvd, staying in the left lanes as you approach Mission Blvd. Bear left onto Mission Blvd. and go 3.5 miles to Garin Ave. Turn left and go 0.9 mile uphill to the entrance kiosk. At the kiosk bear right and proceed to parking areas; park in lowest one if space is available.

From I-580 westbound in Castro Valley, take the Strobridge exit and go 0.2 mile to the first stop sign. Turn right, go 0.1 mile to Castro Valley Blvd., and turn left. Follow Castro Valley Blvd. 0.5 mile to Foothill Blvd., turn left, and follow the directions above.

There are fees for parking and dogs when the entrance kiosk is attended.

**FACILITIES/TRAILHEAD**  A visitor center in a restored barn has displays of antique farm equipment and information about Hayward's ranching and farming history. There are picnic tables, restrooms, phone, and water nearby. The trailhead is on the northeast corner of the lower parking area.

Go east and cross a creek on a bridge, then continue straight on a path into a picnic area. When you come to a gravel road, cross it and begin climbing the High Ridge Loop Trail, a dirt road. Soon you pass a trail, left, to the Newt Pond Wildlife Area. Now the route levels, turns southeast, and meets the Meyers Ranch Trail, right.

Continuing straight, you climb to a notch between two low hills and then reach a junction with the Gossip Rock Trail, left, at about 2 miles. Leaving the junction, the road descends through open grassland dotted with rocks and boulders. Bear right at the next junction, unsigned, and go steeply downhill to a wooded area, where California bay, coast live oak, California buckeye, and blue elderberry thrive.

Spring wildflowers in the park include California poppies, red maids, Ithuriel's spears, and Mariposa lilies.

> **Roots of the Ranch**
> In 1978, EBRPD received a gift of the 1200-acre Dry Creek Pioneer Ranch from the three Meyers sisters, granddaughters of settlers who came here in 1884.

Fremont/Hayward

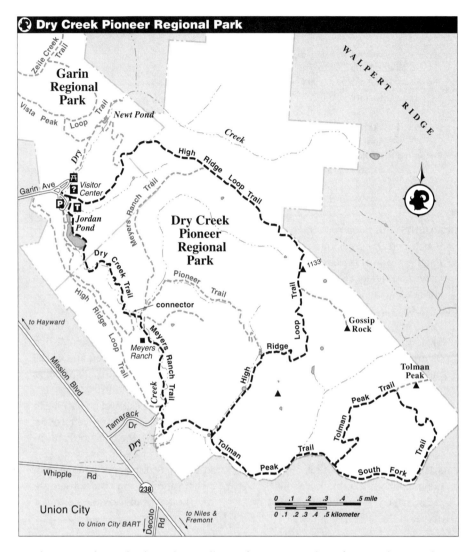

## Dry Creek Pioneer Regional Park

The route descends through a valley, passes the Pioneer Trail, right, and arrives at a T-junction. Here you turn left on the Tolman Peak Trail. (To shorten this route by omitting the hike to Tolman Peak, turn right and follow the directions below to the parking area.)

You pass a stock pond and walk through Black Creek Valley, a lowland area of sycamore, eucalyptus, willow, and bigleaf maple. Past a cattle pen, left, there is a shady place to sit and rest. Now you follow a creek, which may flood the trail and in places

force you to hop from rock to rock. At about 4.4 miles, the Tolman Peak Trail turns left, but you continue straight, now on the South Fork Trail. Just before reaching the regional park boundary, the South Fork Trail, now a single track, turns left and climbs across a steep hillside.

Ahead the trail may be completely overgrown and reduced to a line of matted grass. Where the grades eases, you leave the single-track trail and regain a dirt road, heading northwest. As you begin to descend, you pass a trail post with a sign for

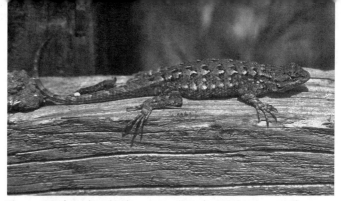
The western fence lizard is the most commonly seen Bay Area reptile.

the Tolman Peak Trail, a short path to a wooded summit. You wind downhill on a moderate and then steep grade to the South Fork Trail. Here, about 6.5 miles, you turn right and retrace your route through Black Creek Valley.

When you return to the junction with the High Ridge Loop Trail, continue straight. Soon an unsigned road heads left, but you turn sharply right and descend to a fork. Angle right to a junction, then leave High Ridge Loop Trail by going straight on the Meyers Ranch Trail, at about 7.8 miles. Dry Creek, which flows into San Francisco Bay via Alameda County's flood-control channel, is on your right, and you are walking upstream.

True to its name, the trail passes the site of Meyers Ranch, where antique farm equipment lies beside the trail. Planted poplars and fruit trees show this was once a homestead.

After leaving the ranch site, turn left on a connector to the Dry Creek Trail and cross Dry Creek on a narrow bridge. About 150 feet ahead, you go through a gate and then come to a T-junction with the Dry Creek Trail, a single track. Turn right, toward Jordan Pond and the visitor center. Along this part of the Dry Creek Trail, you will see numbered markers for the park's self-guiding nature trail, a great excursion for children and parents. (A booklet keyed to the numbers can be bought or borrowed at the visitor center.)

Your route now winds through forest and makes three bridged crossings of the creek. At a T-junction beside Jordan Pond, you turn right and curve around the pond's east side. As you near the north end of the pond, you come to a fork. Bear right and close the loop at the foot of the High Ridge Loop Trail. Turn left and retrace your route to the parking area.

## TRIP 2 Pleasanton Ridge Regional Park

| | |
|---|---|
| **Distance** | 12.3 miles, Semi-loop |
| **Hiking Time** | 6 to 8 hours |
| **Elevation Gain/Loss** | ±3000 feet |
| **Difficulty** | Very Difficult |
| **Trail Use** | Mountain biking allowed, Leashed dogs |
| **Best Times** | Fall through spring |
| **Agency** | EBRPD |
| **Recommended Map** | *Pleasanton Ridge Regional Park* (EBRPD) |

**HIGHLIGHTS** The hike along Pleasanton Ridge, combining the Oak Tree, Ridgeline, Bay Leaf, Sinbad Creek, Thermalito, and Olive Grove trails, while the longest and perhaps most challenging in this book, is also one of the most rewarding. The views are outstanding, extending from Pleasanton, San Ramon, and Mt. Diablo to Sunol Valley, the Sunol/Ohlone Wilderness, and Mission Peak. The terrain is varied — dense woodland, open grassland, and even a restored olive orchard — and bird and plant life flourish in this relatively undeveloped park.

**DIRECTIONS**  From I-680 in Pleasanton, take the Sunol Blvd./Castlewood Dr. exit and go southwest on Castlewood Dr., staying straight where Pleasanton – Sunol Road bends left. After 0.3 mile, you reach Foothill Road. Turn left and go south 1.6 miles to the Oak Tree staging area, right.

**FACILITIES/TRAILHEAD**  There are picnic tables, water, and a toilet beside the parking area; there are several water fountains along the route. The trailhead is on the west side of the first parking area, just beyond the water fountain and information board.

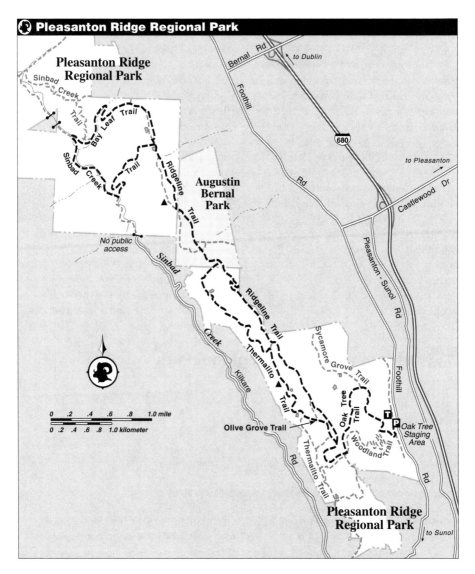

Go west on a dirt road, through a cattle gate, and then left on the Oak Tree Trail, also a dirt road. The climb is moderate at first, as the route passes through alternating areas of open grassland and oak woodland —mostly valley oaks and coast live oaks.

After several hundred yards, you pass the Woodland Trail, a single track closed to bicycles. (This trail is an alternate way to reach the ridgecrest, and although it switchbacks steeply at first, most of the climbing is in the shade.) The route continues its ascent, passing the Sycamore Grove Trail, right. The road makes a 180-degree bend and passes a junction with a grass-covered road, left, which is closed to bicycles.

At about 1.3 miles, you emerge from a wooded area at a four-way junction near a barbed-wire fence, with the Woodland Trail joining from the left. Here you turn right on the Oak Tree Trail and go through an opening in the fence. About 30 feet beyond the fence is a trail post, and a choice of three dirt paths. Take the middle one, the Ridgeline Trail. Great views of Mission Peak and the Sunol/Ohlone Wilderness reward you for climbing so far.

The Ridgeline Trail makes a 180-degree bend to gain the ridgetop, passing an unsigned path, right. Bending left, the route reaches a fork marked by a trail post, where you stay right. About 125 feet past the fork,

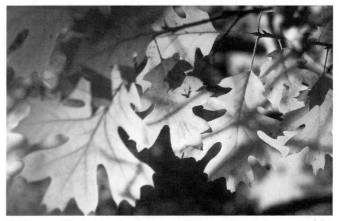

The leaves of black oak, a deciduous species, turn yellow and orange in fall.

you pass a junction, right, with a rough dirt road that runs along a barbed-wire fence. The Ridgeline Trail, also a dirt road, parallels this fence, climbing past an olive grove on a moderate grade. Just beyond the grove is a drinking faucet, a watering trough for animals, and another fork, where you continue straight.

Now you pass the Olive Grove Trail, which merges sharply from the left. The road crests a hill, then drops to a four-way junction, where a short connector to the Thermalito Trail goes left, and an unsigned path climbs right to a cattle gate. Another connector to the Thermalito Trail is just ahead. The Thermalito Trail takes its name from the Thermal Fruit Company, which was active nearby from 1904 until the 1930s.

---

**That Knock-Knock Sound**

Where there are oaks in the East Bay you are likely to find the acorn woodpecker, a dark bird, slightly smaller than a robin, with a black-and-white face, red crown, white rump, and white wing patches. As its name implies, this woodpecker gathers acorns in the winter—it dines on insects in the summer—and often stores them in holes it drills in oak trees.

---

**Olive Groves**

The olive groves atop Pleasanton Ridge were planted here between about 1890 and the 1920s. No record exists of who planted the trees, which are currently being restored by the Regional Parks District and a private concessionaire.

---

You roller-coaster over several more hills, then descend to a forest of California bay, coast live oak, black oak, and bigleaf maple. Beyond where a trail goes right to a gate, you enter the City of Pleasanton's Augustin

Bernal Park. In a level clearing at about 3.4 miles, you meet the Thermalito Trail, a dirt road, left. There is drinking water and a watering trough for animals a short distance down the Thermalito Trail. (To shorten the route, turn left on the Thermalito Trail and follow the route description below.)

Leaving the clearing, you begin a moderate ascent, soon meeting the Valley View Trail, right, and the Equestrian Trail (no bicycles), left. You go past the other end of the Equestrian Trail, left, and reenter the regional park at a gate.

At a junction, you bear right through an oak savanna, with a fence marking the park boundary on your right. After merging with the road that went straight at the previous junction, you climb into the open and pass a pond, left, which may be full of tadpoles, frogs, or both.

Here the Sinbad Creek Trail, which you will use later, goes left. Your route soon swings west and reaches a junction. You go straight, now on the Bay Leaf Trail, and then wind downhill into a shady, creek-filled ravine. At a junction, you join the Sinbad Creek Trail by going straight. Follow the road downhill to Sinbad Creek, at the bottom of Kilkare Canyon. Step across the creek on rocks and turn left at a T-junction with a dirt road, around 5.8 miles.

After less than a mile of pleasant streamside walking, you reach another T-junction, where you turn left, recross the creek, and begin climbing steeply on the Sinbad Creek Trail, a dirt road. Emerging from dense forest into oak savanna, you cross a notch in the ridgeline at meet the Ridgeline Trail at a T-junction. Turn right and retrace your route to the junction of the Ridgeline and Thermalito trails. Here, at about 8.5 miles, you turn right on the Thermalito Trail, a dirt road, and begin a moderate climb.

A rolling course takes you past a connector, left, to the Ridgeline Trail and then brings you to a T-junction, where you angle right. Passing several stock ponds, you finally leave the Thermalito Trail where it turns right by going straight on a connector to the Olive Grove Trail. After 100 yards or so, you come to a junction with the Olive Grove Trail, about 10.6 miles. Continue straight to the next junction, where the Olive Grove Trail swings right. Here you go straight on a connector to the Ridgeline Trail. When you reach the Ridgeline Trail, bear right and retrace your route to the parking area.

## TRIP3 Coyote Hills Regional Park

| | |
|---|---|
| **Distance** | 1.5 miles, Loop |
| **Hiking Time** | 1 hour or less |
| **Elevation Gain/Loss** | ±350 feet |
| **Difficulty** | Moderate |
| **Trail Use** | Mountain biking allowed[1], Leashed dogs |
| **Best Times** | All year |
| **Agency** | EBRPD |
| **Recommended Map** | *Coyote Hills Regional Park* (EBRPD) |
| **Notes** | [1]Bicycles are not allowed on the Quail Trail, and must instead use the Bayview and Tuibun trails to complete the trip) |

**HIGHLIGHTS** Combining parts of the Bayview, Nike, Red Hill, Soaproot, and Quail trails, this short loop over the summits of Red and Glider hills offers more scenery per calorie expended than any other hike in the East Bay. Besides open summits, which provide 360-degree views that extend from San Francisco to the Santa Cruz Mountains, this park contains an extensive brackish marsh, habitat for waterfowl and shorebirds.

**DIRECTIONS** From Highway 84 at the east end of the Dumbarton Bridge in Fremont, take the Thornton Ave./Paseo Padre Pkwy. exit, and go north 1.1 miles on Paseo Padre Pkwy. to Patterson Ranch Road. Turn left, and go 0.5 mile to the entrance kiosk. Another 1.0 mile brings you to the parking area for the visitor center. There are fees for parking and dogs.

**FACILITIES/TRAILHEAD** A visitor center, picnic tables, water, and a toilet are near the parking area. The trailhead is on the west end of parking area, at its entrance.

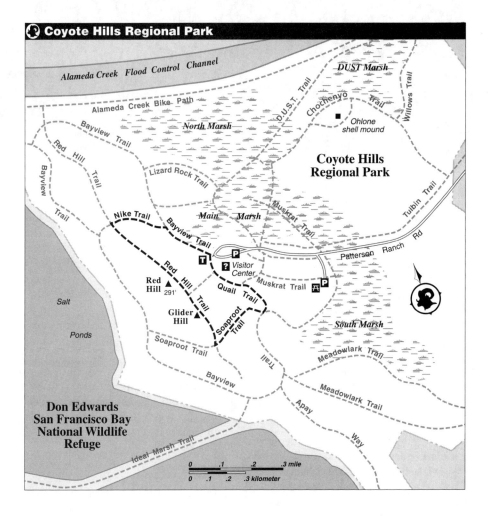

From the west end of the parking area, where the entrance road makes a 180-degree bend, head northwest on the paved Bayview Trail, passing the Quail Trail, a dirt road, left. The Bayview Trail is gated just beyond the parking area; after passing the gate you have the Main Marsh on your right

and beautiful grassy hills rising up on your left. Bear left on the Nike Trail and climb moderately.

Soon you reach a flat spot—a saddle between Red Hill and an unnamed hill to the north—and a four-way junction. Turning left here onto the Red Hill Trail, a

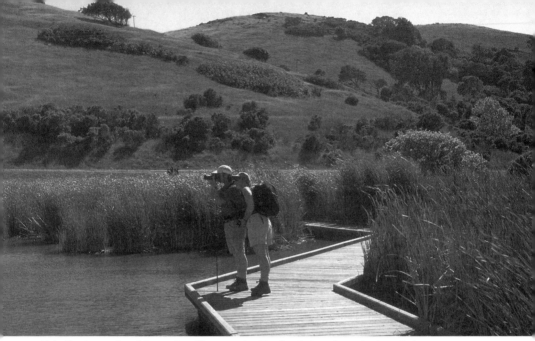

Main Marsh, near the visitor center, offers opportunities for photgraphy and nature study.

dirt road, you continue your ascent over open terrain. A short, steep pitch leads to the rock-studded summit. In terms of scenery per calorie, Red Hill tops the list, being a relatively easy summit to attain, and commanding a superb vantage point. The views from Red Hill take in San Francisco, Mt. Tamalpais, Oakland, Mt. Diablo, Mt. Hamilton, and the Santa Cruz Mountains.

After crossing the level summit, you descend steeply to a saddle between Red Hill and Glider Hill, the next rise south. Just as the route begins to climb once more, you arrive at a four-way junction.

Continuing your climb over moderate and then steep ground, you soon reach the top of Glider Hill, which even has a convenient picnic table. Now a short, steep descent brings you to another saddle and a four-way junction.

Here the Red Hill Trail, which continues straight, is crossed by the Soaproot Trail, a dirt road. Turn left and begin curving moderately downhill to a junction with the Bayview and Quail trails. Turn left onto the hiking-only Quail Trail, a wide dirt road. Just after the road crosses a rise, a single-track trail, right, offers you an easy side trip to Castle Rock, a jumble of pinnacles made from the same red chert as Red Hill.

Following the Quail Trail downhill, you may see and hear its namesake, the California quail. You pass the Hoot Hollow Trail, left, and the Hoot Hollow picnic area.

After the picnic area, you pass an unsigned path heading left up some wooden steps, and a paved path, right, that leads to the visitor center. About 200 feet downhill from these paths, you reach a gate and the entrance to the parking area.

# TRIP 4 Mission Peak Regional Preserve

| | |
|---|---|
| **Distance** | 6.3 miles, Out-and-back |
| **Hiking Time** | 3 to 5 hours |
| **Elevation Gain/Loss** | ±2250 feet |
| **Difficulty** | Difficult |
| **Trail Use** | Mountain biking allowed[1], Leashed dogs |
| **Best Times** | Fall through spring |
| **Agency** | EBRPD |
| **Recommended Map** | *Mission Peak Regional Preserve* (EBRPD) |
| **Notes** | [1]Bicycles are not allowed on the last 0.5 mile of the Peak Trail |

**HIGHLIGHTS** A steady climb of more than 2000 feet in just over 3 miles, most of it on the Hidden Valley Trail, a well-graded dirt road, brings you to the top of Mission Peak. This is one of the East Bay's most dramatic summits, offering views of the entire Bay Area. Not a hike for hot weather, try to do this route just after a winter or spring storm, when the air is clear and the hills green.

**DIRECTIONS** From I-880 in Fremont, take the Mission Blvd./Warren Ave. exit and go northeast on Mission Blvd. 1.8 miles to Stanford Ave. Turn right and go 0.6 mile to a parking area at the end of Stanford Ave.

From I-680 in Fremont, take the Mission Blvd./Warm Springs District exit and follow signs for Mission Blvd. eastbound. Once on Mission Blvd., follow it for 0.6 mile to Stanford Ave. Turn right and go 0.6 mile to a parking area at the end of Stanford Ave.

**FACILITIES/TRAILHEAD** There are water and a toilet near the trailhead, which is on the east side of the parking area.

Take the Hidden Valley Trail, a dirt road, through a gate to a junction with the Peak Meadow Trail. Stay left and follow the road across Agua Caliente Creek to the next junction, where you again stay left. The climb soon becomes moderate. You are joined on the right by a road from the previous junction. At the base of a rocky hill, a road departs to the right, but you stay left.

Your route wanders through a wooded area near a stream, then climbs past the Peak Meadow Trail, right, at about 1.6 miles. Now the road begins a series of switchbacks that will carry you almost to the summit. The terrain becomes more rugged, and ahead you can see the park residence, a collection of several buildings used by EBRPD rangers. Looming above them to the southeast is Mt. Allison, bristling with communication towers.

Just below a band of cliffs you come to a T-junction. Here the A. A. Moore Grove

## Ohlone Trail

The Ohlone Wilderness Regional Trail, a 28-mile trek through some of the East Bay's most scenic and remote territory, begins at the Stanford Ave. parking area and follows the Hidden Valley Trail up the west side of Mission Peak. The emblem for the Ohlone Wilderness Regional Trail, which you may see on trail posts here, is a white oak leaf in a red disk. Numbers on some of the trail posts refer to numbered junctions on EBRPD's *Ohlone Wilderness Regional Trail* map.

Trail goes right, but you turn left and climb steeply toward the skyline ridge. You come to a barbed-wire fence with a gate, beyond which is a four-way junction and the end of the Hidden Valley Trail. Turn right and follow the Peak Trail, a dirt road that is part of the Bay Area Ridge Trail.

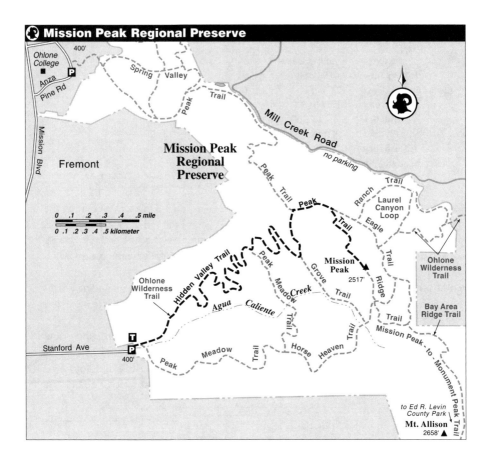

Just as your route veers left away from the fence, you pass a wide path continuing straight. Ahead, the Peak Trail is joined by a dirt road coming sharply from the right. You continue to climb east, toward a flat spot on the skyline ridge. When you crest the ridge, a line of snow-capped Sierra peaks may be visible in the distance, rising behind Livermore and the Altamont Pass. Bear right at a fork to stay on the Peak Trail, soon reaching the end of the road.

From here, several dirt paths head southeast, steeply uphill toward the summit. The final climb is on dirt and rock, past a clever observation device that allows you to identify more than two dozen Bay Area landmarks in a 360-degree circle around Mission Peak. A few more steps bring you at last to the top of Mission Peak. When you have finished enjoy-

ing this exhilarating and hard-won summit, retrace your route to the parking area.

---

**Peak Facts**

Mission Peak (2517') sits atop a long ridge that trends northwest–southeast, towering over the flatlands of Fremont to the west and Sunol Valley to the east. No other earthbound vantage point offers such extensive views this close to San Francisco Bay.

Alfred A. Moore, an early California settler and attorney for the railroad, once owned several thousand acres on Mission Peak, including a ranch with exotic animals, which he used as a weekend retreat for family and friends.

# TRIP 5 Sunol Wilderness: Little Yosemite

| | |
|---|---|
| **Distance** | 3 miles, Loop |
| **Hiking Time** | 2 to 3 hours |
| **Elevation Gain/Loss** | ±600 feet |
| **Difficulty** | Moderate |
| **Trail Use** | Leashed dogs |
| **Best Times** | Fall through spring |
| **Agency** | EBRPD |
| **Recommended Map** | *Sunol Regional Wilderness* (EBRPD) |

**HIGHLIGHTS**  This loop is a fine introduction to Sunol Wilderness, one of EBRPD's gems and, at nearly 7000 acres, one of its largest holdings. A scenic trek along the Canyon View Trail, through oak savanna and grassland, brings you to Little Yosemite, a rocky gorge carved by Alameda Creek. The return part of the loop, Camp Ohlone Road, takes you beside the tree-lined creek, especially lovely in fall.

**DIRECTIONS**  From I-680 southbound in Scotts Corner, take the Calaveras Road exit, and at a stop sign turn left onto Paloma Road. Go back under I-680, stay in the left lane, and at the next stop sign continue straight, now on Calaveras Road. Go 4.2 miles to Geary Road, turn left, and go 1.8 miles to the entrance kiosk. Go 0.1 mile past the kiosk and turn left into a parking area in front of the visitor center, a green barn. (If this parking area is full, there are two more about 100 yards ahead, on both sides of Geary Road.)

From I-680 northbound in Scotts Corner, take the Calaveras Road exit, bear right onto Calaveras Road, then follow directions above.

There are fees for parking and dogs when the entrance kiosk is attended.

**FACILITIES/TRAILHEAD**  There are a visitor center, picnic tables, toilets, phone, and water beside the parking area. The trailhead is in front of the visitor center.

Walk east along a path, paved for the first 150 feet or so, which passes behind two small buildings, the Interpretive Headquarters and the Wilderness Room. Continue east another 200 feet and turn left to cross Alameda Creek via a wood bridge. Now turn right on the Canyon View Trail, a wide dirt path lined with white alder, bigleaf maple, western sycamore, and willow. About 100 feet past the bridge, Hayfield Road climbs left but you go straight.

After crossing Indian Joe Creek, and just as the trail begins to climb, you pass a narrow path that parallels the creek, right. Continue straight as the trail rolls along to a junction with the Indian Joe Creek Trail, left. Stay on the Canyon View Trail, a single track, and climb on a moderate, then steep, grade. After passing through a cattle gate,

you come into the open atop a narrow ridge studded with blue and valley oaks. Groves of oaks here are like islands in a sea of grass, providing shelter and food for a wide variety of birds, including jays, woodpeckers, yellow-billed magpies, western meadowlarks, juncos, brown creepers, and kinglets.

At a four-way junction, cross the McCorkle Trail, a dirt road, and continue on

### Yosemite West?

Little Yosemite features in miniature some of the wonders of its Sierra Nevada namesake, including water rushing through a boulder-strewn gorge, sheer cliffs, forested hillsides, and towering rock formations. Stands of western sycamore add color in the fall.

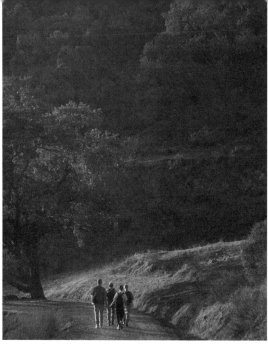

Camp Ohlone Road leads from the visitor center to Little Yosemite and beyond.

to a gully, possibly muddy, and crossing a small plank bridge, you traverse an open expanse of grass dotted with rock outcrops, which are tinged orange by lichen.

In a rocky area shaded by valley oaks, you come to a trail post and a junction with a faint trail, left. Continue straight through an open field to a four-way junction with Cerro Este Road. Turn right and follow the dirt road to Camp Ohlone Road and the area along Alameda Creek called Little Yosemite.

After exploring to your heart's content, head southwest on Camp Ohlone Road and follow a gently rolling course to a wood bridge that takes you across Alameda Creek. Beyond the creek, you follow a paved road through a large parking area and past the Leyden Flats picnic area, left, until you reach the visitor center and the main parking area.

the Canyon View Trail, climbing moderately across a grassy hillside. The route now skims the edge of a steep hillside that drops about 200 feet to Alameda Creek. After descending

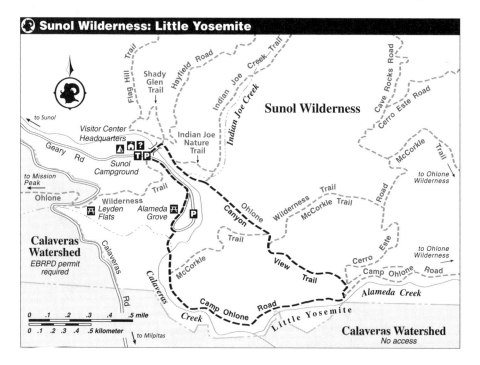

# TRIP 6 Sunol Wilderness: Vista Grande

|  |  |
|---|---|
| **Distance** | 6.1 miles, Loop |
| **Hiking Time** | 3 to 4 hours |
| **Elevation Gain/Loss** | ±1600 feet |
| **Difficulty** | Difficult |
| **Trail Use** | Leashed dogs |
| **Best Times** | Fall through spring |
| **Agency** | EBRPD |
| **Recommended Map** | *Sunol Regional Wilderness* (EBRPD) |

**HIGHLIGHTS** High vantage points and great views reward hikers who tackle this loop, which uses the Canyon View, Indian Joe Creek, Eagle View, and Flag Hill trails, along with parts of Eagle View, Flag Hill, and Vista Grande roads. Climbing from tree-lined Alameda Creek through oak woodland to the high ground of Vista Grande Road and then Flag Hill, you experience a wide variety of terrain and plant life. Best on a clear, windless day, the route crosses some very steep hillsides, where caution is advised.

**DIRECTIONS** From I-680 southbound in Scotts Corner, take the Calaveras Road exit, and at a stop sign turn left onto Paloma Road. Go back under I-680, stay in the left lane, and at the next stop sign continue straight, now on Calaveras Road. Go 4.2 miles to Geary Road, turn left, and go 1.8 miles to the entrance kiosk. Go 0.1 mile past the kiosk and turn left into a parking area in front of the visitor center, a green barn. (If this parking area is full, there are two more about 100 yards ahead, on both sides of Geary Road.)

From I-680 northbound in Scotts Corner, take the Calaveras Road exit, bear right onto Calaveras Road, then follow directions above.

There are fees for parking and dogs when the entrance kiosk is attended.

**FACILITIES/TRAILHEAD** There are a visitor center, picnic tables, toilets, phone, and water beside the parking area. The trailhead is in front of the visitor center.

Walk east along a path, paved for the first 150 feet or so, which passes behind two small buildings, the Interpretive Headquarters and the Wilderness Room. Continue east another 200 feet and turn left to cross Alameda Creek via a wood bridge. Now turn right on the Canyon View Trail, a wide dirt path. About 100 feet past the bridge, Hayfield Road climbs left but you go straight.

After crossing Indian Joe Creek, the trail rolls along to a junction. Here you bear left on the Indian Joe Creek Trail, descending a single track. The route follows the creek northeast, past a junction where the self-guiding Indian Joe Nature Trail goes left across the creek. Continuing straight, you go through a cattle gate, cross the creek's shallow water on rocks, then walk upstream in a narrow, shrub-filled canyon. In fall, sycamore and bigleaf maple add gold and orange to this wonderful area.

You wander back and forth across the creek as the canyon steepens. Finally topping out on a ridge, you pass a connector to Hayfield Road, left, and an unofficial trail, right. Your route continues straight to Indian Joe Cave Rocks, a fantastic jumble of cliffs and boulders towering next to Indian Joe Creek. From here, switchbacks take you to the top of another ridge, with grand views.

Soon the Indian Joe Creek Trail ends, and you turn right on Cave Rocks Road, a dirt road, and climb moderately to a junction. Here you turn left on Eagle View Road and continue your moderate, sometimes steep climb on a rutted dirt road. Around 2

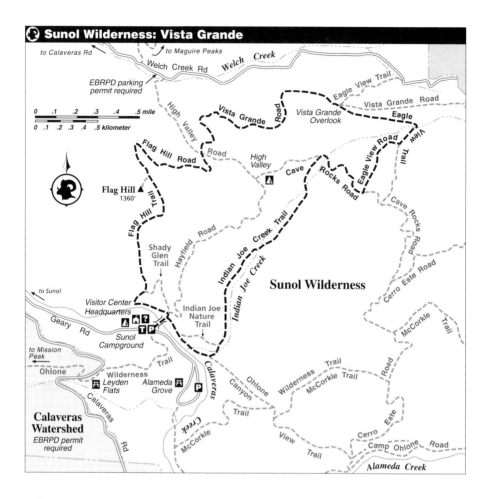

### Sunol Wilderness: Vista Grande

to Calaveras Rd · to Maguire Peaks · Welch Creek Rd · Welch Creek

EBRPD parking permit required

0 .1 .2 .3 .4 .5 mile
0 .1 .2 .3 .4 .5 kilometer

High Valley · Vista Grande Road · Eagle View Trail · Vista Grande Road · Vista Grande Overlook · Eagle View Road · Eagle · Eagle View Trail

Flag Hill Road · Road · High Valley · Cave · Rocks Road · Cave Rocks Road

Flag Hill ▲ 1360'

Flag Hill Trail

Shady Glen Trail · Hayfield Road · Indian Joe Creek Trail · Indian Joe Creek · **Sunol Wilderness** · Cerro Este Road

to Sunol · Visitor Center Headquarters · Indian Joe Nature Trail · McCorkle Trail

Geary Rd · Sunol Campground

to Mission Peak · Ohlone · Trail · Wilderness · Leyden Flats · Alameda Grove · Calaveras Creek · Ohlone · Canyon · Wilderness · Trail · McCorkle Trail · Road

**Calaveras Watershed** · EBRPD permit required · Calaveras Rd · McCorkle · View · Trail · Cerro Este · Camp Ohlone · Road

*Alameda Creek*

miles, Eagle View Road ends at a T-junction with the Eagle View Trail. Turn left and descend a single-track trail into a wooded ravine holding the upper reaches of Indian Joe Creek.

After crossing the creek on rocks, the trail turns sharply left and begins a moderate climb out of the ravine, then cuts across a very steep, shrubby hillside. Use caution here, and keep your eye on the trail. Finally you reach Vista Grande Overlook, a level area and important junction, giving you a place to relax and take in the stunning 360-degree views.

From here, you bear left on Vista Grande Road and descend west on a moderate grade. The route follows a curvy, rolling

**Leaf Lore**

Gazing at the leaf litter on the trail, you may notice a peculiar fact, namely that a leaf's size is unrelated to the size of the tree that produces it. For example, valley oak and western sycamore are both large trees, ranging from 40 to 80 or 100 feet tall. Yet the valley oak's leaf, 2 to 4 inches in size, is dwarfed by the sycamore's 6- to 9-inch leaf.

course before descending steeply to an old homestead in High Valley. This bucolic area, with its large barn, windmill, water tower, and grazing cows, is used by EBRPD as an outdoor campsite. Some planted trees

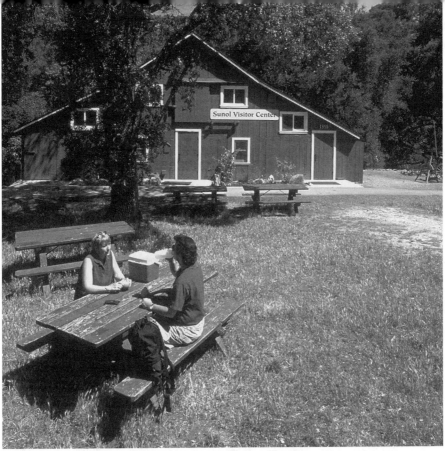

Trip to Vista Grande begins at the Sunol Visitor Center, a beautifully restored barn.

here include almond, eucalyptus, fig, and peppertree.

When you reach a four-way junction with High Valley Road, cross it and then bear left on Flag Hill Road, a dirt road heading southeast and uphill through a cattle gate. Now on atop a ridge, you travel

**Two Views**

- Visible from Vista Grande Overlook are Mt. Diablo (north), Maguire Peaks (northwest), and Apperson Ridge (northeast), site of an environmental battle in the late 1960s and early 1970s over a proposed rock quarry.
- The sweeping view from Flag Hill takes in Calaveras Reservoir, Alameda Creek canyon, Camp Ohlone Road, Mission Peak Regional Preserve, and Maguire Peaks.

south to a junction and a stone marker, at about 4.5 miles. To visit Flag Hill, named for an American flag displayed here by a picnicking family on July 4th, 1903, continue straight. From where the road ends in a few hundred feet at a turnaround, follow a dirt path to the edge of a steep, rocky promontory—use caution!

From the summit of Flag Hill, return to the stone marker and begin a moderate descent southeast on the Flag Hill Trail, a single track. The trail crosses steep, open hillsides and descends through mixed woodland. You pass through a cattle gate and fence guarding a grove of trees near Alameda Creek. The trail winds downhill to a barbed-wire fence with a turnstile. When you reach a T-junction near the creek, turn left on a wide dirt path and then close the loop at the bridge. Now cross bridge, turn right, and retrace your route to the parking area.

# Chapter 7
# San Jose/Santa Clara

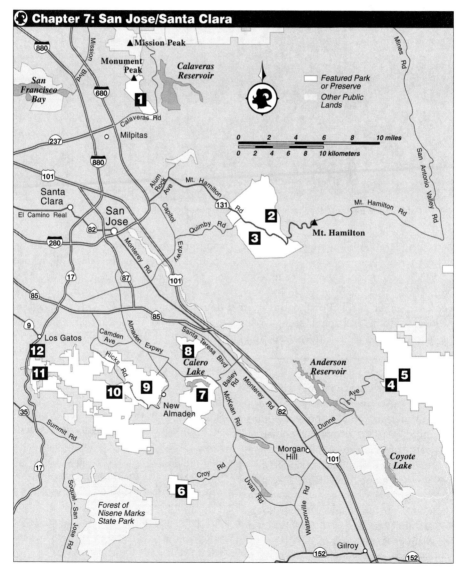

Mines Rd

▲Mission Peak

Monument
Peak ▲

Calaveras
Reservoir

880

Mission Blvd

San
Francisco
Bay

680

Calaveras Rd

Featured Park
or Preserve

Other Public
Lands

**1**

237

Milpitas

0   2   4   6   8   10 miles

0   2   4   6   8   10 kilometers

880

San Antonio Valley Rd

101

Santa
Clara

Alum Rock Ave

Mt. Hamilton

El Camino Real

Capitol Expwy

131

Rd

**2**

Mt. Hamilton Rd

San
Jose

82

Quimby Rd

**3**

▲ Mt. Hamilton

280

Monterey Rd

17

87

101

85

85

9

Los Gatos

Camden Ave

Almaden Expwy

Santa Teresa Blvd

**8**

Anderson
Reservoir

**12**

Hicks Rd

Calero
Lake

Bailey Rd

Ave

**4** **5**

**11**

**10** **9**

**7**

Monterey Rd

McKean Rd

35

New
Almaden

82

Dunne

Coyote
Lake

Summit Rd

Morgan
Hill

101

17

Croy Rd

Uvas Rd

**6**

Watsonville Rd

Soquel - San Jose Rd

Forest of
Nisene Marks
State Park

Gilroy

152

152

# TRIP 1 Ed R. Levin County Park

| | |
|---|---|
| **Distance** | 7.8 miles, Semi-loop |
| **Hiking Time** | 4 to 6 hours |
| **Elevation Gain/Loss** | ±2800 feet |
| **Difficulty** | Difficult |
| **Best Times** | Fall through spring |
| **Agency** | SCCP&R |
| **Recommended Map** | *Ed R. Levin County Park* (SCCP&R) |

**HIGHLIGHTS** Explore the high ground on the border of Alameda and Santa Clara counties via this aerobic route, which uses the Tularcitos, Agua Caliente, and Monument Peak trails, and you will be rewarded with great views and the chance to spot aerial hunters such as hawks, falcons, and even golden eagles. Open grasslands dominate here, but you also cross wooded canyons holding Calera and Scott creeks.

**DIRECTIONS** From I-680 in Milpitas, take the Calaveras Blvd./Milpitas exit and go east 1.9 miles to Downing Road. Turn left and after 0.5 mile come to an entrance kiosk and self-registration station. Go another 0.9 mile to a paved parking area just north of Sandy Wool Lake.

**FACILITIES/TRAILHEAD** There are picnic tables, restrooms, and water beside the parking area. There is a phone beside a locked gate about 0.3 mile back on Downing Road. The trailhead is at the end of Downing Road, about 100 yards northeast of the parking area.

You climb east on the Tularcitos Trail, a dirt road closed to bicycles and dogs. At the second of two closely spaced junctions, you turn left on the Agua Caliente Trail, also a dirt road. There are a number of cattle gates on this route: make sure you close each one after passing through it. The terrain here is open, giving you views of San Francisco Bay's south end—extensively engineered with levees and ponds for salt production—and of the Santa Cruz Mountains.

The road follows a rolling course, sometimes pitching steeply upward. After passing a hang-gliding area, left, you come to a four-way junction. Continue straight and then begin a series of switchbacks, which climb on a grade that alternates between moderate and steep. Resuming its rolling course, the trail wanders through groves of coast live oak and fragrant California bay. Now you descend to a shady, wooded ravine that holds a tributary of Calera Creek, fenced to keep out cattle.

As you work your way uphill from this drainage, you are joined on the right by two unsigned dirt roads, not shown on the park map. California buckeyes, which produce spikes of white flowers in late spring, stand beside the trail. At about 1.5 miles, leave the Agua Caliente Trail and veer right on the Monument Peak Trail. Just ahead is

**Historical Snapshot**

The name of this park honors a Santa Clara County supervisor, who in the 1960s, before his death in 1966, was instrumental in getting the county to purchase nearly 500 acres of state-owned land in Laguna Valley. In the early 1800s, the present-day park's 1500 acres were divided among three Mexican ranchos. The land has retained its rural character and today forms a buffer of open space between busy Milpitas and the rugged terrain surrounding Calaveras Reservoir.

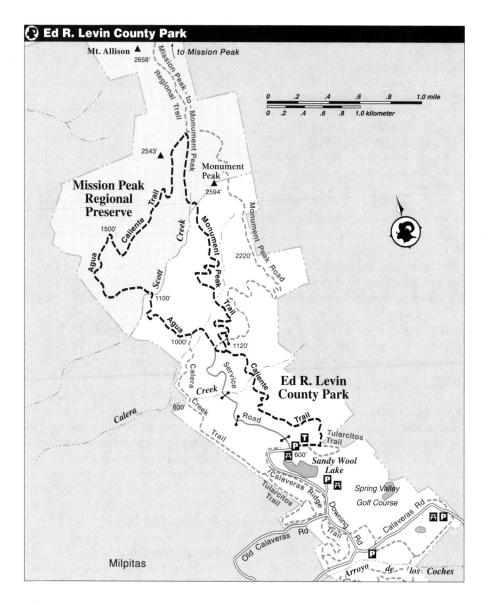

## Ed R. Levin County Park

Mt. Allison ▲
2658'

to Mission Peak

Mission Peak - to - Monument Peak
Regional Trail

0   .2      .4      .6      .8      1.0 mile

0   .2   .4   .6   .8   1.0 kilometer

2543' ▲

Monument
Peak ▲
2594'

Mission Peak
Regional
Preserve

Caliente
Trail

1500'

Scott Creek

Monument Peak Road

2220'

Monument Peak Trail

Agua

1100'

Agua

1000'

1120'

Caliente

Ed R. Levin
County Park

Calera Creek

Service

Calera Creek
600'

Road

Trail

Calera

Trail

Tularcitos
Trail

T
P

A  600'

Sandy Wool
Lake

P   A

Spring Valley
Golf Course

Calaveras Ridge

Tularcitos
Trail

Downing

A  P

Calaveras Rd

Old Calaveras Rd

Trail

Rd

P

Milpitas

Arroyo  de  los  Coches

a four-way junction with Monument Peak Road. Here you continue straight, passing a watering trough for horses and then a dirt road heading downhill, both left.

Climbing steeply on an eroded and rocky track, you meet a dirt road joining sharply from the right. Soon the trail comes to Calera Creek, which you may need to cross on rocks. North of the creek, the trail finds level ground, and you begin to see the

communication towers atop Monument Peak, which is uphill and right. The valley holding Scott Creek, which forms part of the boundary between Santa Clara and Alameda counties, is to your left.

Soon the trail swings right and begins a steep, winding ascent. As you gain elevation, look for Mt. Hamilton, topped with white observatory domes, to the southeast. Slightly southwest of Monument Peak's summit, you

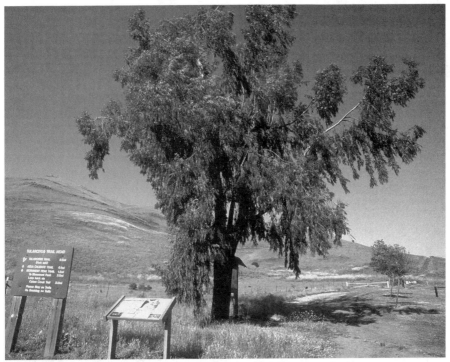

This trailhead is the start point for trips to the high ground near Monument Peak.

leave Santa Clara County and enter the East Bay Regional Park District's Mission Peak Regional Preserve. A nearly level walk takes you past the headwaters of Scott Creek. With a communication tower looming overhead, you join a dirt-and-gravel road and head straight for a saddle and a four-way junction.

Here you turn left on the Agua Caliente Trail, a multi-use dirt road that is part of the Bay Area Ridge Trail. Climbing gently, you soon reach today's high point, only about 50 feet lower than the summit of Monument Peak (2594'). From this vantage point, around 4 miles, on a clear day many familiar Bay Area landmarks are visible. Skirting a communication facility, the road veers left and descends on a grade that shifts between moderate and steep.

Soon the grade eases, and you make a winding descent into the wooded canyon holding Scott Creek. After crossing the creek and climbing steeply out of its drainage,

the road bends sharply left and descends on a moderate and then steep grade. At about 6 miles, the Calera Creek Trail turns right, but you continue straight to the next junction, closing the loop. From here, simply angle right and retrace your route to the parking area.

---

**Look! Up in the Sky!**

- You may see aerial acrobats, both avian and human: the park is one of the Bay Area's best places for hang gliding, and is home of the Wings of Rogallo hang-gliding club.

- Also look for birds, especially hawks, falcons, kites, eagles, and other airborne hunters.

- Northern flickers, western scrub-jays, black phoebes, and goldfinches are among the common songbirds found in the skies (and the trees) in this park.

# TRIP2 Joseph D. Grant County Park: Antler Point

| | |
|---:|:---|
| **Distance** | 9.8 miles, Semi-loop |
| **Hiking Time** | 4 to 6 hours |
| **Elevation Gain/Loss** | ±1650 feet |
| **Difficulty** | Difficult |
| **Trail Use** | Mountain biking allowed |
| **Best Times** | Fall through spring |
| **Agency** | SCCP&R |
| **Recommended Map** | *Joseph D. Grant County Park* (SCCP&R) |

**HIGHLIGHTS** Following a mostly rolling, ridgetop course on the Canada de Pala and Pala Seca trails, you enjoy views that extend from the Diablo Range, crowned by nearby Mt. Hamilton, to the distant Santa Cruz Mountains. After visiting Antler Point, the trail dips to Deer Camp and then a marshy meadow, but soon resumes its quest of high places.

**DIRECTIONS** From I-680 in San Jose, take the Alum Rock exit, go northeast 2.2 miles to Mt. Hamilton Road, and turn right. At 7.7 miles you reach the entrance to the park's main area. Continue another 3.4 miles to a paved parking area, left, for the Twin Gates Trailhead.

**FACILITIES/TRAILHEAD** There are campgrounds, restrooms, picnic tables, phone, and water in the park's main area. There is a toilet at the trailhead, which is on the west side of the parking area.

You go through a metal gate and then climb moderately on the Canada de Pala Trail, a dirt road. The road bends right and gains the top of a ridge. This ridge overlooks Halls Valley, the site of most park facilities, several lakes, and a network of trails. Mt. Hamilton, a hulking giant topped by 4373-foot Copernicus Peak, rises to the east. The white domes clustered around Mt. Hamilton's summit belong to the University of California's Lick Observatory.

A grove of valley oaks nearby shows evidence of resident acorn woodpeckers—the trunks are riddled with holes. True to their name, these woodpeckers collect acorns and store them in the perforated bark of trees.

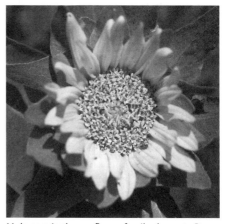

Mule ears, in the sunflower family, decorate Bay Area grasslands in spring.

**Traveling Leaves**

Don't be surprised to see black oak and western sycamore leaves on the ground. Although the area around you is treeless, wooded ravines can be found on the ridge's lower slopes. Wind whipping across the ridge picks up leaves and deposits them here.

Soon the grade eases, and you enjoy a rolling course over mostly open, grassy terrain, perfect for songsters such as western meadowlarks and horned larks. Your route starts at an elevation of 2350 feet and stays above that for its entire length. If the Santa Clara Valley is foggy, you may still be reveling under clear skies, enjoying views of the Santa Cruz Mountains to the west. But with the

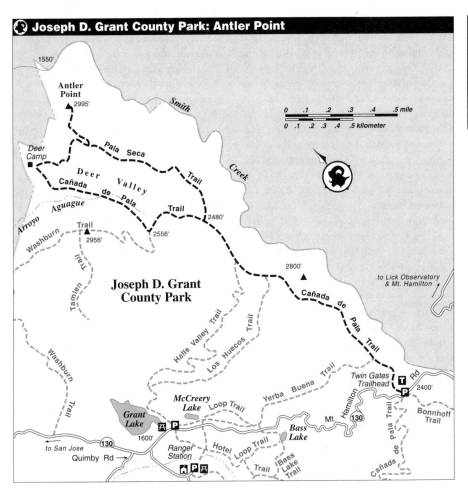

## Joseph D. Grant County Park: Antler Point

altitude comes the possibility of cool temperatures and blustery winds.

At a junction with the Yerba Buena Trail, left, you continue straight. An occasional gray pine or venerable valley oak dots the landscape. Now you pass a rest bench and a stock pond, both left. Beyond a cattle gate, you descend an eroded stretch of road to a junction, left, with the Los Huecos Trail, a dirt road. Steadily losing elevation, you reach the Halls Valley Trail, left, and then a saddle in the ridge you've been following.

Climbing on a moderate grade, you come to a barbed-wire fence and a cattle gate. Just ahead, the grade eases as the road bends right. Around 2.6 miles, the Canada

de Pala Trail bends left, but you continue straight, now on the Pala Seca Trail. This trail, also a dirt road, climbs moderately and then steeply, still following a ridgecrest.

A rest bench, right, invites you to stay awhile and enjoy the seemingly endless parade of ridges and canyons marching east toward the Central Valley. To the southwest are double-humped Loma Prieta and its neighbor Mt. Umunhum, topped by a concrete-block building once used by the Air Force. The road levels, curves right, and then begins to descend. Twin summits are just ahead, the right one being Antler Point. You reach it via the Antler Point Trail, a single track angling right.

This trail wanders across a hillside and soon reaches an unsigned fork. You bear right and climb gently to a rest bench at the end of the trail, around 4.4 miles. The view northward takes in a rugged ensemble of canyons, ravines, and ridges that make up some of the wildest land in the Bay Area. Monument Peak, bristling with communication towers, is in the distance to the northwest. After enjoying this invigorating scene, retrace your route to the Pala Seca Trail.

---

**Birds & Beasts**

Western scrub-jays, yellow-billed magpies, and dark-eyed juncos are some of the birds to look for here. Also keep an eye peeled for coyotes and bobcats, and an ear out for frogs.

---

Turn sharply right on the dirt road, pass a rest bench, and begin to descend via S-bends over rocky, eroded, and perhaps muddy ground. After losing elevation, you climb on a gentle grade to a barbed-wire fence and a cattle gate. Ahead is Deer Camp, site of a renovated cabin. Here the Pala Seca Trail ends and you join the Canada de Pala Trail, which at this point is unsigned.

Resuming the descent, you drop steeply to a ravine, where the creek you crossed earlier is confined to a culvert. Climbing out of this drainage, you traverse a ridge and enter beautiful, wide Deer Valley. A creek, right, creates a marshy tract of sedges and rushes. California bay, coffeeberry, bush monkeyflower, and gooseberry grow beside the road. A culvert carries the creek under the road and puts it on your left.

A wet meadow, left, marks the head of the creek, with an extensive ground squirrel colony nearby. After meeting the Washburn Trail, a dirt road heading right, you continue straight and climb out of the valley at its south end. Soon you reach a cattle gate and then close the loop at the Pala Seca Trail. From here, at about 7 miles, bear right and retrace your route to the parking area.

## TRIP 3 Joseph D. Grant County Park: Ridgetop Ramble

| | |
|---|---|
| **Distance** | 7.1 miles, Loop |
| **Hiking Time** | 3 to 4 hours |
| **Elevation Gain/Loss** | ±1400 feet |
| **Difficulty** | Difficult |
| **Trail Use** | Mountain biking allowed[1] |
| **Best Times** | Spring and fall |
| **Agency** | SCCP&R |
| **Recommended Map** | *Joseph D. Grant County Park* (SCCP&R) |
| **Notes** | [1]Bicycles are not allowed on parts of the San Felipe Trail, and must instead use the Corral and Hotel (or Lower Hotel) trails to complete the trip |

**HIGHLIGHTS**  This vigorous loop, using the Dairy, Dutch Flat, Brush, and San Felipe trails, takes you to through oak woodlands and wildflower meadows to a high ridge where a picnic table and 360-degree views reward the sometimes steep climbing.

**DIRECTIONS**  From I-680 in San Jose, take the Alum Rock exit, go northeast 2.2 miles to Mt. Hamilton Road, and turn right. At 7.7 miles you reach the entrance to the park's main area, where you turn right. After several hundred feet you come to an entrance kiosk and a self-registration station. Continue straight for about 0.5 mile to the Stockman's group picnic/parking area.

**FACILITIES/TRAILHEAD**  There are campgrounds, restrooms, picnic tables, phone, and water in the park's main area. The trailhead is on the northwest corner of the parking area.

## Joseph D. Grant County Park: Ridgetop Ramble

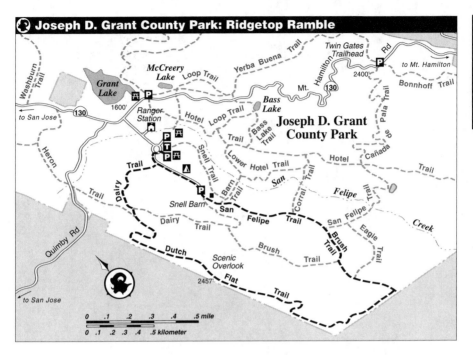

Turn left on a paved road that skirts the north side of the parking area. After about 100 yards, you come to an equestrian area, left, and the start of the Dairy Trail, on the right. You climb gently on the Dairy Trail, a multi-use dirt road. The park's main area sits in Halls Valley, beside San Felipe Creek. You are climbing toward the ridge that forms the valley's west wall. To the east rises another high ridge, which you can explore by following the route description for "Antler Point" on p. 178.

As you gain elevation over eroded ground, Mt. Hamilton, with its white observation domes, comes into view. Valley oaks and coast live oaks offer some shade, but much of the climb is in the open. Leave the Dairy Trail where it goes left, and continue through a gate on the Dutch Flat Trail. (To shorten the trip, bear left on the Dairy Trail, follow it down to the San Felipe Trail, and then go straight.)

Curving uphill on a moderate grade, you meet the Heron Trail joining from the right. The Heron Trail and the next 3.5 miles of the Dutch Flat Trail are part of the Bay Area Ridge Trail. Finally gaining the ridgetop, you are rewarded by fine views of the Santa Clara Valley and the Santa Cruz Mountains.

---

**Flora and Fauna Watch**

- This park boasts an impressive array of spring wildflowers, including lupine, blue-eyed grass, fiddleneck, bluedicks, scarlet pimpernel, owl's-clover, mule ears, Johnny jump-up, checkerbloom, California buttercup, yarrow, Chinese houses, winecup clarkia, California poppy, and popcorn flower.
- Here also is a population of wild pigs, and beside the trail you may see evidence of their destructive rooting.
- This park is one of a few places in the Bay Area to find yellow-billed magpies, a large member of the crow family. Also here are western bluebirds, oak titmice, California towhees, northern flickers, and wild turkeys.

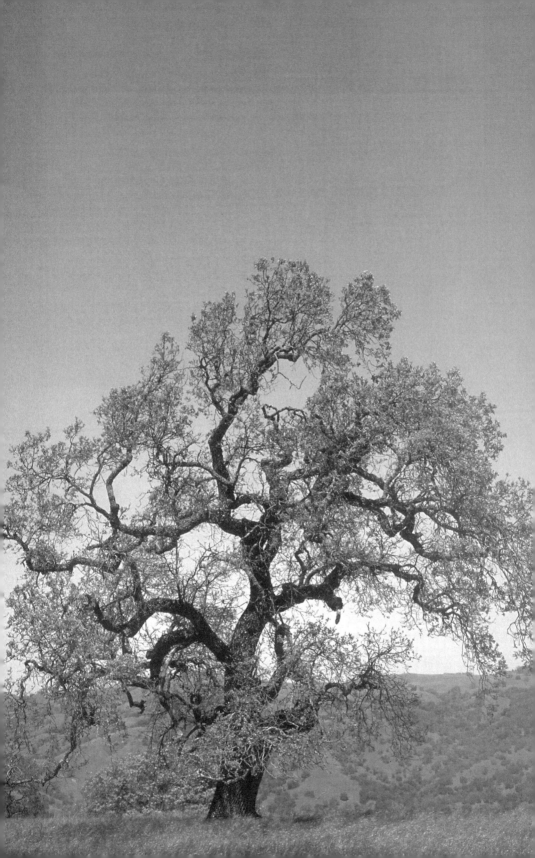

The sight of sprawling San Jose underscores the value of protecting open space.

Around 2 miles, a picnic table atop the ridge welcomes you to the Scenic Overlook (2437'), and indeed it is! (A sign here that robs you of 433 hard-won feet is curious.) Beyond the overlook, the road descends on a moderate, then steep, grade and soon enters a woodland of black oak and valley oak. After passing through a seasonally wet area, the route follows a rolling course along the ridgecrest. In spring, the park's verdant grasslands, decorated with colorful wildflowers, are lovely.

Several sweeping bends help you descend to a level area holding two ponds, separated by a fence marking the park boundary. Nearby is a granary tree, a large valley oak riddled with holes and used by acorn woodpeckers to store their namesake food. Climbing over a rise, you resume your descent, in places over steep, eroded ground. Passing a dirt road, right, at around 4 miles, you enjoy a mostly level course that soon reaches a junction with the Eagle Trail, right.

You continue straight across a huge, possibly wet, meadow. The Dutch Flat Trail ends at a junction, where you bear right on the Brush Trail. At the next junction, angle left on the San Felipe Trail, a dirt road. A ravine, left, bordered by valley oaks draped with lace lichen, holds a seasonal creek. At about 5.8 miles, the Corral Trail goes right, but you go through a gate and stay on the San Felipe Trail, from here closed to bicycles. Climbing on a gentle grade, you pass Snell Barn, which is right.

A dirt road, not shown on the park map, departs left. Ahead, a road goes sharply right to the barn. You continue straight, passing a gate and junctions with the Snell Trail, right, and the Dairy Trail, left. About 75 feet ahead, the road becomes paved. Just beyond the next gate is a four-way junction with a dirt road, left, and a paved road, right. You go straight, finding a path paralleling the road on its left side. The path soon ends, and now you follow the paved road back to the parking area.

## TRIP 4 Henry W. Coe State Park: Forest Trail

| | |
|---|---|
| **Distance** | 3.7 miles, Semi-loop |
| **Hiking Time** | 2 to 3 hours |
| **Elevation Gain/Loss** | ±350 feet |
| **Difficulty** | Moderate |
| **Trail Use** | Good for kids |
| **Best Times** | Spring and fall |
| **Agency** | CSP |
| **Recommended Map** | *Henry W. Coe State Park* (Pine Ridge Association) |

**HIGHLIGHTS**  This enjoyable semi-loop uses the Corral, Forest, and Springs trails to explore part of Pine Ridge, near park headquarters. The Forest Trail is a self-guiding nature path, and printed guides available at its start describe many of the area's trees and shrubs.

**DIRECTIONS**  From Highway 101 in Morgan Hill, take the East Dunne Ave./Morgan Hill exit and go northeast on East Dunne Ave. At 11.7 miles you reach the Coe Ranch entrance and the overflow parking area (a short trail leads from here to the main entrance). At 12.3 miles you reach the main entrance. There are fees for parking and camping; backpackers must register at the visitor center.

Majestic valley oaks grace many Bay Area parks; elsewhere they are being lost to development.

**FACILITIES/TRAILHEAD** The park's visitor center—open weekends fall and winter, and Friday through Sunday spring and summer—has books, maps, snacks, and cold drinks. A campground, restrooms, picnic tables, phone, and water are available. The trailhead is about 100 feet east of the visitor center, across the entrance road.

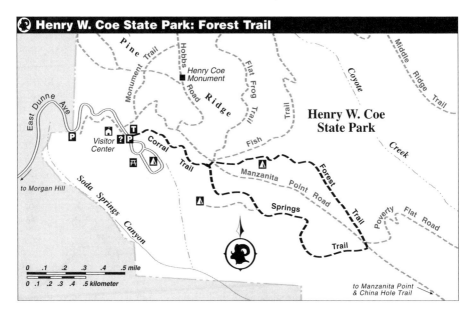

**Henry W. Coe State Park: Forest Trail**

Pine Trail · Monument Trail · Hobbs Road · Henry Coe Monument · Flat Frog Trail · Ridge · Trail · Middle Ridge Trail · Coyote · Henry W. Coe State Park · Creek · East Dunne Ave · P · Visitor Center · P · Corral Trail · Fish · Soda Springs Canyon · Manzanita · Point Road · Forest · Springs · Trail · Poverty · Flat Road · to Morgan Hill · Trail · to Manzanita Point & China Hole Trail

0　.1　.2　.3　.4　.5 mile
0　.1　.2　.3　.4　.5 kilometer

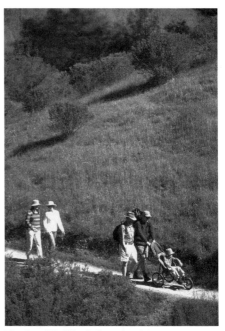

escend a few wood steps and turn left on the Corral Trail, which soon turns right to cross a bridge and then wanders beside a creek. A shady forest soon gives way to open hillsides of chaparral and a savanna of mostly valley oaks, where damage from the park's large population of wild pigs is especially evident. At a four-way junction, you turn left on a short trail to Manzanita Point Road. Across the road is an information board. Just beyond it, you bear right on the Forest Trail, a self-guiding nature path. Just ahead is a box with printed guides keyed to numbered markers along the trail. (Return them to a box at the end of the trail.)

The trail, a single track closed to bicycles and horses, crosses a little gully and then swings sharply left. Tall California bays, gray pines, ponderosa pines, and magnificent manzanitas line the route. Skirting a very steep hillside that drops left, the trail climbs on a gentle grade and wanders into a

The Corral Trail leads from the visitor center to the self-guiding Forest Trail, a nature path.

rocky canyon. Crossing a plank bridge over a seasonal creek, the trail bends left and then passes a rest bench. The views north from this trail take in a stunning expanse of wilderness, including the canyon holding Little Fork Coyote Creek, the high ground of Middle Ridge, and then Blue Ridge on the horizon.

Cresting a ridgetop, you pass a box for trail guides and then reach Poverty Flat Road, at about 1.8 miles. Cross it, and then cross Manzanita Point Road to find the Springs Trail. You wind your way to a gully,

cross it, and then make a rising traverse across a grassy, oak studded hillside. Following the southwest side of Pine Ridge, the trail cuts into canyons and wraps around ridges, passing several springs along the way. Passing a rest bench, right, you descend via switchbacks to a creek bridged by a wood plank.

Staying straight at a junction, you pass a rest bench atop a ridge, and then close the loop at a four-way junction. From here, continue straight and retrace your route to the parking area.

## TRIP 5 Henry W. Coe State Park: Middle Ridge

| | |
|---|---|
| **Distance** | 6.3 miles, Loop |
| **Hiking Time** | 3 to 4 hours |
| **Elevation Gain/Loss** | ±1950 feet |
| **Difficulty** | Difficult |
| **Trail Use** | Backpacking option |
| **Best Times** | Spring and fall |
| **Agency** | CSP |
| **Recommended Map** | *Henry W. Coe State Park* (Pine Ridge Association) |

**HIGHLIGHTS** This loop, using the Monument, Frog Lake, Middle Ridge, Fish, and Corral trails, and Manzanita Point and Hobbs roads, samples only a small corner of northern California's largest state park, but it should be enough to whet your appetite for further exploration of this magnificent area's rugged canyons, oak-studded ridges, and sky-scraping slopes.

**DIRECTIONS** From Highway 101 in Morgan Hill, take the East Dunne Ave./Morgan Hill exit and go northeast on East Dunne Ave. At 11.7 miles you reach the Coe Ranch entrance and the overflow parking area (a short trail leads from here to the main entrance). At 12.3 miles you reach the main entrance. There are fees for parking and camping; backpackers must register at the visitor center.

**FACILITIES/TRAILHEAD** The park's visitor center—open weekends fall and winter, and Friday through Sunday spring and summer—has books, maps, snacks, and cold drinks. A campground, restrooms, picnic tables, phone, and water are available. The trailhead is about 100 feet east of the visitor center, across the entrance road.

Climbing moderately on paved Manzanita Point Road, you soon reach a gate and a junction. Here you angle left on the Monument Trail, a single track closed to bicycles and horses. Switchbacks help you gain elevation to a four-way junction with the Ponderosa Trail. The Henry W. Coe

monument is about 0.1 mile to your right, just across Hobbs Road.

Continue on the Monument Trail to its merger with Hobbs Road, where you veer left. Making a long descent on a moderate and then steep grade, you eventually step across Little Fork Coyote Creek and then

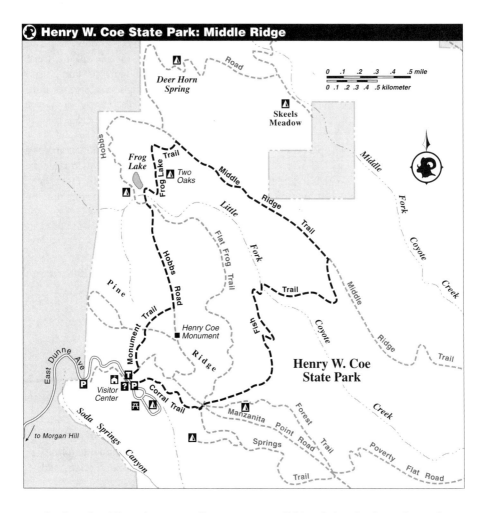

reach a junction. Here, about 1.4 miles, you turn sharply right onto the Frog Lake Trail, a single track closed to bicycles and horses. After a few tight switchbacks, you meet Hobbs Road at Frog Lake. Turning right, you cross an earthen dam, pass a trail that circles the lake, and then start to climb by switchbacking right.

This park has fine stands of ponderosa pines, a rarity in the Bay Area. Usually found in mountains, these stately trees are the most common pine in North America.

Passing a trail to Two Oaks Camp, right, you wind your way gently uphill to a T-junction with the Middle Ridge Trail. Turning right, you climb gently across an open field and then begin to descend on a moderate grade through stands of gray pine and blue oak. Beyond a saddle, the trail rises steeply, then descends through a corridor of chaparral that includes giant manzanitas.

### Sada's Gift

In 1953, Henry Coe's daughter, Sada Coe, gave Santa Clara County the former Pine Ridge Ranch, more than 12,000 acres of land that had belonged to her father and uncle. Today, at more than 86,000 acres, this is the largest state park in Northern California, and the second largest in California.

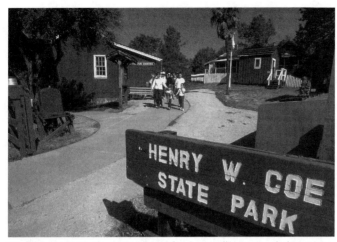

The visitor center is the starting point for short walks or extended trips into the park's backcountry.

over open and then forested ground puts you in a narrow canyon that holds a tributary of Little Fork Coyote Creek.

Leaving the canyon, the trail climbs to a broad ridgetop and several junctions with a welter of trails, at about 5.7 miles. First is a four-way junction with the self-guiding Forest Trail, left, and the Flat Frog Trail, right. Then, past an information board, you come to Manzanita Point Road and a short connector, just across it, to the Corral Trail. Cross the road, and in a few hundred feet you reach the Corral Trail, where you turn right.

This park is infested with wild pigs, and beside the trail you may see evidence of their destructive rooting.

Around 3.8 miles, you leave Middle Ridge and turn right on the Fish Trail. In places the trail is merely a ledge cut in the hillside, so use caution. A rolling course brings you to Little Fork Coyote Creek, which you step across on rocks. Now the trail zigzags uphill and then contours across a hillside that slopes left. After passing a seasonal creek in a mossy, fern-filled ravine, you climb steeply via switchbacks to a saddle. A gentle descent

You enjoy a level walk across a forested hillside that drops steeply left to Soda Springs Canyon. The trail ducks into and swings out of ravines cut into the hillside. Climbing on a gentle grade, you reach open ground, curve left, and cross a bridge over a creek. Just ahead is the parking area at park headquarters.

## TRIP 6 Uvas Canyon County Park

| | |
|---|---|
| **Distance** | 3 miles, Loop |
| **Hiking Time** | 2 to 3 hours |
| **Elevation Gain/Loss** | ±800 feet |
| **Difficulty** | Moderate |
| **Trail Use** | Leashed dogs |
| **Best Times** | Fall through spring |
| **Agency** | SCCP&R |
| **Recommended Map** | *Uvas Canyon County Park* (SCCP&R) |

**HIGHLIGHTS**  Waterfalls, at their best during winter and early spring, especially right after a rainstorm, draw visitors to this secluded park, which is tucked in a canyon on the east side of the Santa Cruz Mountains. This loop, requiring sturdy footwear to negotiate slippery rocks and slopes, uses the Waterfall Loop Foot Path, and the Waterfall Loop, Contour, and Alex Canyon trails.

**DIRECTIONS** From Highway 85 in San Jose, take the Bernal Road exit and go south 1.1 miles to Santa Teresa Blvd. Turn left, go 3 miles to Bailey Ave., and turn right. Go 2.3 miles to McKean Road and turn left. At 2.4 miles from Bailey Ave., McKean Road becomes Uvas Road. At 6.2 miles, turn right on Croy Road. Go 4.5 miles, through the private resort of Sveadal (drive slowly), to the park entrance, where there are a self-registration station and a phone. Go another few hundred feet to a parking area, right.

**FACILITIES/TRAILHEAD** Camping is available. There are picnic tables, restrooms, and water near the trailhead, which is on the northwest corner of the parking area.

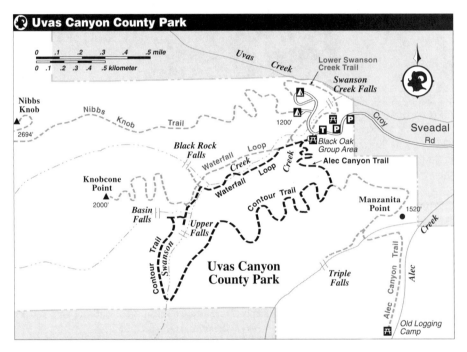

Climb a set of steps and then follow a paved path that goes just right of a restroom. Angle left, pass an information board, and join the paved park road, which you follow uphill and right (watch for cars). After several hundred feet the road forks, and you bear left. Just past the Black Oak Group picnic area, the pavement ends at a gate.

Beyond the gate, you follow the road, now dirt, moderately uphill. The soothing sound of water rushing in Swanson Creek, downhill and right, may provide an auditory accompaniment. Where the road forks, you bear right, following a sign for the Waterfall Loop Trail. One of the park's waterfalls is downhill and right.

Passing two trails, right, that lead to the campground, you soon come to Swanson Creek and cross it on a bridge. A steep climb leads to a junction, where you turn left on the Waterfall Loop Foot Path, a single-track trail. Wood steps lead down to the creek, which you cross.

Now the trail turns right and takes you upstream through a narrow, steep-walled canyon. Bay trees arch over the trail, which rises on a grade that alternates between gentle and moderate. Wood planks help you across a tributary, and then you wander back and forth across Swanson Creek on several bridges. A scenic waterfall on the right vies with the narrowing trail for your

> **Woody Duo**
>
> Two trees uncommon in the Bay Area, California nutmeg and knobcone pine, are found in this park, along with more common species such as Douglas-fir, coast redwood, western sycamore, California bay, bigleaf maple, tanbark oak, canyon oak, and madrone.

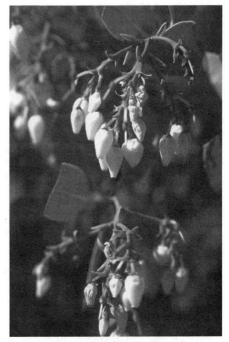

Various manzanitas are found in the park; some species bloom as early as December.

attention, and soon you ascend a set of stone steps.

Now on a rolling course, you once again cross the boulder-strewn creek on a bridge. Several short trails angle right, to the Waterfall Loop Fire Road, but you stay beside the creek. Passing a flat spot with picnic table, you arrive at a junction beside the Waterfall Loop Fire Road. You veer slightly left, cross a bridge over a tributary, and after about 50 feet, come to the next junction. From here, short trail goes straight to a viewpoint for Upper Falls, a beautiful cascade splashing down a sheer rocky face.

After enjoying Upper Falls, return to the junction and turn left. Just ahead, a trail to Basin Falls goes straight, and the Contour Trail, signed for Alec Canyon, swings sharply left. Go straight about 100 yards to view Basin Falls, which tumbles over a mossy cliff and coats the nearby rocks with slippery spray. The trail ends at the base of the falls, in a narrow canyon graced by coast redwoods. Now retrace your route to the previous junction. (To shorten the route, retrace a bit farther and descend via the Waterfall Loop Fire Road.)

> **Side Trip**
>
> For an invigorating side trip of a little more than 2 miles, turn right at the junction of the Contour and Alec Canyon trails to visit Manzanita Point, Triple Falls, and the site of an old logging camp.

Bear right at the junction and climb steeply on the Contour Trail. Soon you have

a bird's-eye view of Upper Falls from a precarious stretch of trail—use caution! As you proceed upstream along Swanson Creek, the scene becomes more wild and rugged. Debris—rocks and tree limbs—from the steep hillsides above collects in the creek bed and in places interrupts the rushing water, forming miniature waterfalls and glistening pools.

Now you embark on a roller-coaster ride beside the creek. After crossing the water on rocks, you climb steeply through a rough and rocky area that may be wet. The trail, which here may be obscure, hugs the creek bank and continues upstream. At a junction, an unofficial trail goes straight, but you turn sharply left to stay on the Contour Trail. True to its name, the trail follows a mostly level course across a very steep hillside that drops to the creek—use caution!

Back on the roller coaster, you enter a brighter zone, where chaparral plants thrive. Now you descend on a moderate grade to a bridge that spans a seasonal stream. At about 1 mile, your trail ends at a T-junction with the Alec Canyon Trail, a dirt road. Turn left and follow the road, rocky and eroded in places, downhill on a gentle grade that eventually becomes steep. Losing elevation via tight turns, you pass a water tank and soon meet the Waterfall Loop Trail, left. From here, retrace your route to the parking area.

# TRIP 7 Calero County Park

| | |
|---|---|
| **Distance** | 7.9 miles, Loop |
| **Hiking Time** | 3 to 4 hours |
| **Elevation Gain/Loss** | ±1200 feet |
| **Difficulty** | Difficult |
| **Best Times** | Fall through spring |
| **Agency** | SCCP&R |
| **Recommended Map** | *Calero County Park* (SCCP&R) |

**HIGHLIGHTS** Birds and wildflowers are the main attractions of this route, which uses the Los Cerritos, Figueroa, and Pena trails, along with the Javelina Loop, to make an extended figure-eight through the rolling backcountry south of Calero Reservoir.

**DIRECTIONS** From Highway 85 in San Jose, take the Bernal Road exit and go south 1.1 miles to Santa Teresa Blvd. Turn left, go 3 miles to Bailey Ave., and turn right. Go 2.3 miles to McKean Road and turn left. Go 0.6 mile to the park entrance, turn right, and go 0.2 mile to a large dirt parking area, right.

**FACILITIES/TRAILHEAD** There are picnic tables, water, and toilets beside the parking area. The trailhead is about 200 feet south of the parking area, on the west side of the entrance road.

You follow a dirt road south through open country to a junction, where you turn left on the Los Cerritos Trail. A short stroll brings you to the Figueroa Trail, also a dirt road, which you join by angling right. Soon you cross a creek flowing through a culvert, and then the road bends right and stays level through a wooded area punctuated by wildflower meadows. The next creek crossing is on rocks, and now you emerge from forest into an expanse of rolling hills.

Beyond where the Vallecito Trail departs right, you climb gently through a blue oak savanna. The road swings sharply left to cross the creek, then climbs on a moderate grade to a junction, about 2.2 miles. (To shorten the route, turn right on the Pena Trail and follow the route description below.)

Here you turn left on the Javelina Loop and go past two roads leading left to a closed area. A rolling course, in places steep, brings you ever-improving views. After crossing a saddle, you descend moderately

---

**On the Ground & in the Air**

- The park is home to a variety of shrubs, such as toyon, coffeeberry, snowberry, gooseberry, blue elderberry, California sagebrush, bush monkeyflower, chamise, and black sage.
- Enjoy the spring wildflowers, including Johnny jump-up, lupine, fiddleneck, checkerbloom, California poppy, yarrow, California buttercup, Ithuriel's spear, bluedicks, blue-eyed grass, and shooting stars.
- Golden eagles have been spotted here, and check the ponds and the reservoir for egrets, herons, ducks, geese, and shorebirds.

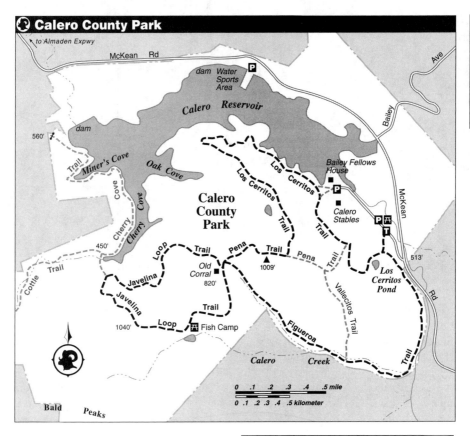

**Calero County Park**

to Almaden Expwy

McKean Rd

dam Water Sports Area

Calero Reservoir

dam

560'

Miner's Cove

Oak Cove

Cove

Cherry Cove

Cherry Cove

Los Cerritos

Los Cerritos

Los Cerritos

Bailey Fellows House

Calero Stables

**Calero County Park**

450'

Loop Trail

Trail

Pena

Trail

Pena

Trail

Pena

Vallecitos Trail

513'

*Los Cerritos Pond*

Cottle

Trail

Javelina

Old Corral 820'

1009'

Javelina

Trail

Trail

1040'

Loop

Fish Camp

Figueroa

Trail

Calero Creek

Bald Peaks

0  .1  .2  .3  .4  .5 mile

0 .1 .2 .3 .4 .5 kilometer

to Fish Camp, where an observation deck and several picnic tables overlook an artificial pond. The pond is home to the endangered red-legged frog, along with California newts, western pond turtles, red-winged blackbirds, and wood ducks.

A steep climb takes you to a serpentine rock garden, decorated in spring with California poppies and goldfields. Cresting a rise, you can admire Mt. Umunhum and the Sierra Azul, a vast area administered by the Midpeninsula Regional Open Space District. A very steep descent drops you to a junction, where you stay on the Javelina Loop by turning right. Rolling for a while, the road next climbs steeply to the Calera Bat Inn, a 512-cubic-foot structure where spotted bats and Yuma bats "hang out."

Now you descend, curve left, and close the loop at a four-way junction, at about 4.8

**Fellows House**

Future plans for the Bailey Fellows house, built by Boargenes Bailey around 1870 and later owned by Judge Edward Fellows, include a visitor center, museum, and special-event area.

miles. Go about 50 feet to the junction of the Figueroa and Pena trails, then straight on the Pena Trail. Climbing steeply, then moderately, you come to a T-junction where you turn left and enjoy a level stroll with fine views of the Santa Clara Valley and the Diablo Range. At a junction, you turn left on the Los Cerritos Trail. (To shorten the route, go straight on the Pena Trail to the Los Cerritos Trail, then follow the route description below.)

Turn left and descend moderately, then steeply, along a grassy ridgetop. Beyond a

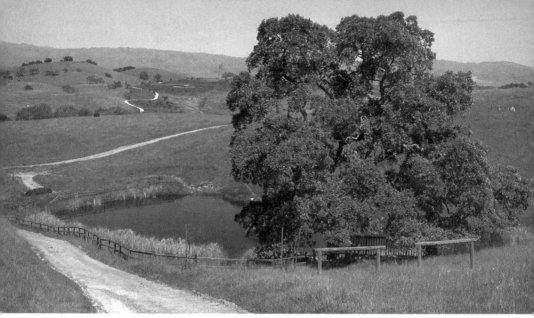

Los Cerritos Pond provides habitat for wildlife, including birds and amphibians.

fence with a gate, you roll along toward Calero Reservoir, then curve right and finally find level ground, near the reservoir's shore. An unsigned road departs, then rejoins, on the left. Where a road goes left to the historic Bailey Fellows house, at about 7 miles, you turn right to stay on the Los Cerritos Trail.

More ups and downs take you past a junction, right, with the Pena Trail, and then through a valley with a creek. At Los Cerritos Pond, an observation deck with rest benches offers a place to relax. Just ahead is a T-junction where you close the loop. From here, retrace your route to the parking area.

## TRIP 8 Santa Teresa County Park

| | |
|---|---|
| **Distance** | 3.4 miles, Loop |
| **Hiking Time** | 2 to 3 hours |
| **Elevation Gain/Loss** | ±750 feet |
| **Difficulty** | Moderate |
| **Trail Use** | Mountain biking allowed |
| **Best Times** | Fall through spring |
| **Agency** | SCCP&R |
| **Recommended Map** | *Santa Teresa County Park* (SCCP&R) |

**HIGHLIGHTS** Spring wildflowers are the prime attraction here, although this scenic loop, using the Mine, Rocky Ridge, Coyote Peak, and Hidden Springs trails, is enjoyable in all but the hottest months.

**DIRECTIONS** From Highway 85 in San Jose, take the Bernal Road exit and go south, then southwest, 2.7 miles to the park entrance. Turn left and go 0.7 mile to a large paved parking area at the end of the road.

**FACILITIES/TRAILHEAD** Picnic tables, restrooms, and water are near the trailhead, which is on the southwest end of the parking area.

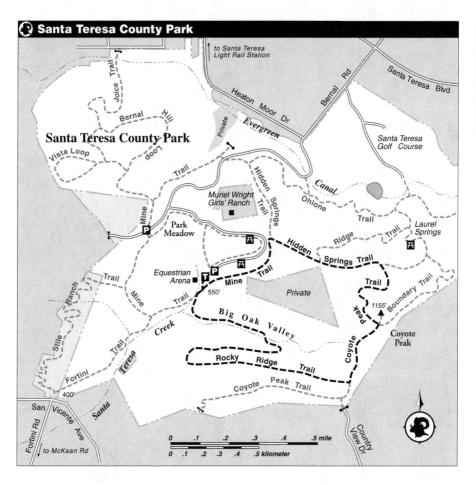

### Santa Teresa County Park

to Santa Teresa
Light Rail Station

Joice Trail

Bernal Rd

Santa Teresa Blvd

Heaton Moor Dr

Bernal Hill

Private

Evergreen

Santa Teresa
Golf Course

Santa Teresa County Park

Vista Loop

Loop

Trail

Canal

Hidden Springs Trail

Ohlone

Muriel Wright
Girls' Ranch

Trail

Laurel
Springs

Mine

Park
Meadow

Hidden Springs Trail

Ridge

Trail

Equestrian
Arena

Mine Trail

550'

Private

Trail

1155'

Boundary Trail

Trail

Ranch

Mine

Trail

Big Oak Valley

Creek

Coyote
Peak

Stile

Trail

Teresa

Rocky Ridge Trail

Coyote Peak

Fortini

400'

Coyote Peak Trail

San Vicente Ave

Santa

Fortini Rd

County View Dr

to McKean Rd

0   .1   .2   .3   .4   .5 mile

0   .1   .2   .3   .4   .5 kilometer

You pass an information board and head southwest on the Mine Trail, a multi-use dirt road. Where the Mine Trail veers right, you continue straight on the Rocky Ridge Trail. Soon the trail curves left into Big Oak Valley, following a tributary of Santa Teresa Creek. A steep climb brings you to a barbed-wire fence, which you cross through a gap. Beyond, the trail narrows and descends through chaparral to the tributary, which you cross on a plank bridge.

Once across, angle left, ignoring an unofficial trail that goes straight. You climb moderately on a rough, rocky track that soon switchbacks right. On a rolling course in the open, you have views of both the Diablo Range (east), crowned by Mt.

Hamilton, and the Santa Cruz Mountains (west), topped by the twin summits of Loma Prieta. The large building in the distance is IBM's Almaden Research Center.

The trail makes a sharp bend left as it rises toward a wildflower-strewn ridgetop. Topping a rise, you are rewarded by fine views of the Santa Clara Valley. At about 1.7 miles, you reach a T-junction with the Coyote Peak Trail, a gravel road, and turn left. Descending and then climbing on moderate and steep grades, you come to a four-way junction. A dirt road goes slightly left to the nearby summit of Coyote Peak (1155'), a hilltop from where you can almost reach out and touch the planes zooming toward San Jose International Airport.

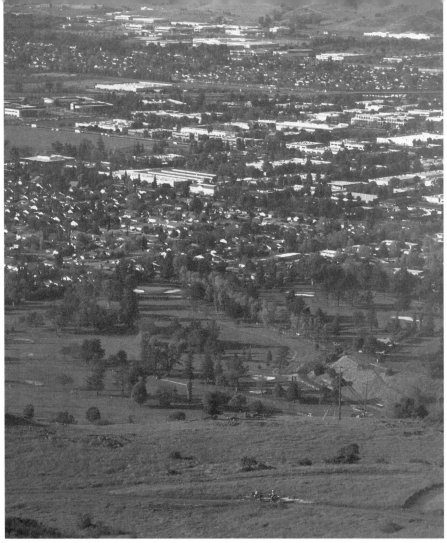

Santa Teresa County Park is an island of open space in the busy Santa Clara Valley.

You turn left to stay on the Coyote Peak Trail, a dirt road that winds downhill on a gentle, then moderate, grade. At a T-junction, you turn left on the Hidden Springs Trail, which descends gently past a hillside of black sage, when in bloom a favorite of bees. Passing a pond, left, you wander through a woodland of California bay, coast live oak, and leather oak, a shrub that grows on serpentine soil.

After the Ridge Trail departs right, you reach level ground among blue oaks, and then come to a junction just beyond a gate. Here you veer left on a short path that connects to the Mine Trail, a dirt road. Turning

### Santa Teresa Flowers

Visit this park in spring, and you may find blue-eyed grass, checkerbloom, California buttercup, Ithuriel's spear, yarrow, California poppy, bluedicks, fiddleneck, shooting stars, tidytips, goldfields, popcorn flower, owl's-clover, linanthus, red maids, and Chinese houses.

left, you follow the road as it skirts a parking area and restrooms, then heads through a corral to close the loop at a junction close to the trailhead. From here, turn right and return to the parking area.

# *TRIP9* Almaden Quicksilver County Park

|  |  |
|---|---|
| **Distance** | 7 miles, Semi-loop |
| **Hiking Time** | 3 to 5 hours |
| **Elevation Gain/Loss** | ±1750 feet |
| **Difficulty** | Difficult |
| **Trail Use** | Leashed dogs |
| **Best Times** | Fall through spring |
| **Agency** | SCCP&R |
| **Recommended Map** | *Almaden Quicksilver* (County of Santa Clara Parks & Recreation) |

**HIGHLIGHTS** Travel back in time on this strenuous route through one of the Bay Area's most famous mining areas, where cinnabar ore was once hauled out of the earth and converted to mercury in fiery brick furnaces. Today, oak woodlands, grasslands, and chaparral are the main attractions of this rugged and remote park. This extended tour uses the Hacienda, Capehorn Pass, Randol, Day Tunnel, Great Eastern, April, Mine Hill, San Cristobal, Buena Vista, and New Almaden trails.

**DIRECTIONS** From Highway 85 in San Jose, take the Almaden Expressway exit and go south 4.4 miles to Almaden Road. Turn right, go 0.5 mile, then turn right on Mockingbird Hill Lane and go 0.4 mile to a paved parking area, left.

**FACILITIES/TRAILHEAD** There are restrooms, picnic tables, and water near the trailhead, which is on the south corner of the parking area.

Follow a wide, dirt path south about 30 feet to a four-way junction. Here the New Almaden Trail goes straight, but you turn right on the Hacienda Trail and are soon joined by another trail from the parking area. Now you begin climbing on a moderate and then steep grade. After a short climb you meet the New Almaden Trail, which crosses your route. Continuing straight, you wind uphill through an oak savanna, with ever-improving views.

The wide track climbs relentlessly, tops a rise, and then begins a roller-coaster ride to a junction with the Capehorn Pass Trail (shown incorrectly on the park map). Here you turn right and descend on a moderate and then gentle grade. Soon you come to a junction with the Randol Trail, named for James B. Randol, president of the Quicksilver Mining Company from 1870 to 1892. Turn right and contour across a north-facing hillside on a multi-use dirt road.

Piles of red rock beside the trail are mine tailings hauled out of nearby Day Tunnel,

whose entrance is no longer visible. At about 2 miles, you reach a shady picnic area beside a spring (non-potable water). Just beyond the picnic area, the Day Tunnel Trail, a single-track, veers left and climbs. (To shorten the route, you can omit the following side-trip, which visits several mine sites.)

Following the Day Tunnel Trail, a single track, you climb on a mostly moderate

---

### Trees & Shrubs & Things That Fly

- This parks features a wide variety of trees, including California bay, coast live oak, blue oak, valley oak, black oak, and California buckeye.
- Leather oak, found nearby in company with other chaparral shrubs, indicates the presence of serpentine, the California state rock.
- Northern flickers, scrub jays, golden-crowned sparrows, ruby-crowned kinglets, and dark-eyed juncos are some of birds you may find along the route.

## Almaden Quicksilver County Park

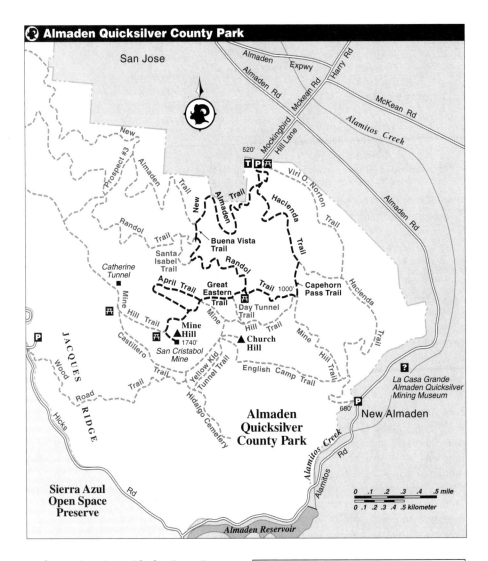

grade to a junction with the Great Eastern Trail, unsigned. Turn right and continue uphill to a T-junction with the April Trail. Turning right on the April Trail, a dirt road, you descend gently, then curve left and climb. Ahead is a trestle, part of the system used to transport ore dug from the April tunnel to the Hacienda reduction works, located about a mile to the southeast.

Follow the trail past a replica of an old powder house, a building used to store explosives. When you reach the Mine Hill Trail, a dirt road, turn sharply right and

### Day Tunnel

This tunnel, dug to vent toxic gases from New Almaden's quicksilver mines, was named for engineer and mine supervisor Sherman Day. Eventually the tunnel itself was used as a mine shaft. In the 1870s, Day Tunnel provided the main route for the company's many tons of cinnabar ore—from which mercury, or quicksilver, is extracted—to reach the surface.

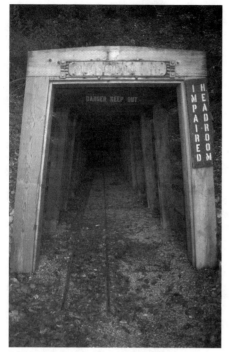

San Cristobal Tunnel, atop Mine Hill, was once part of New Almaden Quicksilver Mines.

climb across a forested hillside to a junction with the San Cristobal Trail. Turn left and climb to the San Cristobal Tunnel, gated to prevent public access, and the top of Mine Hill. A picnic table here commands a gorgeous view of San Jose, the Santa Clara Valley, and the summits of Mission and Monument peaks.

Now retrace your route to the junction of the Mine Hill and April trails, at about 4 miles. From here, follow the Mine Hill Trail as it curves right. Where the Great Eastern Trail goes left, use it and then the Day Tunnel Trail to retrace your route to the Randol Trail.

Turning left on the Randol Trail, you follow the dirt road on a level but curvy course that wanders past a large pile of mine tailings. At a junction with the Santa Isabel Trail, you stay right, following the Randol Trail as it descends. Soon you meet the Buena Vista Trail, where you turn right. The trail, a rocky single track, for hiking only, cuts a narrow swath through vast thickets of manzanita and leather oak as it descends on a gentle grade.

When you reach a junction with the New Almaden Trail, at about 5.8 miles, turn right. This trail, also for hiking only, drops to a creek, which you cross on a plank bridge. A picnic table here awaits weary walkers. A rolling course takes you across several more seasonal creeks, and then the trail snakes uphill to close the loop at a four-way junction with the Hacienda Trail. Continue straight and follow a series of S-bends down to the parking area.

## TRIP 10 Sierra Azul Open Space Preserve: Woods Trail

| | |
|---|---|
| **Distance** | 5.4 miles, Out-and-back |
| **Hiking Time** | 2 to 3 hours |
| **Elevation Gain/Loss** | ±900 feet |
| **Difficulty** | Moderate |
| **Trail Use** | Mountain biking allowed |
| **Best Times** | Fall through spring |
| **Agency** | MROSD |
| **Recommended Map** | *Sierra Azul Open Space Preserve* (MROSD) |

**HIGHLIGHTS** This out-and-back stroll along the Woods Trail to its junction with Barlow Road lets you sample some of what MROSD's largest and most remote preserve has to offer. From the forested canyon holding Guadalupe Creek to chaparral-clad slopes of serpentine soil in the shadow of Mt. Umunhum, this botanically rich route will delight

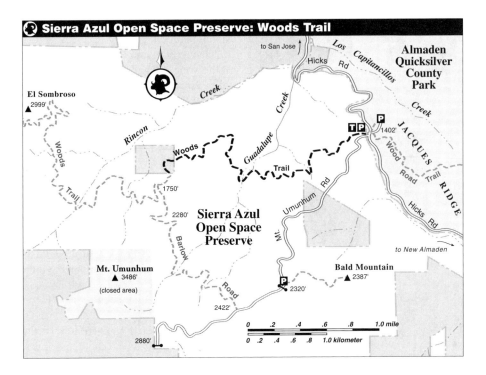

## Sierra Azul Open Space Preserve: Woods Trail

to San Jose

Hicks Rd

Los Capitancillos Creek

Almaden Quicksilver County Park

El Sombroso
▲ 2999'

Creek

Rincon

Woods Trail

Woods

1750'

Guadalupe

Trail

2280'  **Sierra Azul Open Space Preserve**

Mt. Umunhum Rd

Umunhum Rd

1402'

Wood Road

Trail

JACQUES RIDGE

Hicks Rd

to New Almaden

Mt. Umunhum
▲ 3486'

(closed area)

Barlow Road

2422'

2880'

Bald Mountain
▲ 2387'

2320'

| 0 | .2 | .4 | .6 | .8 | 1.0 mile |
| 0 | .2 | .4 | .6 | .8 | 1.0 kilometer |

native-plant enthusiasts. A connection with other Sierra Azul trails offers opportunities for long-distance travel. A trailhead on the east side of Hicks Road provides access to Almaden Quicksilver County Park.

**DIRECTIONS**  From Highway 85 in San Jose, take the Camden Ave. exit and go south on Camden Ave. At 1.7 miles turn right on Hicks Road. Go 6.4 miles to Mt. Umunhum Road and turn right. There is a parking area immediately on your right, with space for 14 cars. (There is another parking area nearby, on the east side of Hicks Road, which serves Almaden Quicksilver County Park.)

**FACILITIES/TRAILHEAD**  There is a toilet on the west side of the parking area near the trailhead, which is at gate SA06.

Go past a gate and follow the Woods Trail, a dirt road. The rolling hills to the right of the road drop steeply to the canyon holding Guadalupe Creek. The creek, which starts high on Mt. Umunhum, eventually flows through San Jose on its way to San Francisco Bay. Hugging the 1400-foot contour line, the road curves back and forth to follow the terrain. Soon you reach the head of a ravine holding a seasonal tributary of Guadalupe Creek. Curving downhill on a gentle grade, you come to Guadalupe Creek itself, which flows under the road through a culvert.

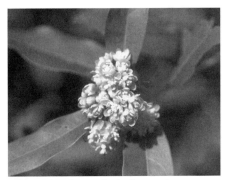

California bay, known for its fragrant leaves, blooms in late winter.

This botanically rich preserve is home to a variety of trees, including coast live oak, interior live oak, canyon oak, scrub oak, tanbark oak, California buckeye, Douglas-fir, California bay, madrone, California nutmeg, and bigleaf maple.

Beyond the creek, at about 1.3 miles, the road swings sharply right and climbs on a moderate, then gentle, grade. The route alternates between wooded areas and hillsides of chaparral, and the scenery is dominated by the rugged north face of Mt. Umunhum (3486'), topped by a concrete radar tower left over from the Cold War but still off-limits to the public. The mountain may take its name from the Ohlone word for hummingbird, or "the resting place of hummingbirds."

Now in shade, you enjoy a level walk that soon brings you to a junction with Barlow Road. From here, retrace your route to the parking area.

## TRIP 11 Sierra Azul Open Space Preserve: Limekiln–Priest Rock Loop

| | |
|---|---|
| **Distance** | 5.2 miles, Loop |
| **Hiking Time** | 2 to 3 hours |
| **Elevation Gain/Loss** | ±1300 feet |
| **Difficulty** | Moderate |
| **Trail Use** | Mountain biking allowed, Leashed dogs |
| **Best Times** | Fall through spring |
| **Agency** | MROSD |
| **Recommended Map** | *Sierra Azul Open Space Preserve* (MROSD) |

**HIGHLIGHTS** This loop, which starts and ends in Lexington Reservoir County Park, uses the Limekiln and Priest Rock trails and a short stretch of Alma Bridge Road to visit the northwest corner of MROSD's largest, most remote preserve. Much of the journey is over serpentine soil, which gives rise to a fascinating community of shrubs and wildflowers.

**DIRECTIONS** From Highway 17 northbound, exit at Alma Bridge Road south of Los Gatos. At 0.7 mile you pass a parking area, right, for Lexington Reservoir. At 1.2 miles, stay right at a fork with the entrance road to Lexington Quarry. Roadside parking is just ahead on the right side of Alma Bridge Road.

From Highway 17 southbound, take the Bear Creek Road exit south of Los Gatos. After 0.1 mile you come to a stop sign at a four-way junction. Turn right, cross over Highway 17, and turn left to get on Highway 17 northbound. Go 0.4 mile to Alma Bridge Road, and then follow the directions above.

**FACILITIES/TRAILHEAD** There are no facilities at the trailhead, which is at gate SA22, on the southeast side of Alma Bridge Road, across from the parking area.

From the trailhead, you begin climbing northeast on the Limekiln Trail, a formerly paved road that is part of Lexington Reservoir County Park's trail system. You climb the rough and rocky road on a moderate grade. A creek flows through Limekiln Canyon, which is downhill and left. Still climbing, now on a gentle grade, you follow a winding course up a hillside that drops steeply left.

Now the road turns left and crosses a creek that drains into Limekiln Canyon. The road here, which goes across a landslide-prone area, may be very wet and muddy. After climbing out of the slide area, the road swings right. Now you descend

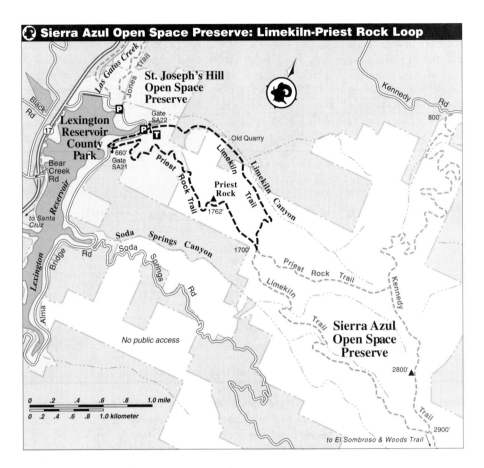

**Sierra Azul Open Space Preserve: Limekiln-Priest Rock Loop**

into a cool and shady forest. Soon you reach the preserve boundary and begin a moderate-to-steep climb over very rocky ground. Through openings in the trees, left, you can see the Lexington Quarry, a massive limestone quarry.

You continue your uphill trek to a junction, at about 2.3 miles. Here the Limekiln Trail continues straight, and the Priest Rock Trail, a dirt road, goes left and right. (To extend the route by adding a 6.1-mile loop, turn left on the Priest Rock Trail and climb nearly 1000 feet to a junction with the Kennedy Trail. From there, turn right onto the Kennedy Trail and right again onto the Limekiln Trail.)

Turn right on the Priest Rock Trail and climb past an unsigned dirt road, left, and then a short trail to a viewpoint, right.

### What's Green in the Blues

The Sierra Azul, or "Blue Mountains" in Spanish, boasts a rich array of chaparral shrubs, including chamise, manzanita, scrub oak, leather oak, mountain mahogany, chaparral pea, buckbrush, toyon, silk tassel, hollyleaf cherry, spiny redberry, and bush monkeyflower. The plant world here, where the climate is mild, sometimes seems out of synch with the calendar. For example, some early-flowering shrubs such as manzanita and chaparral currant are true harbingers of spring, blooming in December. Herbs like black sage may sprout new leaves around Christmas.

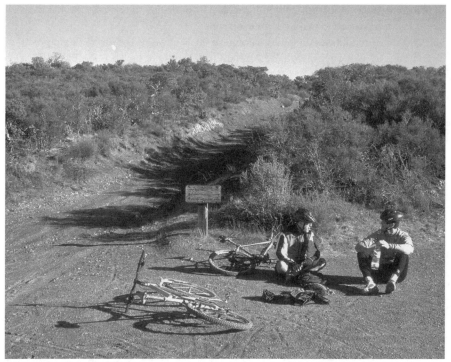

The junction of the Limekiln and Priest Rock trails makes a perfect rest spot.

Ahead, Priest Rock, a modest formation half hidden in the chaparral, rises behind a fence to the right. The road snakes its way downhill to gate SA23 and the preserve boundary. Now in Lexington Reservoir County Park, you follow the road to its end at gate SA21. Here you turn sharply right to meet paved Alma Bridge Road. Cross it carefully, turn right, and walk northeast along the road shoulder, about 0.4 mile to the parking area.

 ## St. Joseph's Hill Open Space Preserve

| | |
|---|---|
| **Distance** | 4.4 miles, Semi-loop |
| **Hiking Time** | 2 to 3 hours |
| **Elevation Gain/Loss** | ±800 feet |
| **Difficulty** | Moderate |
| **Trail Use** | Mountain biking allowed[1], Leashed dogs |
| **Best Times** | Fall through spring |
| **Agency** | MROSD |
| **Recommended Map** | *St. Joseph's Hill Open Space Preserve* (MROSD) |
| **Notes** | [1]Bicycles are not allowed on the Flume Trail, and must instead use the Jones Trail |

**HIGHLIGHTS** Surrounded by development, this compact urban preserve is a triumph of open space protection. And don't let its diminutive size fool you. The botanical diversity you encounter on this route, which uses the Flume, Jones, Novitiate, and

Manzanita trails, is superb, ranging from dense woodlands to open slopes that once held vineyards used to make communion wine.

**DIRECTIONS** From Highway 17 in Los Gatos, take the Highway 9/Los Gatos/Saratoga exit and go southeast on Saratoga Ave. After 0.4 mile turn right on Los Gatos Blvd., which soon becomes E. Main St. At 0.7 mile turn left onto College Ave., go 0.4 mile and turn right on Jones Road. After 0.1 mile, park along the right side of Jones Road, just ahead of a gated entrance to Novitiate Park.

**FACILITIES/TRAILHEAD** There are no facilities at the trailhead, which is at gate SJ01, at the south end of Jones Road.

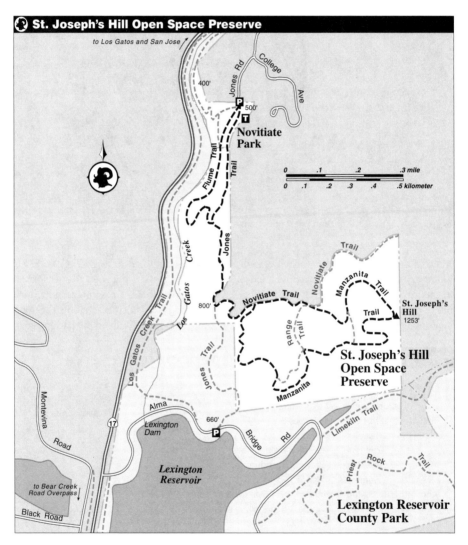

You follow a dirt road straight past an information board to a fork. The multi-use Jones Trail, which you will be on later, is left. For now, veer right on the Flume Trail, for hiking only. This trail, a triumph of trail-building ingenuity, takes its name

### One Tough Shrub

Flowering in early winter and continuing through spring, manzanitas are at home throughout California. Their small, tough leaves are designed to reduce moisture loss and optimize photosynthesis. Manzanitas are adapted to fire, and some species can reproduce by sprouting new shoots from an underground burl.

from a waterway that once ran parallel to, but high above, Los Gatos Creek. The trail climbs on a moderate, then gentle, grade on a narrow ledge, through dense forest, and across sheer rock cliffs.

Meeting the Jones Trail, a multi-use dirt road, you bear right. Level at first, the road soon ascends on a gentle and then moderate grade. When you reach the Novitiate Trail, turn left and climb moderately beside a metal fence topped with barbed wire.

Behind the fence, and also lining the road, is an extensive manzanita forest, one of the most beautiful in the entire Bay Area.

Where one end of the Manzanita Trail departs right, you go straight. At the next junction, angle right on the Manzanita Trail and follow it uphill through dense forest that soon gives way to open slopes. Ahead is your goal, St. Joseph's Hill, topped with a solitary cypress. Passing the Serpentine Trail, left, and the Upper Brothers Bypass, right, you continue to summit. From this vantage point, you have 360-degree views that take in many of the Bay Area's tallest peaks, as well as the bayside communities from San Jose to San Francisco.

Continue across the top of St. Joseph's Hill and then begin to wind your way downhill. Beyond the Upper Brothers Bypass, right, an almost unbroken sea of manzanita awaits, at around 2 miles. At a four-way junction with the Range Trail and

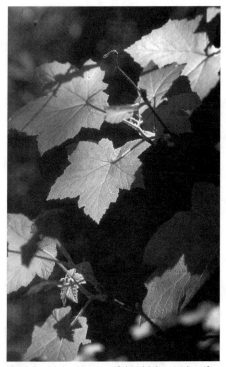

The broad, lobed leaves of thimbleberry identify this shade-loving shrub

### Raptor Rapture

Red-tailed hawks, American kestrels, and northern harriers are among the avian hunters that visit this preserve. The northern harrier is one of only a few raptors that shows a pronounced difference in coloration between male and female. The female northern harrier is brown, whereas the male is light gray, similar to a gull.

an unnamed trail, you stay on the Manzanita Trail by turning left and continuing to descend, now over rough ground.

Soon the unnamed trail you just passed joins sharply from the right. Now the trail curves downhill to meet the Novitiate Trail. Here you turn left and retrace your route to the Jones Trail. Turn right on the Jones Trail —staying right as a courtesy to bicyclists— and retrace your route to its junction with the Flume trail. Continue straight on the Jones Trail and follow it downhill to Novitiate Park. Then simply continue straight to the roadside parking area along Jones Road.

# Chapter 8
## *Palo Alto/Sunnyvale*

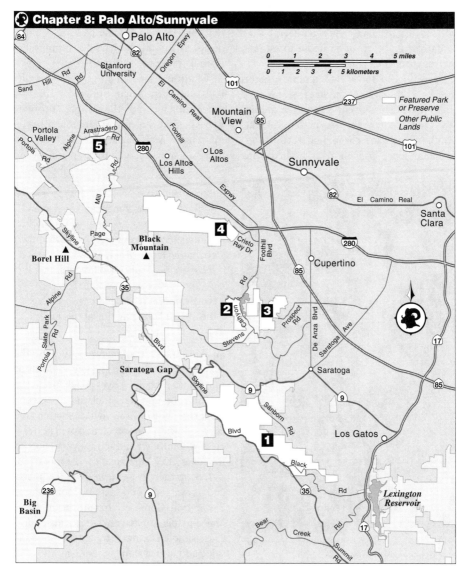

Palo Alto

Stanford University

Sand Hill Rd

Oregon Epwy

El Camino Real

Mountain View

Portola Valley

Arastradero Rd

Alpine

Portola Rd

Foothill

Los Altos

Los Altos Hills

Sunnyvale

Santa Clara

El Camino Real

Mill

Page

Skyline

Black Mountain

Borel Hill

Cristo Rey Dr

Foothill Blvd

Cupertino

Alpine Rd

Canyon Rd

Stevens

Prospect Rd

De Anza Blvd

Saratoga Ave

Portola State Park Rd

Saratoga Gap

Skyline

Blvd

Saratoga

Sanborn Rd

Los Gatos

Black

Lexington Reservoir

Big Basin

Bear

Creek

Rd

Summit Rd

0  1  2  3  4  5 miles
0  1  2  3  4  5 kilometers

Featured Park or Preserve

Other Public Lands

# TRIP 1  Sanborn County Park

| | |
|---:|:---|
| **Distance** | 5 miles, Out-and-back |
| **Hiking Time** | 2 to 3 hours |
| **Elevation Gain/Loss** | ±550 feet |
| **Difficulty** | Moderate |
| **Best Times** | All year |
| **Agency** | SCCP&R |
| **Recommended Map** | *Sanborn County Park* (SCCP&R) |

**HIGHLIGHTS** The San Andreas fault slices through this park, which is home to towering redwoods and Douglas-firs. This out-and-back stroll along the John Nicholas Trail takes you past Lake Ranch Reservoir, said to have emptied much of its water during the 1906 earthquake.

**DIRECTIONS** From Highway 85 in Saratoga, take the Saratoga Ave. exit and go southwest. Approaching 0.5 mile, get in the extreme right lane and continue straight. At 1.9 mile, Saratoga Ave. becomes Highway 9. At 4.5 miles from Highway 85, turn left on Sanborn Road. At 1 mile you pass the park entrance, right. Go another 0.8 mile to a small road-side parking area, on the right.

**FACILITIES/TRAILHEAD** The park's main area, where a vehicle entry fee is charged, has camping, picnic tables, restrooms, phone, and water. There are no facilities at the trail-head, which is several hundred feet south of the parking area, just across a bridge over a creek, on the right side of the road.

Take the John Nicholas Trail, a steeply rising dirt road, through a shady canyon that holds an unnamed tributary of Sanborn Creek, which is right and down-hill. After an overgrown dirt road joins sharply from the left, the grade eases and you enjoy a gentle uphill stroll. Now the road bends left and the grade changes to moderate. An earthen dam, left, signals your approach to Lake Ranch Reservoir, which is uphill and hidden from view. Welcome shade on the first part of the route is provided by Douglas-firs, tanbark oaks, black oaks, canyon oaks, California buck-eyes, bigleaf maples, and California bays.

Just before reaching the reservoir, the road makes a 180-degree bend to the left. At this bend is a junction with a road joining from the right (not shown on the park map). Also here is a picturesquely situated picnic table. The road crosses the earthen dam, then forks. You bear right, skirting the northeast side of the reservoir. Passing a

road that joins sharply from the left (also not on the park map), you soon reach the reservoir's southeast end, at about 1 mile. Here, with a picnic table on your left, the road bends right, crosses an earthen dam, and then bends left.

You follow the John Nicholas Trail, still a dirt road, into dense forest. A creek, left, flows through ever-deepening Lyndon Canyon on its way to Lexington Reservoir. The road stays mostly level as it winds in

---

**Sanborn Park Denizens**
- Some of the reservoir's residents include great blue herons, ducks, coots, and killdeer; deer and bobcats reside nearby.
- The park's woodland habitat favors songbirds, and among those you may see and hear are chestnut-backed chickadees, dark-eyed juncos, and Steller's jays.

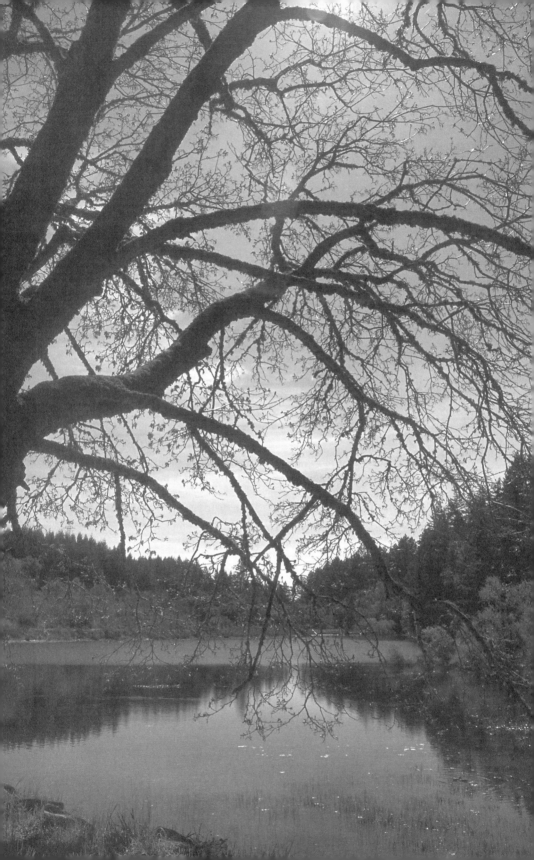

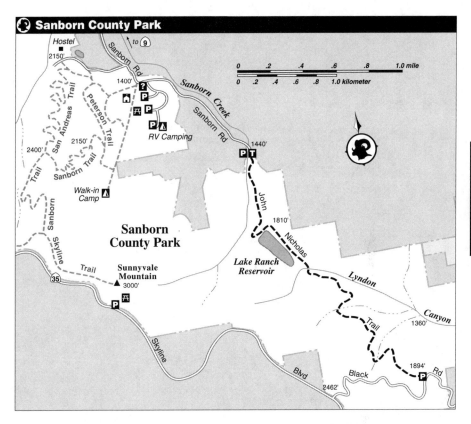

and out of three stream-filled side canyons. In the last of these, where water flows through a rocky defile and then spills across the road, there are coast redwoods. Now the road meanders and descends gently to a gate beside Black Road. From here, retrace your route to the parking area.

## TRIP2 Picchetti Ranch Open Space Preserve

|  |  |
|---|---|
| **Distance** | 3.3 miles, Semi-loop |
| **Hiking Time** | 1 to 2 hours |
| **Elevation Gain/Loss** | ±550 feet |
| **Difficulty** | Moderate |
| **Trail Use** | Good for kids (to shorten the route, omit the out-and-back segment of the Zinfandel Trail) |
| **Best Times** | All year |
| **Agency** | MROSD |
| **Recommended Map** | *Picchetti Ranch Open Space Preserve* (MROSD) |

**HIGHLIGHTS** This route, using the Zinfandel, Orchard Loop, Bear Meadow, and Vista trails, combines an easy semi-loop through an old orchard and up a scenic hill with a more

The John Nicholas Trail skirts Lake Ranch Reservoir, near the San Andreas fault.

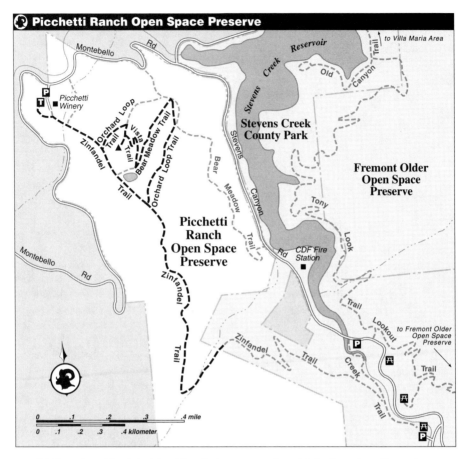

athletic out-and-back trek beside a lush canyon where bigleaf maples offer autumn hues. Along the way, the trail passes a seasonal pond where you may find California newts and frogs during the rainy season.

**DIRECTIONS** From I-280 at the Cupertino–Los Altos border, take the Foothill Expressway/Grant Road exit and go south on Foothill Blvd. At 1.6 miles this becomes Stevens Canyon Road. At 3.3 miles you turn right on Monte Bello Road. Go 0.6 mile to a parking area on the left.

**FACILITIES/TRAILHEAD** There are no facilities at the trailhead, but there are restrooms about 0.1 mile ahead, adjacent to the winery. The trailhead is about 100 feet south of the parking area, on the right side of the dirt road to the winery.

Pass through a gap in a wood fence and follow a single-track trail, which soon merges with the Zinfandel Trail, a dirt road. The historic winery, well worth a visit, is to the left (as are restrooms). The Zinfandel Trail wanders past an old orchard. Plums, apricots, and pears once flourished on this ranch, which also produced grapes for wine. There are still some 100-year-old Zinfandel vines growing on a hillside below Monte Bello Road. The appropriately named Orchard Loop Trail circles the high hill to your left, and you meet one branch of the trail just ahead on your left. Ignoring it for now, you continue straight, passing the Bear Meadow Trail, which also departs left —you will meet this trail again too.

Now the road descends and curves right, bringing you alongside a seasonal pond. Magnificent valley oaks and madrones add to the picturesque scene. An unofficial trail, left, wanders over to the pond. Where the Orchard Loop Trail (second time you meet it) curves left, you continue straight on the Zinfandel Trail, now a single track, for hiking only.

After about 25 feet, you cross a wood bridge over a seasonal creek. After passing through a gap in a wooden fence, you follow a rolling course through a shady forest and across an open hillside. Now descending on a ledge that has been notched from a steep slope, you enter a cool, shady forest of mostly bay trees. Ferns—and not much else—thrive on the slanting forest floor, which is dimly lit even during the day.

Reaching a tributary of Stevens Creek set in a deep canyon, you cross it on a wooden bridge, then turn sharply left and begin to climb. Above you tower bigleaf maples, colorful in fall. Climbing on a moderate and then gentle grade, the trail hugs a hillside

> **Ranch Life**
> - The preserve boasts an interesting assortment of native plants, including California nutmeg, silk tassel, hollyleaf cherry, pitcher sage, mountain mahogany, and wind poppy, which sports four bright orange petals spotted with purple.
> - Birds in residence here include California quail, spotted towhees, olive-sided flycatchers, wrentits, northern flickers, and chestnut-backed chickadees.

that falls dizzyingly left. The route soon bends right and reaches the preserve boundary at about 1.2 miles. (Ahead the trail enters Stevens Creek County Park and descends about 400 feet in 0.6 mile to Stevens Canyon Road.)

From here, simply retrace your route to the previous junction and turn right on the Orchard Loop Trail. Meeting the Bear Meadow Trail at a four-way junction, you turn left and follow a single track for about 100 yards to where it rejoins the Orchard

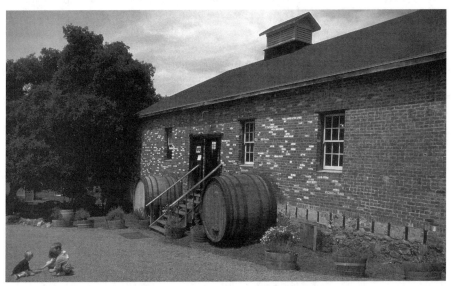

Visiting the historic Picchetti Winery is part of the fun at this open space preserve.

Loop Trail. At the next junction, turn sharply left onto the Bear Meadow Trail, a rising single track.

With the seasonal pond ahead and left, you come to a four-way junction, where you turn sharply right on the Vista Trail. After a short climb, you arrive atop the high hill mentioned earlier. Just ahead is a T-junction. Here a short trail leads left about 100 feet to a viewpoint, where you can look out over the preserve, the old orchard, and the winery.

Back at the T-junction, you continue straight on the remaining 150 or so feet of the Vista Trail, enjoying views of Silicon Valley, the southern reaches of San Francisco Bay, and the East Bay hills. At a T-junction with the Orchard Loop Trail, you turn left. A short, moderate descent soon eases, and you find level ground amid old fruit trees. When you reach a T-junction with the Zinfandel Trail, go right and retrace your route to the parking area.

## TRIP 3  Fremont Older Open Space Preserve

| | |
|---|---|
| **Distance** | 3.7 miles, Semi-loop |
| **Hiking Time** | 2 to 3 hours |
| **Elevation Gain/Loss** | ±800 feet |
| **Difficulty** | Moderate |
| **Trail Use** | Mountain biking allowed[1], Leashed dogs |
| **Best Times** | Spring and fall |
| **Agency** | MROSD |
| **Recommended Map** | *Fremont Older Open Space Preserve* (MROSD) |
| **Notes** | [1]Bicycles are not allowed on the Creekside Trail, and must instead descend via the Cora Older Trail |

**HIGHLIGHTS**  Reaching Maisie's Peak is just one of the attractions of this aerobic loop, which uses the Cora Older, Hayfield, Coyote Ridge, Toyon, and Creekside trails to explore the southern part of this preserve, named for a crusading newspaper editor who, with his wife, Cora, lived here for many years. In spring, the preserve's grasslands host a colorful array of wildflowers.

**DIRECTIONS**  From Highway 85 at the Cupertino–San Jose border, take the De Anza Blvd. exit, go south 0.5 mile to Prospect Road, and turn right. After 0.4 mile you come to a stop sign, where you stay on Prospect Road by turning left and crossing a set of railroad tracks. When you reach the junction of Prospect Road and Rolling Hills Road, follow Prospect Road as it bends sharply left. At 1.8 miles, you reach the preserve entrance and the parking area, which is left. (The parking area is adjacent to Saratoga Country Club, and a sign here warns you to beware of flying golf balls and to park at your own risk.)

**FACILITIES/TRAILHEAD**  There is a toilet beside the parking area. The trailhead is on the north side of Prospect Road, across from the parking area.

Follow the Cora Older Trail uphill and right, past two information boards. Turning left and crossing an open hillside, you soon reach a T-junction. Here you go right on a dirt road and after several hundred feet arrive at another junction, this one with the Seven Springs Trail, right.

Turning left, you go several hundred feet to a T-junction with the Hayfield Trail, a dirt road. Again turning left, you descend, curve right, and then find level ground amid stands of walnut trees, some riddled with woodpecker holes. Soon the road bends left and climbs to a junction, left,

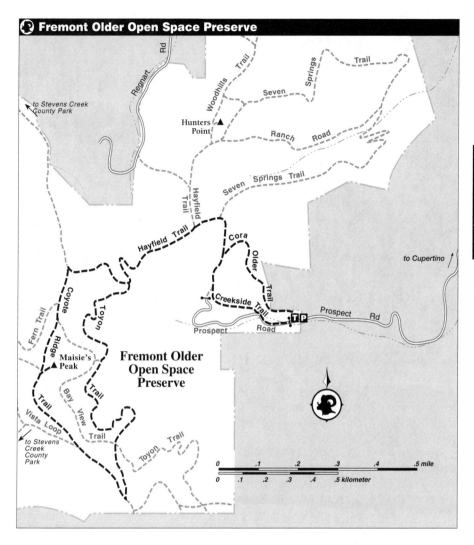

**Fremont Older Open Space Preserve**

Regnart Rd

Woodhills Trail

Seven Springs Trail

Trail

to Stevens Creek County Park

Hunters Point

Ranch Road

Seven Springs Trail

Hayfield Trail

Hayfield Trail

Cora

Older Trail

to Cupertino

Coyote Ridge

Fern Trail

Toyon

Creekside Trail

Prospect Road

Prospect Road

Rd

Maisie's Peak

**Fremont Older Open Space Preserve**

Bay View Trail

Trail

Vista Loop Trail

Trail

to Stevens Creek County Park

Toyon Trail

| 0 | .1 | .2 | .3 | .4 | .5 mile |
| 0 | .1 | .2 | .3 | .4 | .5 kilometer |

with the Toyon Trail, at about the 1-mile point.

You stay on the Hayfield Trail as it switchbacks right and becomes steep. Winding your way uphill, you reach a T-junction with the Coyote Ridge Trail. Turning left, you spy Maisie's Peak ahead. An unofficial trail that climbs to a viewpoint joins sharply from the left, and then you come to a junction with the Fern Trail, right. Staying on the Coyote Ridge Trail, you cling to a ridgetop that climbs and bends left.

Passing the Bay View Trail, left, and the Vista Loop Trail, right, you turn sharply left

**Shoots and Leaves**

- The preserve's grasslands sport a stunning selection of spring wildflowers, including blue-eyed grass, Ithuriel's spear, bluedicks, California poppy, mule ears, lupine, and owl's-clover.
- Chamise, scrub oak, hollyleaf cherry, toyon, and mountain mahogany grow on the open hillsides.

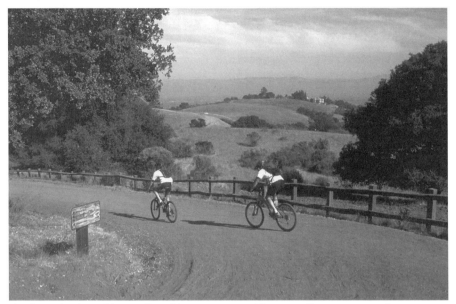

Bicyclists enjoy the multi-use trails at this preserve, named for a crusading newspaper editor.

and climb steeply to Maisie's Peak, at about 1.5 miles. A screen of trees and low shrubs circle the summit, but a few gaps offer views to other parts of the preserve. After enjoying this airy perch, retrace your route to the previous junction.

Turn left on the Coyote Ridge Trail and descend moderately, rewarded with fine views to the left of the Santa Clara Valley, Mt. Hamilton, and the East Bay hills. Now you meet the Vista Loop Trail joining sharply from the right, and soon reach a junction with the Bay View Trail, a dirt road. Here you turn left and then meet the Toyon Trail at a four-way junction.

Angling slightly right to get on the Toyon Trail, you pass a fence with a gate that prevents access by bicycles and horses during wet weather. The trail's namesake plant is abundant nearby, bearing bright green leaves and, in fall, red berries that are food for birds. You follow a rolling course through a wet area drained by culverts. Passing another seasonal gate, you arrive at a junction where a short connector jogs left to the Bay View Trail.

**Who's Maisie?**

The preserve's highest point is named for Maisie Garrod, who, with her brother, bought the surrounding lands in 1910 and used them for pasture, orchards, and hay growing. The land remained in the Garrod family until it was purchased by MROSD in 1980.

Stay on the Toyon Trail, descending gently and then traversing a hillside of chaparral. Soon you are back at the junction with the Hayfield Trail. Now you retrace your route to the junction with the Cora Older Trail (here bicycles must turn left). From here, stay on the dirt road, following it downhill and right to a junction with the Creekside Trail, a single track. Turning left, you soon enter a lovely forest of oak, bay, and California buckeye.

The Fremont Older house is uphill and right, hidden from view. An unsigned trail that descends left via wood steps leads to the Olders' pet cemetery, where you will find markers for some of their pets, including

Gretel, Melitta, and Sylvie. Fremont Older himself was buried here until the death of his wife, Cora. Now descending on a moderate grade, the trail winds its way down to a bridge over a creek. After crossing the bridge, you soon reach paved Prospect Road. Turn left and follow the road about 0.1 mile to the parking area.

## TRIP 4 Rancho San Antonio Open Space Preserve

| | |
|---|---|
| **Distance** | 4.8 miles, Semi-loop |
| **Hiking Time** | 2 to 3 hours |
| **Elevation Gain/Loss** | ±600 feet |
| **Difficulty** | Moderate |
| **Best Times** | Fall through spring |
| **Agency** | MROSD |
| **Recommended Map** | *Rancho San Antonio Open Space Preserve* (MROSD) |

**HIGHLIGHTS** This aerobic semi-loop uses the Rancho San Antonio, Permanente Creek, Lower Meadow, Farm Bypass, Rogue Valley, and Wildcat Loop trails to explore the east half of one of MROSD's few urban preserves, near the heart of Silicon Valley. The rustic buildings at Deer Hollow Farm hark back to an earlier era, and the riparian corridor along a tributary of Permanente Creek is lush with native plants. This route is popular with runners, so be alert. (Rancho San Antonio is MROSD's busiest preserve and parking may be unavailable. Please have an alternate destination in case the parking areas are full.)

**DIRECTIONS** From I-280 at the Cupertino–Los Altos border, take the Foothill Expwy./Grant Road exit and go south on Foothill Blvd. 0.1 mile to Cristo Rey Dr. Turn right, go 0.8 mile to a traffic circle, and continue on Cristo Rey Dr. by going half-way around the circle. At 1 mile, turn left into Rancho San Antonio County Park. Bear right and go 0.3 mile to two parking areas, one on each side of the road.

**FACILITIES/TRAILHEAD** There are restrooms, phone, and water beside the parking areas. The trailhead is on the northwest corner of the northwest parking area.

Take the county park's Rancho San Antonio Trail, a paved hiking and bicycling path, and bear left. Almost immediately you cross a bridge over Permanente Creek and then come to a four-way junction. Here you turn right on the Permanente Creek Trail, a dirt path signed FOOT PATH, DEER HOLLOW, ST. JOSEPH AVENUE. Just past a set of tennis courts is a fork, where you bear right. After several hundred feet you come to another fork and angle left. After about 75 feet is a paved road. Turning left, you reach a four-way junction in about 100 feet.

Here you meet another paved road, and just across it is the preserve boundary and the start of the Lower Meadow Trail, your route. With a fence and a paved road immediately right, you follow the hiking-only dirt track. Soon you merge briefly with the paved road you've been walking beside, then veer right into a dirt, permit-only parking area. The Lower Meadow Trail continues from the northwest corner of the parking area, just to the right of a wood fence.

A tributary of Permanente Creek is downhill and right, and your trail soon turns right, descends slightly, and crosses it on a wooden bridge. The paved road you have been following is now on your left, and soon the Mora Trail, a dirt road, is to your right. At about 0.8 mile from the trailhead, a potentially confusing junction requires

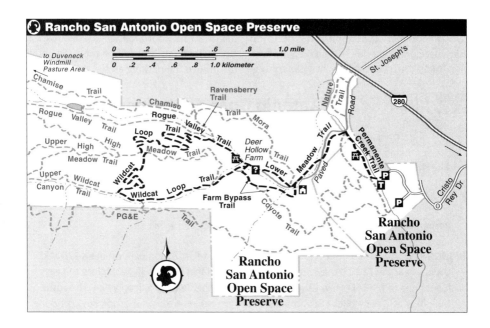

some attention. Your trail meets the paved road just where the road begins to bend to the right. Bear left across the road and get on the Farm Bypass Trail.

After about 30 feet, you cross a bridge over a tributary of Permanente Creek and then follow the trail as it turns right. Coast redwoods grow beside the tributary, as do blue elderberry, hazelnut, poison oak, and tangles of berry vines. Climbing on a gentle grade, and shaded by valley oaks, you begin to notice the buildings of Deer Hollow Farm, downhill and right.

This preserve is home to large flocks of California quail, the state bird. You may hear them rustling in the underbrush, clucking furtively to each other, or giving their unmistakable "Chi-ca-go" calls.

Around 1 mile, you meet the Coyote Trail, joining on the left. Stay on the Farm Bypass Trail by angling right. After several hundred feet, the trail turns right, crosses a culvert, and then bends sharply right. Now you descend gently to a junction where you leave the Farm Bypass Trail and angle sharply right. Still descending, you reach a T-junction in about 100 yards. Here you turn right. There are toilets on the right and a covered picnic area ahead.

After several hundred feet, you come to another T-junction, where you turn left on the Rogue Valley Trail, following a line of willows that hides the tributary of Permanente Creek you crossed earlier. Your route, a dirt road, passes the Ravensbury Trail, right, and then meets the Wildcat Loop Trail, where you turn left. (At some junctions, preserve signs refer to the Wildcat Loop Trail as the Wildcat Canyon Trail.)

---

**Trip Extension**

To add an approximately 5-mile out-and-back extension, continue on the Rogue Valley Trail, then turn right on the Chamise Trail and follow it to the Duveneck Windmill Pasture Area.

---

Now on a single-track trail, you climb through a corridor of shrubs into a forest of bay and coast live oak. In places, openings in the dense foliage give you an opportunity to admire the surrounding scenery. At one vantage point, you are rewarded with terrific

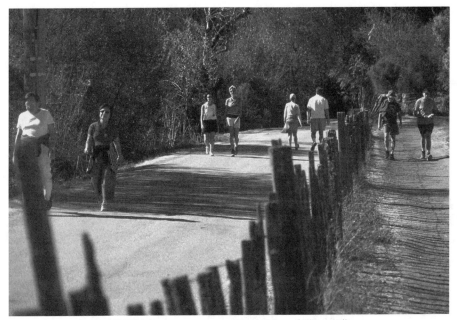

Rancho San Antonio is MROSD's busiest preserve, set in the heart of Silicon Valley.

views of familiar Bay Area summits—Mt. Tamalpais, Mt. Diablo, and Mission Peak. On a clear day, you can also pick out San Francisco, Oakland, Palo Alto, and the bridges that cross San Francisco Bay. Just north of the preserve, in Los Altos Hills, housing developments crowding up to the preserve boundary offer strong testimony in favor of preserving open space.

At a T-junction with the High Meadow Trail, you turn left and walk about 50 feet to a four-way junction. Here the High Meadow Trail veers left, and a short trail going straight climbs a grassy hill, where more great views await. Your route, signed WILDCAT CANYON TRAIL, goes right. The trail, a single track, descends on a gentle, winding course through forest to meet the Upper Wildcat Canyon Trail, right, around 3 miles. Here you turn sharply left to stay on the Wildcat Loop Trail, which follows a tributary of Permanente Creek downstream to Deer Hollow Farm.

Ahead, you cross the tributary on a wooden bridge. Now in the bottom of a cool, shady canyon, you enjoy a level walk through groves of fragrant bay trees and tall bigleaf maples. Where a trail signed COUNTY PARK departs to the right, you continue straight, passing through a gap in a fence. Now the tributary flows under the trail, through two large culverts, and reappears on your right. Three more bridges help you across the tributary at various points. Then the canyon widens, and soon you reach another fence with a gap, and then a junction.

Continue straight on the Wildcat Loop Trail and follow it to a T-junction with the

**Down on the Farm**
Deer Hollow Farm is managed as an old-fashioned homestead and funded by the City of Mountain View, MROSD, and Santa Clara County, with support from Friends of Deer Hollow Farm. The oldest remaining building on the farm is the two-room Grant Cabin, originally a single room, built in the 1850s. In 1996, the interior of the cabin was restored and furnished with artifacts.

Rogue Valley Trail, closing the loop. Here you turn right on the Lower Meadow Trail and enter Deer Hollow Farm. A large covered barn with picnic tables is on your right, as is a garden of herbs, vegetables, and flowers. Ahead there are more farm buildings and livestock, including sheep, goats, pigs, rabbits, ducks, chickens, geese, and a cow. Drinking water is on your left.

After crossing a tributary of Permanente Creek on a bridge, you reach a junction. A paved road continues straight, but you angle left onto the hiking-only Lower Meadow Trail. In late spring, you may notice the sweet aroma of black locust trees in bloom. These East Coast natives are in the pea family and produce dangling clusters of fragrant white flowers. Traveling parallel to the paved road, you soon cross the Mora Trail, then veer left onto the continuation of the Lower Meadow Trail and retrace your route to the parking area.

## TRIP 5  Arastradero Preserve

| | |
|---|---|
| **Distance** | 2.8 miles, Semi-loop |
| **Hiking Time** | 1 to 2 hours |
| **Elevation Gain/Loss** | ±300 feet |
| **Difficulty** | Easy |
| **Trail Use** | Mountain biking allowed, Leashed dogs, Good for kids |
| **Best Times** | All year |
| **Agency** | PADCS |
| **Recommended Map** | *Arastradero Preserve* (PADCS) |

**HIGHLIGHTS**  This easy route uses the Gateway, Juan Bautista de Anza, Arastradero Creek, Acorn, and Meadowlark trails to wander through oak-and-bay woodlands and across wildflower-dotted hillsides, all within earshot of busy I-280.

**DIRECTIONS**  From I-280 in Los Altos Hills, take the Page Mill Road/Arastradero Road exit and go south 0.3 mile to Arastradero Road. Turn right and go 0.5 mile to a parking area, right.

**FACILITIES/TRAILHEAD**  There are toilets, phone, and water near the trailhead, which is on the east end of the parking area.

Follow the Gateway Trail, a dirt-and-gravel path that parallels Arastradero Road and skirts a lovely meadow decorated with spring wildflowers. After several hundred yards the trail bends right to meet Arastradero Road, which you cross carefully. On the other side, the trail crosses a culvert holding Arastradero Creek and then enters Gate A of the preserve. You join the Juan Bautista de Anza Trail, a wide dirt path, and soon pass the Wild Rye Trail, left. A level walk brings you to a bridge over willow-lined Arastradero Creek.

Ahead is a fork, where the Juan Bautista de Anza Trail goes left and the Meadowlark Trail, which you will use later, heads right. Stay left, climb on a moderate grade, and then enjoy a level stroll beside Arastradero Creek. At a junction with the Paseo del Roble Trail, which crosses the earthen dam forming Arastradero Lake, you continue straight, now on a dirt road. The small lake, bordered by cattails and rushes, is home to fish, reptiles, and birds.

Soon you veer left on the Arastradero Creek Trail, also a dirt road. Leaving the lake behind, you follow Arastradero Creek through forest, then climb moderately to meet the Acorn Trail. Here you turn sharply right and follow a single track that rises gently across a sloping hillside. In a large grassy clearing you come to a four-way junction (shown incorrectly on the preserve map).

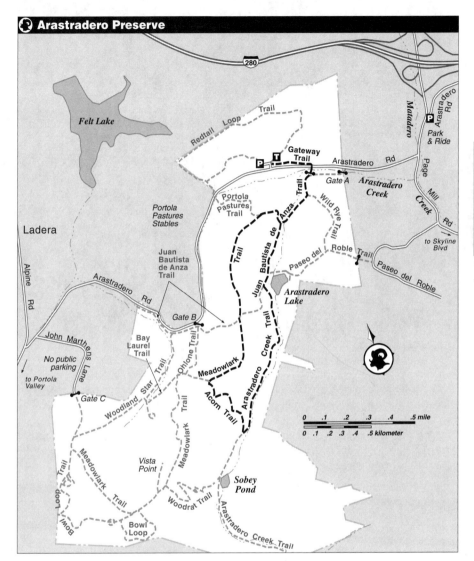

**Arastradero Preserve**

Felt Lake

Redtail Loop Trail

Gateway Trail

Arastradero Rd

Gate A

Arastradero Creek

Portola Pastures Trail

Juan Bautista de Anza Trail

Wild Rye Trail

Paseo del Roble Trail

to Skyline Blvd

Ladera

Portola Pastures Stables

Juan Bautista de Anza Trail

Paseo del Roble

Matadero

Arastradero Rd

Page Mill Rd

Park & Ride

Arastradero Creek

Alpine Rd

Arastradero Rd

Gate B

Arastradero Lake

John Marthens Lane

Bay Laurel Trail

Ohlone Trail

Meadowlark

Arastradero Creek Trail

No public parking

to Portola Valley

Gate C

Woodland Star Trail

Acorn Trail

Meadowlark Trail

0  .1  .2  .3  .4  .5 mile
0  .1  .2  .3  .4  .5 kilometer

Bowl Loop Trail

Meadowlark Loop Trail

Vista Point

Sobey Pond

Woodrat Trail

Bowl Loop

Arastradero Creek Trail

Here the Meadowlark Trail goes straight and right, and an unsigned trail goes left. Turning right, you descend an open slope that affords an expansive eastward view sweeping from Mt. Diablo to Mt. Hamilton. This vantage point also lets you appreciate the value of protecting open space from encroaching development. A moderate descent leads to a patch of level ground. Look left from here, and you can see the San Francisco skyline through a gap in the trees on a distant ridge.

At a four-way junction, you cross the Juan Bautista de Anza Trail, here a paved road, and continue on the Meadowlark

**Bloomers**

The preserve's grasslands host a colorful array of spring bloomers, including California poppy, lupine, blue-eyed grass, bluedicks, California buttercup, and fiddleneck.

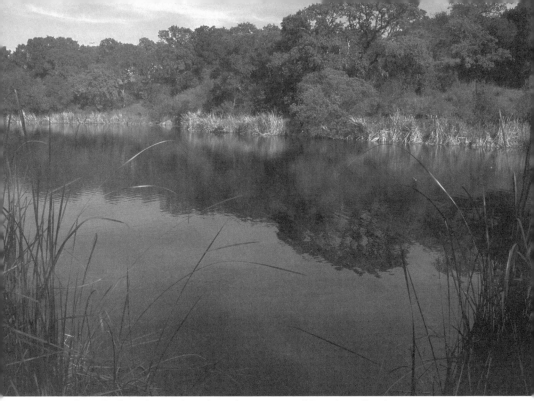

Arastradero Lake, formerly a ranch stock pond, is an easy stroll from the trailhead.

Trail. Soon you come to a trail, left, not shown on the preserve map, that climbs to a viewpoint. Continuing on the Meadowlark Trail, you reach a junction with the Portola Pastures Trail, left, and an unofficial trail, straight. Turn right to stay on the Meadowlark Trail, and descend the steep and eroded track. The grade eases, and now you close the loop at a junction with the Juan Bautista de Anza Trail. From here, retrace your route to the parking area.

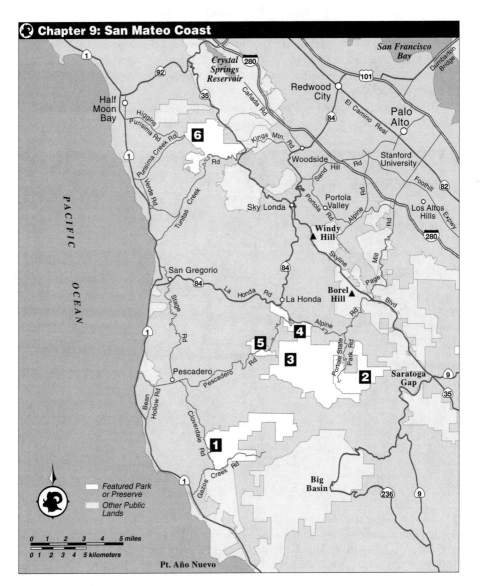

## Chapter 9
# *San Mateo Coast*

San Francisco Bay

Dumbarton Bridge

Crystal Springs Reservoir

280

92

Cañada Rd

Redwood City

101

El Camino Real

Palo Alto

Half Moon Bay

35

Higgins Purisima Rd

84

**6**

Purisima Creek Rd

Rd

Kings Mtn. Rd

Woodside

Sand Hill Rd

Stanford University

Foothill

82

Verde Rd

Tunitas Creek

Sky Londa

Portola Rd

Portola Valley

Alpine Rd

Los Altos Hills

PACIFIC

San Gregorio

84

84

La Honda Rd

La Honda

Windy Hill ▲

280

OCEAN

Borel Hill ▲

Skyline

Page

Mill Rd

Stage Rd

Alpine

Blvd

**4**

**5**

**3**

Portola State Park Rd

**2**

Saratoga Gap

9

Pescadero

Pescadero Rd

35

Bean Hollow Rd

Cloverdale Rd

**1**

Gazos Creek Rd

Big Basin

236

9

**Featured Park or Preserve**
**Other Public Lands**

0  1  2  3  4  5 miles
0  1  2  3  4  5 kilometers

Pt. Año Nuevo

# TRIP 1  Butano State Park

| | |
|---|---|
| **Distance** | 5.5 miles, Loop |
| **Hiking Time** | 2 to 3 hours |
| **Elevation Gain/Loss** | ±1250 feet |
| **Difficulty** | Moderate |
| **Best Times** | All year |
| **Agency** | CSP |
| **Recommended Map** | *Butano State Park* (CSP) |

**HIGHLIGHTS** This vigorous loop uses the Six Bridges, Año Nuevo, Goat Hill, and Little Butano Creek trails, along with the Olmo Fire Road, to explore the west part of this botanically rich park, nestled in the coastal hills midway between San Francisco and Santa Cruz.

**DIRECTIONS** From the intersection of Highway 1 and Pescadero Road, go east 2.5 miles to Cloverdale Road and turn right. Go 4.3 miles to the park entrance and turn left. At about 0.2 mile are the entrance kiosk and visitor center. Go another 0.2 mile to a small paved parking area, right.

**FACILITIES/TRAILHEAD** Camping is available. There are picnic tables, restrooms, and water near the trailhead, which is on the east corner of the parking area.

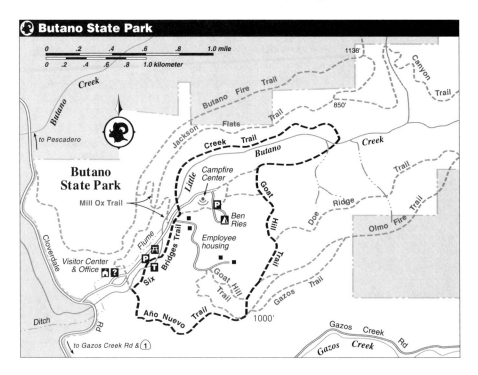

Follow a single track about 125 feet through a narrow corridor of shrubs and vines to a junction with the Six Bridges Trail. Here you bear right and after about 50 feet cross a bridge over Little Butano Creek, which is home to trout, crayfish, and red-legged frogs, the latter federally listed as a threatened species. Your route, a single-track trail, climbs on a gentle grade and soon passes a trail, left, signed BAT HABITAT. Descending gently, the Six Bridges Trail ends and you merge with the Año Nuevo Trail by continuing straight.

A moderate but relentless climb brings you to a zone that is lighter and more open than the densely vegetated creek bed. At about 1 mile, the trail begins to wind its way past massive Douglas-firs with sturdy limbs, which radiate from the trunk like spokes from a hub. Gaining elevation via a series of switchbacks, you begin to get expansive views northwest across the coastal hills toward the Pacific Ocean. A short trail, right, leads to a nearby rest bench.

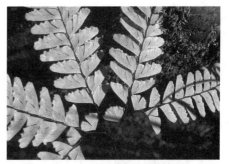

Fivefinger fern, a lover of damp and shade, is one of the plants at home in a coast redwood forest.

---

**Butano Greenery**

- This park hosts a rich variety of trees and shrubs, including coast redwood, Douglas-fir, coast live oak, tanbark oak, madrone, red alder, bigleaf maple, red elderberry, toyon, hazelnut, cream-bush, blue blossom, thimbleberry, twinberry, osoberry, gooseberry, and evergreen huckleberry.

- Moisture-loving plants such as elk clover, skunk cabbage, colt's-foot, fairy bells, fetid adder's-tongue, fat Solomon, slim Solomon, and clintonia thrive beside Little Butano Creek.

---

The grade finally eases as you near a ridgetop and then turn left to gain the ridge, where another bench awaits. Leaving the ridgecrest and wandering across its northwest-facing slope, you soon merge with the Olmo Fire Road by angling right. Rising to meet an unsigned trail, right, the road then plunges steeply and curves left. At the next junction, signed GOAT HILL TRAIL CON-NECTOR, you leave the road and follow a sin-gle-track trail that descends steeply and then gently through forest.

At a junction with the Goat Hill Trail, you go straight on a single track carpeted with Douglas-fir needles, most from trees

that are dead or dying. Where a trail signed OLMO FIRE TRAIL CONNECTOR heads right, you stay on the Goat Hill Trail by bearing left. Watch for poison oak and stinging nettles here—both are to be avoided! At a junction with the Doe Ridge Trail, you follow the Goat Hill Trail as it bends left. Descending across a fern-covered hillside, you soon enter a grove of awe-inspiring coast red-woods, most of them reaching skyward, some reclining on the forest floor. Redwood companions such as wood rose, trillium, trail plant, and redwood sorrel grow nearby.

Where a trail to the Ben Ries Campground goes left, at about 3 miles, you continue straight, soon reaching a T-junc-tion with a dirt-and-gravel road. Here you turn right, following a sign that reads LITTLE BUTANO CREEK TRAIL. The road parallels Little Butano Creek, which is left and downhill at the bottom of a deep canyon. A snaking descent on a moderate and then steep grade brings you to a wood bridge over the creek. Just past the bridge is the start of the Little Butano Creek Trail (called the Creek Trail on the park map).

Heading straight, you climb steeply to a switchback. This abrupt turn puts you on a hillside that drops steeply to the creek, which is now on your left. The trail is merely a ledge etched out of the hillside. A wild, jungle-like feeling pervades this red-wood forest, which is dampened by sum-mer fog and drenched by winter rains. The rolling course gives you a taste of grades from gentle to steep.

Now you descend to the creek. An unstable bridge takes you across a side channel, and then you step across the creek on rocks. Once across, look for a narrow trail angling left between two logs, and then curving right. You enjoy a level walk beside the burbling creek, which is spanned at various points by bridges. After the final bridge, the trail rises to meet the park's main road, which is paved. There is a roadside parking area here.

Cross the paved road and turn right, walking along its edge. After several hundred yards, you come to dirt road on your left. From here, you can simply follow the paved road for about 0.5 mile to the parking area, or you can turn left to find the Six Bridges Trail. If you opt for the trail, follow the dirt about 100 yards to where it inter-

> **Bygone Days**
> Large stumps testify to the area's logging days, when a shingle mill operated on Little Butano Creek. Across the creek is an old flume, a remnant left by early settlers, who lived and worked in this canyon.

sects the trail. Turn sharply right and begin a roller-coaster ride along a steep hillside.

Crossing a dirt road that leads to employee homes, you continue on the Six Bridges Trail, marked by a sign that may be partially hidden. A bridge takes you across Little Butano Creek, and now you make your way through a tunnel of shrubs and vines. (The park map has the creek here on the wrong side of both the paved road and the trail.) After closing the loop at a junction signed SIX BRIDGES TRAIL, bear right and retrace your route to the parking area.

# TRIP2 Portola Redwoods State Park

| | |
|---|---|
| **Distance** | 5 miles, Loop |
| **Hiking Time** | 2 to 3 hours |
| **Elevation Gain/Loss** | ±1100 feet |
| **Difficulty** | Moderate |
| **Trail Use** | Backpacking option[1] |
| **Best Times** | All year |
| **Agency** | CSP |
| **Recommended Map** | *Portola Redwoods State Park* (CSP) |
| **Note** | [1]at Slate Creek Trail Camp, 1.1 miles from junction of the Slate Creek and Summit trails. |

**HIGHLIGHTS**  Using the Coyote Ridge, Slate Creek, and Summit trails, along with a service road, this redwood-shaded loop explores rolling terrain on both sides of Peters Creek, a tributary of Pescadero Creek. This Santa Cruz Mountain state park is an important link in a chain of open space that connects Silicon Valley with the San Mateo coast. (If you have time, also visit the Sequoia Nature Trail, a self-guiding route that starts beside the visitor center.)

**DIRECTIONS**  From the intersection of Skyline Blvd. (Highway 35) and Page Mill Road/Alpine Road, go west 3.4 miles on Alpine Road to Portola State Park Road. Follow Portola State Park Road 3 miles to the entrance kiosk (if the kiosk is unattended, pay day-use and camping fees at the visitor center, ahead). Go another 0.4 mile to the Madrone picnic/parking area, left.

**FACILITIES/TRAILHEAD**  There are family and group campsites in the park. Reservations are always required for group camps and are required mid-May through Labor Day for family campsites; call (800) 444-7275. The Slate Creek trail camp is 1.1 miles northeast of the Slate Creek Trail/Summit Trail junction; call (831) 338-8861 (Big Basin Redwoods State Park) for reservations. The park is closed to all camping December–March.

Just past the parking area is the park office/visitor center, with displays, books, maps, and helpful staff. Restrooms, phone, and water are nearby. There are picnic tables and restrooms beside the parking area. The trailhead is on the west side of Portola State Park Road, opposite the entrance to the parking area.

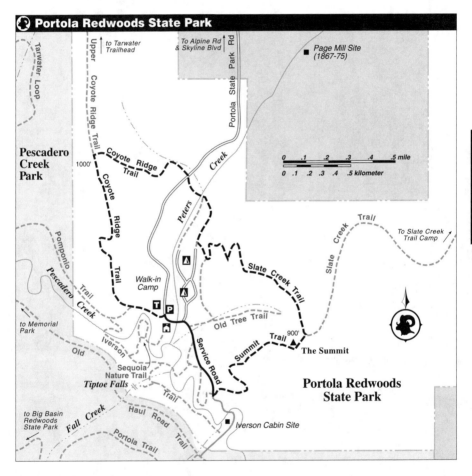

The Iverson Trail, a wide dirt path, leads you northwest through a lush corridor of evergreen huckleberry. After about 100 feet, a fence forces you to turn right, and you climb on a moderate grade until the route soon levels. Where the Iverson Trail turns left, you go straight, on the Coyote Ridge Trail. When you reach a paved road,

cross it and regain the single-track trail. Your route zigzags its way uphill and then teeters on the edge of a steep slope that drops left.

Gaining a ridgetop, the trail heads north and climbs moderately to a junction, at about 1.2 miles, with the Upper Coyote Ridge Trail. Here you stay on the Coyote

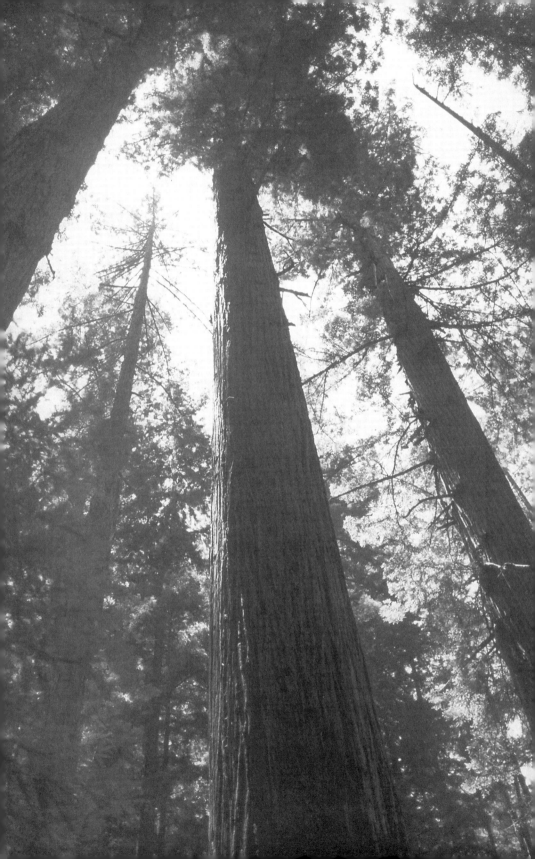

Ridge Trail by bearing right. Now you descend and curve right, leaving the ridgetop. The trail, in places steep, drops into a ravine holding a tributary of Peters Creek. You cross the tributary on a plank bridge, then turn right and walk downstream. When you reach paved Portola State Park Road, cross it and find the continuation of the Coyote Ridge Trail on the other side.

Walking down a set of steps (slippery when wet!), you turn left on a level dirt path. Peters Creek is to your right, behind a screen of shrubs. Bigleaf maples sway overhead, in the fall decorating the scene with their colorful leaves. Trillium and redwood sorrel, two shade-loving plants, thrive in the moist soil beside the trail. Where a set of steps rises left to the paved road, you turn right and cross a bridge spanning Peters Creek. Beyond the creek, find the Slate Creek Trail, which angles left.

---

### Park Trees & Critters

- Take time to admire the coast redwoods and equally impressive Douglas-firs towering overhead; the trail may be littered with their cones and twigs. Other common coastal trees, such as coast live oak, California bay, and madrone thrive here as well.
- Listen for the raucous braying call of the acorn woodpecker, a species named for its habit of storing acorns in holes drilled in tree trunks; these so-called granary trees can contain thousands of acorns, and serve a community of woodpeckers.
- Fire-hollowed redwood stumps were sometimes used by early settlers to keep domestic geese and other animals, hence their name, goosepens; today they are used as den sites by mammals ranging in size from bats to bears.

---

### Sawing Logs

In 1867, William Page began operating a sawmill on Peters Creek, just outside the park's present-day boundaries. In 1875, the mill was moved to a site on Slate Creek, upstream from where the Slate Creek Trail Camp is now located. The road used to haul lumber over the summit and down to Palo Alto was named Page Mill Road. Part of that historic alignment may exist today as the Old Page Mill Trail, which descends about 500 feet in a little less than 2 miles, from Alpine Pond in Skyline Ridge Open Space Preserve.

---

Now you follow a road that alternates between paved and dirt. At the next junction, leave the road by turning left and climbing a few steps. From here, the Slate Creek Trail is a single track wandering among impressive redwoods, some of them fire-scarred. Gaining elevation on a gentle and then moderate grade, you arrive at a junction. The Slate Creek Trail to Old Tree Trail goes straight, but your route, the Slate Creek Trail to the Slate Creek Trail Camp, goes left.

The trail is tucked in the folds of a ridge that rises steeply to the left. A tributary of Peters Creek is downhill and right, and during the rainy season it collects water spilling through gullies that cross the trail. In a clearing atop a ridge, at about 3.6 miles, you meet the Summit Trail on your right. (The Slate Creek Trail continues for several more miles until it meets Ward Road, providing a connection with Long Ridge Open Space Preserve. Along the way, it passes Slate Creek trail camp and then the second site of Page's sawmill.)

Your route veers right on the Summit Trail, skirting a hill called The Summit on the park map. A right-hand switchback helps you gain a ridgetop, but you hold the high ground for only a short while before

San Mateo Coast

---

Coast redwoods are among the world's tallest trees and also among the fastest growing.

descending across a steep, southwest-facing slope. Several switchbacks and a set of steps help you downhill, past two water tanks, to a dirt road. This road curves downhill to a junction with a paved road, called Service Road on the park map. From here, turn right and follow the paved road about 0.6 mile to the parking area, which will be on your right just past the park office.

# TRIP3 Pescadero Creek Park

| | |
|---|---|
| **Distance** | 9.1 miles, Loop |
| **Hiking Time** | 4 to 6 hours |
| **Elevation Gain/Loss** | ±1550 feet |
| **Difficulty** | Difficult |
| **Trail Use** | Backpacking option |
| **Best Times** | Spring through fall |
| **Agency** | SMCP&R |
| **Recommended Map** | *Pescadero Creek Park* (SMCP&R) |

**HIGHLIGHTS**  This extended trek uses the Old Haul Road and Pomponio trails, along with the Brook Trail Loop and the Towne Fire Road, to climb from redwood-lined Pescadero Creek to a high ridge of grasses and coastal scrub that borders Sam McDonald Park. This route requires two crossings of Pescadero Creek. Bridges over the creek are removed during the rainy season, so check first with the park supervisor, (650) 879-0601, to see if the route is passable. There is a trail camp just off the route at Shaw Flat —first come, first served; register at Memorial Park. There is also a hikers "hut," actually a full-service cabin, near the route's high point. Reservations are through the Sierra Club's Loma Prieta chapter, www.lomaprieta.sierraclub.org or (650) 390-8411.

**DIRECTIONS**  From the intersection of Highway 84 and Pescadero Road in La Honda, go southeast on Pescadero Road, and after 1 mile turn right to stay on Pescadero Road at its intersection with Alpine Road. Go another 4.3 miles to Wurr Road, turn left, and go 0.2 mile to a dirt parking area, on the left, for the Hoffman Creek Trailhead. Overnight parking requires a permit, obtainable at Memorial Park.

**FACILITIES/TRAILHEAD**  Memorial Park, just west, has camping, picnic tables, phone, and water, along with a visitor center, camp store, and restrooms (all open seasonally). There are no facilities at the trailhead, which is on the southeast corner of the parking area.

Take the Old Haul Road Trail past a metal gate and over a bridge that spans Hoffman Creek, a tributary of Pescadero Creek. Picnic tables and an information board, with an enlarged map of the park, are left. The dirt road follows a rolling course through a forest of coast redwood, where the silence may be broken by the drumming of a pileated woodpecker, and the dense shade pierced by shafts of sunlight. As its name implies, the Old Haul Road trail traces the route of a narrow-gauge railroad once used to haul logs to mills in the Santa Cruz Mountains.

After a road joins sharply from the right, you curve left and descend to a junction with the Pomponio Trail, which you will use later. At the next junction, you turn left on the Towne Fire Road, signed for Shaw Flat trail camp. The road descends, makes a sweeping right-hand bend, and reaches Pescadero Creek, which you cross on a bridge.

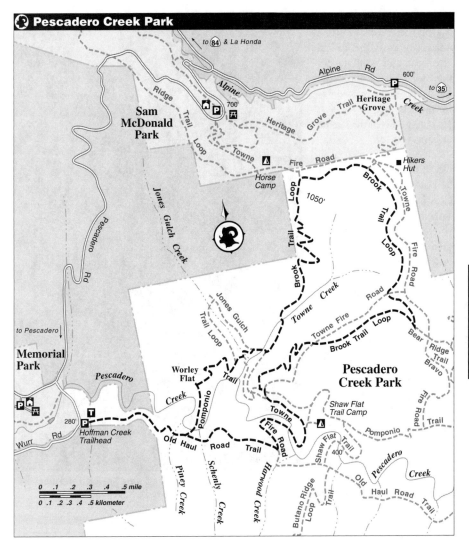

## Pescadero Creek Park

to (84) & La Honda

Alpine Rd   600'

to (35)

Alpine

Ridge

Sam
McDonald
Park

700'

Heritage Grove Trail   Heritage Grove   Creek

Trail Loop

Towne

Fire   Road

Horse
Camp

Hikers
Hut

Jones Gulch Creek

Brook   Towne

1050'

Loop

Trail

Pescadero   Rd

Brook   Trail   Loop

Fire   Road

to Pescadero

Jones Gulch

Towne   Creek

Road

**Memorial
Park**

Trail Loop

Towne Fire   Road

Brook Trail Loop

Bear Ridge Trail Bravo

Worley
Flat   Trail

**Pescadero
Creek Park**

Pescadero

Creek

Pomponio

Towne

Shaw Flat
Trail Camp

Fire Road   Trail

280'

Hoffman Creek
Trailhead

Fire Road

Pomponio   Trail

Wurr   Rd

Old Haul   Road   Trail

Shaw Flat Trail

400'

Pescadero

Creek

Piney Creek   Schenly   Creek   Hammood Creek

Butano Ridge Loop   Trail

Old Haul Road Trail

0  .1  .2  .3  .4  .5 mile

0  .1  .2  .3  .4  .5 kilometer

San Mateo Coast

Pescadero Creek has a run of steelhead trout, federally listed as a threatened species.

Climbing out of the creek canyon at about 2 miles, you pass a road, right, to Shaw Flat trail camp and emerge from dense forest. Where the Jones Gulch Trail angles left, you stay on the Towne Fire Road and climb steeply, but briefly, to meet the Pomponio Trail, a single track gated to block horses during wet weather. Turn left and go about 100 feet to a fork, then veer right on the Brook Trail Loop, also a single

track. Climbing via switchbacks, you merge briefly with a dirt road, then turn left to cross the Towne Fire Road. Neck-craning redwoods tower overhead.

The fire road follows a ridge, and once on its other side, you make a long traverse across a hillside that drops right, to Parke Gulch. Giant redwood stumps stand as mute testimony to the loggers' Herculean efforts, while the surrounding forest counsels the wisdom of preserving open space. Where the Bear Ridge Trail goes right, you stay on the Brook

Trail Loop by turning sharply left. At about 4 miles, you cross the Towne Fire Road and continue on the Brook Trail Loop. Now the drop, extremely steep, is to your left.

With a view of the Pacific Ocean, you cross a sun-drenched hillside of coastal scrub, passing a rest bench beneath a Douglas-fir. Crossing a dirt road (not shown on the park map), you reach an open slope and then a corridor of coyote brush, beyond which is a junction. To visit the Sierra Club hut, turn right, cross the Towne Fire Road, then angle right on a short trail that climbs through forest. Otherwise, go straight to the next junction, signed for the Pomponio Trail, the Old Haul Road Trail, and the Memorial Ranger Station. Here you bear left.

A rolling course takes you past a seasonal horse gate, and then switchbacks aid your descent to Towne Creek and the redwood realm, where some of the most magnificent trees in the Bay Area stand guard over their young. At about 7 miles, you turn left, cross the creek via a bridge, and then turn right and walk downstream. Soon you merge with a dirt road joining sharply from the left. Ahead you meet another road at the apex of a hairpin turn. Turn right, go about 100 yards, and then turn left to stay on the Brook Trail Loop. Beyond a seasonal horse gate, you turn left to cross a bridge over Jones Gulch.

About 75 feet past the bridge, you swing right on the Pomponio Trail. The single track rises gently and passes the Jones

Hikers hut, near the junction of the Towne Fire Road and the Heritage Grove Trail, can be reserved for overnight use.

### The Joy of Trees

Joining the redwoods in this park are Douglas-firs, interior live oaks, tanbark oaks, madrones, hazelnut, blue blossom, and evergreen huckleberry. Coast live oak, California bay, creambush, and gooseberry grow at the park's higher elevations.

Gulch Trail, right. A steady gain of elevation leads you through a forest of Douglas-fir, California bay, tanbark oak, and toyon. Beyond the next seasonal horse gate, you reach a dirt road (not shown on the park map), and angle across it. Now descend to a T-junction with a dirt road, and stay on the Pomponio Trail by turning right. Crossing Worley Flat, a gorgeous meadow, you arrive a the next junction, also a T, and turn left on a dirt road. When you reach Pescadero Creek, cross it via a bridge. Then climb to the Old Haul Road Trail, turn right, and retrace your route to the parking area.

## TRIP4 Sam McDonald Park

| | |
|---|---|
| **Distance** | 4 miles, Loop |
| **Hiking Time** | 2 to 3 hours |
| **Elevation Gain/Loss** | ±700 feet |
| **Difficulty** | Moderate |
| **Trail Use** | Backpacking option |
| **Best Times** | All year |
| **Agency** | SMCP&R |
| **Recommended Map** | *Sam McDonald Park* (SMCP&R) |

**HIGHLIGHTS** Although in the past logging decimated vast swaths of the Santa Cruz Mountains' ancient redwood forests, you can still wander amid magnificent groves that were preserved thanks to the efforts of individuals, groups, and government agencies. This loop uses the Heritage Grove Trail and the Towne Fire Road to visit the Heritage Grove of coast redwoods, and then climb to a grassy ridge where expansive views await. Backpackers will enjoy a hikers "hut," actually a full-service cabin, near the route's high point. Reservations are through the Sierra Club's Loma Prieta chapter, www.lomaprieta.sierraclub.org or (650) 390-8411.

**DIRECTIONS** From the intersection of Highway 84 and Pescadero Road in La Honda, go southeast on Pescadero Road, and after 1 mile turn right to stay on Pescadero Road at its intersection with Alpine Road. Go another 0.6 mile to the park entrance, right. Pay fee at the self-registration station.

**FACILITIES/TRAILHEAD** Group hike-in campsites are available for organized groups by reservation (youth groups have first priority); (650) 363-4020. A ranger station, picnic tables, restrooms, phone, and water are near the trailhead, which is on the northwest corner of the parking area.

The Heritage Grove Trail, a single track, skirts the north side of the parking area and after about 100 yards reaches Pescadero Road. Carefully cross the road and regain the trail beside a metal gate. Your route is a wide dirt path that slopes gently downhill through stands of towering coast redwoods. Occasional Douglas-firs compete with the redwoods in girth and height.

Other members of the redwood-forest community, such as evergreen huckleberry, hazelnut, and tanbark oak, grow beside the trail. Where the redwoods yield

### Redwoods Galore
Redwoods have several means of reproduction, including from seeds and from stumps of cut or fallen trees. This latter method, a form of cloning, commonly produces a so-called family circle of new trees around the remains of their ancestor. Sometimes, however, a new tree will sprout directly from the stump of an old one, and this park has many examples of this type of regeneration.

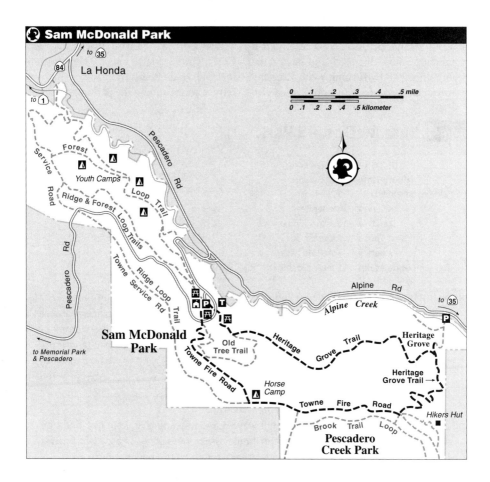

## Sam McDonald Park

and allow more light, you may find madrone, California bay, and interior live oak, and shrubs such as thimbleberry and creambush.

Now the trail swings left and begins a moderate climb. At a junction with the Big Tree Trail, right, you stay on the Heritage Grove Trail and climb on a gentle grade. On a sunny day, shafts of light filter through the forest canopy, highlighting individual trees against a shadowy backdrop.

At a junction, the Heritage Grove Trail, signed HIKERS HUT, turns right. To view the Heritage Grove of redwoods, continue straight for several hundred yards as the trail wanders amid superb specimens that were spared the logger's axe thanks to the fundraising efforts of concerned citizens

and San Mateo County matching funds. (The trail eventually descends to a parking area beside Alpine Road, but the best views of the upper grove come before you lose elevation.)

Springtime flowers here include trillium, clintonia, starflower, redwood sorrel, and forget-me-not. Bigleaf maple trees add color in fall and preside over an understory that includes toyon, pinkflower currant, and blue blossom.

When you have finished enjoying the magnificent trees, return to the junction, bear left, and follow the Heritage Grove Trail uphill on a grade that alternates between gentle and moderate. After a steady ascent, some of it steep, you reach a metal gate which you pass on the left.

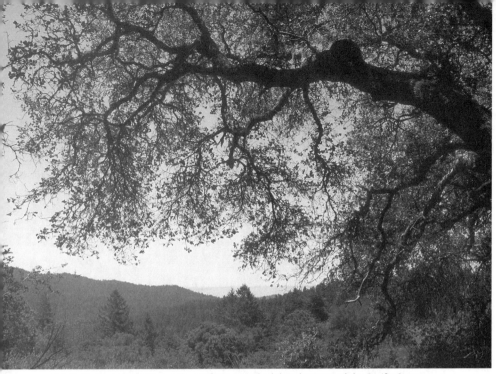

Oak limbs frame the view southwest from near the hikers hut toward the Pacific Ocean.

Suddenly you are out of the woods, crossing a wide, grassy field dotted with California poppies, blue-eyed grass, yarrow, and scarlet pimpernel.

Just ahead, at about 2.5 miles, is a junction. Here the Towne Fire Road goes left and right; a short connector to the Brook Trail Loop goes straight; and a trail to the Sierra Club hut angles sharply left. To spend a few minutes relaxing on the deck of the hikers hut, follow the trail as it crosses open

### Mr. McDonald

This park honors Sam (Emanuel) McDonald, a former Stanford employee, who was born in Louisiana and whose ancestors were slaves. McDonald became superintendent of Stanford's athletic grounds and buildings and was also active in law enforcement. McDonald, who died in 1957, left more than 400 acres to Stanford, requesting that the land be used as a park to benefit youth. San Mateo County acquired the land in 1958 and opened it to the public in 1970.

grassland and then switchbacks uphill through the trees.

From the junction of the Heritage Grove Trail and the Towne Fire Road, head west on the dirt road, which runs atop a ridge. The Brook Trail Loop, popular with equestrians, is left. The road follows a rolling course as it wanders through stands of coast live oak and passes another connector to the Brook Trail Loop, left. Now descending, you enjoy a picturesque scene in the distance—a barn, a wood fence, and a few Fremont cottonwoods, which turn bright gold in fall. At a junction, a dirt road heads right to the Jack Brook Memorial Horse Camp. Your route, the Towne Fire Road, turns left.

About 150 feet ahead, you stay on the Towne Fire Road by veering right at a junction with the Ridge Trail, also a dirt road. Now in a dense forest of redwoods and lichen-draped coast live oaks, you descend moderately beside a ravine, right. Soon the Big Tree Trail departs right, but you follow the road as it makes a winding descent, in places steep. Ahead, you meet two more junctions, also signed for the Big Tree Trail, right. Relief for your knees comes when you reach a fence with a gate and a gap. Just beyond is Pescadero Road, which you carefully cross. Now you find a single-track trail, which soon deposits you back at the parking area.

## *TRIP 5* Memorial Park

| | |
|---|---|
| **Distance** | 3.2 miles, Semi-loop |
| **Hiking Time** | 1 to 2 hours |
| **Elevation Gain/Loss** | ±800 feet |
| **Difficulty** | Moderate |
| **Best Times** | All year |
| **Agency** | SMCP&R |
| **Recommended Map** | *Memorial Park* (SMCP&R) |

**HIGHLIGHTS** This short but enjoyable semi-loop uses the Pomponio Trail to explore a redwood forest, a creek-filled canyon, and a ridge with great views.

**DIRECTIONS** From the intersection of Highway 84 and Pescadero Road in La Honda, go southeast on Pescadero Road, and after 1 mile turn right to stay on Pescadero Road at its intersection with Alpine Road. Go another 4.4 miles to the Memorial Park entrance, on your left. At 0.1 mile there are an entrance kiosk and a self-registration station. Continue straight another 0.1 mile to the Tan Oak Flat picnic/parking area.

**FACILITIES/TRAILHEAD** Camping is available. A visitor center, camp store, and restrooms (all open seasonally) are near the entrance kiosk, along with phone and water. There are picnic tables and restrooms (open seasonally) near the parking area. The trailhead is on the north side of Pescadero Road, opposite the park entrance.

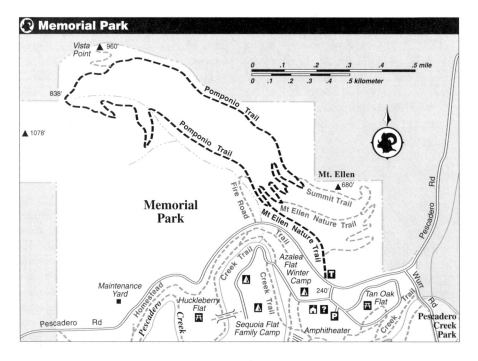

From the trailhead, which serves the Mt. Ellen Nature Trail, the Mt. Ellen Summit Trail, and the Pomponio Trail, you climb gently on a wide dirt-and-gravel path through stands of coast redwood, Douglas-fir, coast live oak, tanbark oak, and fragrant California bay. At a junction, the Mt. Ellen Summit and Nature trails, here joined as one, veer right, but you stay on the Pomponio Trail.

The name Memorial refers to a dedication that took place in 1924 honoring San Mateo County residents killed in World War I. Later, during the Depression, WPA work crews built picnic sites, restrooms, and roads in the park.

The trail climbs moderately via switchbacks, then follows a rolling course across a hillside that drops left. Soon you reach a junction with a trail, right, signed MT. ELLEN SUMMIT TRAIL. This is actually the returning leg of the Pomponio Trail, which you will use later. For now stay left, then merge with a dirt road by bearing right.

Now you climb moderately beside a creek lined with willows and bigleaf maples, colorful in fall. A sharp bend to the left takes you across the creek, which flows through a culvert. The road continues to wind its way uphill on a moderate grade, climbing out of a canyon. At the head of the

---

### Cloud's Clout

Massive redwood stumps here are remnants of the area's logging past, which lasted from 1856 to around 1930. About a dozen mills producing lumber and shingles were active along Pescadero Creek and its tributaries. Many of the trees in present-day Memorial Park were spared this onslaught, thanks to the advocacy of Roy W. Cloud, superintendent of schools for San Mateo County. Impressed by a visit here in the spring of 1923, and with the logger's axe about to fall, Cloud convinced the county board of supervisors to intervene.

---

### Flora

Evergreen huckleberry, hazelnut, and creambush, along with an assortment of flowers and ferns, grow in the park's forested areas. Sunny, open slopes are home to thickets of coyote brush, California sagebrush, blue blossom, coffeeberry, creambush, bush monkeyflower, and poison oak.

---

canyon, the road ends, and you follow a single-track trail that soon crosses a bridge over the creek's uppermost reaches.

At about 1.5 miles, a rest bench, left, provides a place to sit and enjoy the view. California fuchsia, one of the Bay Area's latest-blooming wildflowers and a favorite with hummingbirds, grows nearby. Nearby, a short trail goes left to a viewpoint. Flirting briefly with a forested ridgecrest, the trail soon switchbacks down to a flat area, then climbs moderately beside a precipice where towering Douglas-firs barely cling to the edge.

Now on a gentle descent, you come to a junction

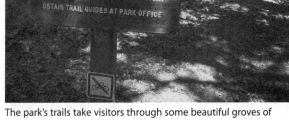

The park's trails take visitors through some beautiful groves of coast redwoods.

with the Mt. Ellen Summit Trail, left. Bear right and continue downhill, dropping into the redwood forest you explored earlier. Where the unsigned Mt. Ellen Nature Trail angles left, you go straight. After a left-hand switchback, you arrive at the junction that closes loop. From here, continue straight and retrace your route to the parking area.

# TRIP 6 Purisima Creek Redwoods Open Space Preserve: Harkins Ridge

| | |
|---|---|
| **Distance** | 7 miles, Loop |
| **Hiking Time** | 3 to 5 hours |
| **Elevation Gain/Loss** | ±1150 feet |
| **Difficulty** | Difficult |
| **Best Times** | All year |
| **Agency** | MROSD |
| **Recommended Map** | *Purisima Creek Redwoods Open Space Preserve* (MROSD) |

**HIGHLIGHTS**  Using the Harkins Ridge Trail, this invigorating loop starts by climbing more than 1000 feet, from the shady confines of redwood-lined Purisima Creek to a ridge with superb views of Half Moon Bay and the surrounding hills. The relaxing return is via the delightful Soda Gulch and Purisima Creek trails, giving you an opportunity to learn about and enjoy the redwood-forest community that still thrives here despite extensive logging in the 19th and early 20th centuries.

**DIRECTIONS**  From the intersection of Highway 1 and Higgins Purisima Road south of Half Moon Bay, take Higgins Purisima Road east 4.5 miles to a parking area, left.

**FACILITIES/TRAILHEAD**  None at the trailhead, which is at gate PC05, on the east side of the parking area. There is a toilet about 100 yards east on the Purisima Creek Trail.

Follow the Purisima Creek Trail, a dirt road, into a dense, secluded forest. After several hundred feet, you turn left, crossing lovely Purisima Creek on a wood bridge, and then come to a T-junction with the Harkins Ridge and Whittemore Gulch trails.

The forest here includes coast redwood, red alder, bigleaf maple, and tanbark oak. The understory is made up of common shrubs such as coffeeberry, thimbleberry, gooseberry, creambush, and elk clover. Growing beside the road are shade-loving wildflowers such as miner's lettuce, hedge nettle, forget-me-not, and two species of fairy bells, Hooker's and Smith's.

A right turn puts you on the gently rolling Harkins Ridge Trail, a dirt road that for a while runs parallel to the redwood-bordered creek. The grade steepens, and soon you begin a series of sweeping switch-backs that bring you to a brighter, more open realm. The view to your right takes in the canyon holding Purisima Creek and the ridge rising just south of the creek to Bald Knob, more than 2000 feet above sea level.

At one of the road's right-hand switch-backs, you have a fine vantage point that looks west toward Half Moon Bay and the

---

**Flower Bonanza**

Various wildflowers associated with redwood forests grow nearby, including redwood sorrel, which has clover-like leaves and pink flowers; columbine, told by its beautiful orange-and-yellow blossoms; starflower, each with a delicate flower held aloft on a thread-like stem; and red clintonia, a member of the lily family that produces clusters of pink blooms in early summer and blue berries later in the year.

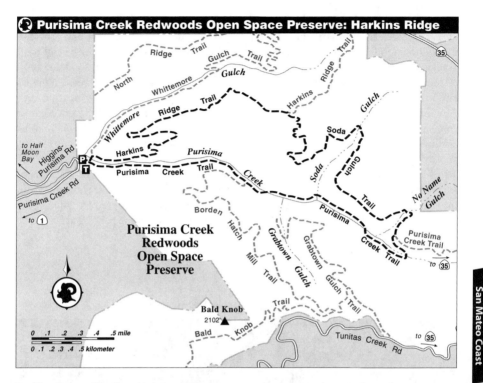

**Purisima Creek Redwoods Open Space Preserve: Harkins Ridge**

Purisima Creek Redwoods Open Space Preserve

Bald Knob 2102'

San Mateo Coast

Pacific Ocean. Finally gaining a ridgetop, you follow it uphill over rough ground. In places the grade is very steep, stretching your calf muscles to their limit. Otherwise it is a long, steady climb on a moderate grade. At about 2.1 miles, you meet the Soda Gulch Trail, part of the Bay Area Ridge Trail. Here you turn right and follow the single-track trail, closed to bicycles and horses, across an open slope of coastal scrub.

Now descending via switchbacks, you pass a beautiful stand of coast live oaks, their twisted, gnarled limbs draped with lace lichen. A sudden transition brings you into the realm of the redwoods. A rest bench, left, invites you to spend a few minutes contemplating these towering giants in cool and shady surroundings. Some of the trees are fire-scarred, and some grow in so-called family circles around a fallen ancestor.

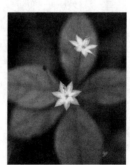

Starflower, which blooms from April to July, is found on the floor of shady forests.

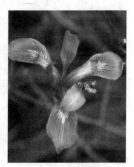

Douglas iris is one of the Bay Area's loveliest wildflowers, ranging from cream to lavender.

As you continue to lose elevation on a gentle grade, you pass a second rest bench and several seasonal creeks. Soda Gulch, another tributary of Purisima Creek, is downhill and right. When you reach Soda Gulch, turn sharply right to cross a bridge that spans the creek bed. Soon the route emerges briefly onto an open hillside before ducking back into the redwoods. You descend to an unnamed tributary of Purisima Creek and cross it on a bridge, then zigzag uphill meet the Purisima Creek Trail, a dirt road, at about 4.7 miles.

Join the road by bearing right, then follow it downhill to Purisima Creek, which flows under the road through a culvert. You enjoy a level walk through a riparian corridor lush with red alder, hazelnut, elk clover, and red elderberry. Soon a bridge takes you across Purisima Creek, which is now on your left. The creek from Soda Gulch joins from the right, and you cross it on the next bridge. Look here for tiger lilies in late spring.

On the left is a remnant of a bridge that once spanned Purisima Creek and provided a link with the Grabtown Gulch Trail until it was washed out during a flood. Descend on a moderate grade to the creek and cross it on a bridge, soon passing a junction with the Borden Hatch Mill Trail, left. One of Purisima Canyon's many lumber mills stood in a nearby clearing. At about 7 miles, you pass a toilet, left, and then close the loop at the connector to the Whittemore Gulch and Harkins Ridge trails, right. From here, go straight and retrace your route about 100 yards to the parking area.

The Soda Gulch Trail wanders downhill through a beautiful redwood forest

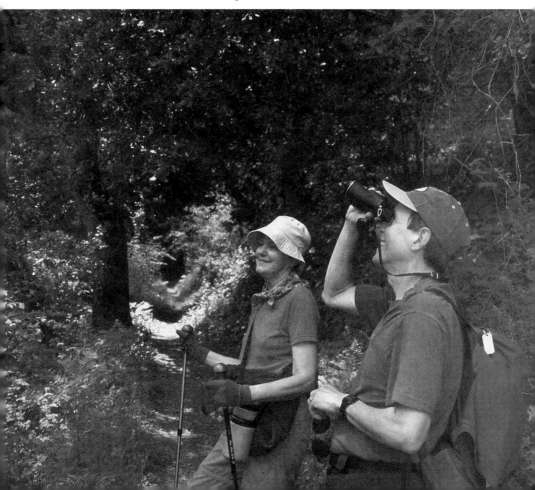

*Chapter 10*

# Peninsula

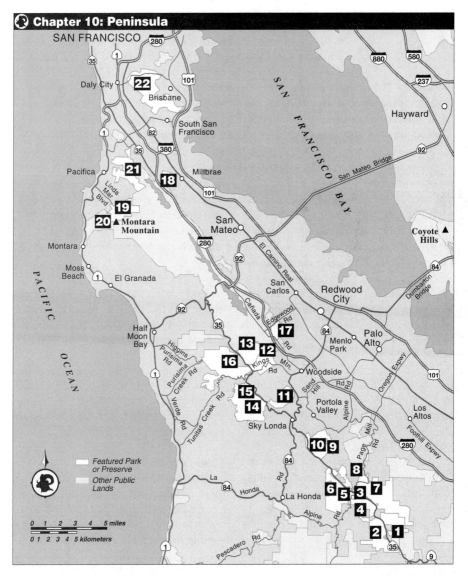

SAN FRANCISCO

Daly City

Brisbane

South San Francisco

Hayward

Pacifica

Millbrae

Linda Mar Blvd

Montara Mountain

San Mateo

Coyote Hills

Montara

Moss Beach

El Granada

San Carlos

Redwood City

Palo Alto

PACIFIC

Half Moon Bay

Higgins Purisima Rd

Purisima Creek Rd

Menlo Park

Woodside

OCEAN

Kings Rd

Portola Valley

Los Altos

Tunitas Creek Rd

Verde Rd

Sky Londa

Sand Hill Rd

Alpine Rd

Page Mill Rd

Oregon Expwy

Foothill Expwy

La Honda Rd

La Honda

Alpine Rd

Pescadero Rd

Featured Park or Preserve

Other Public Lands

0  1  2  3  4  5 miles

0 1 2 3 4 5 kilometers

San Mateo Bridge

Dumbarton Bridge

El Camino Real

Cañada Rd

Edgewood Rd

Mtn.

SAN FRANCISCO BAY

PACIFIC OCEAN

# TRIP 1 Upper Stevens Creek County Park/Long Ridge Open Space Preserve

| | |
|---:|:---|
| **Distance** | 10.2 miles, Loop |
| **Hiking Time** | 4 to 6 hours |
| **Elevation Gain/Loss** | ±2000 feet |
| **Difficulty** | Very difficult |
| **Trail Use** | Mountain biking allowed[1] |
| **Best Times** | Spring through fall |
| **Agency** | MROSD, SCCP&R |
| **Recommended Map** | *South Skyline Region* (MROSD) |
| **Notes** | [1]Bicycles are not allowed on the unnamed hiking-only trail, and are allowed going only uphill on the Table Mountain Trail and Charcoal Road. Thus, bicyclists must follow the loop in the opposite direction, and ascend from the Canyon Trail via the Table Mountain Trail and Charcoal Road. |

**HIGHLIGHTS**  This grand tour through Upper Stevens Creek County Park and Long Ridge Open Space Preserve uses the Table Mountain, Canyon, Grizzly Flat, Peters Creek, and Hickory Oaks trails, along with Ward Road and an unnamed hiking-only trail. It descends from Skyline Blvd. to Stevens Creek and back again, and then to climbs to the heights of Long Ridge, where views of the Pacific Ocean await. (Crossing Stevens Creek may be difficult and dangerous in wet weather.)

**DIRECTIONS**  From the intersection of Skyline Blvd. (Highway 35) and Page Mill Road/Alpine Road south of Palo Alto, take Skyline Blvd. southeast 5.1 miles to a road-side parking area on the left. If this area is full, turn around and go back about 100 yards on Skyline Blvd. to another parking area, right.

**FACILITIES/TRAILHEAD**  There are no facilities at the trailhead, which is on the northeast side of the parking area, near its midpoint.

Angle right (east) into dense forest on the Saratoga Gap Trail, part of the Bay Area Ridge Trail. This trail is popular with mountain bicyclists, so be alert. Losing elevation via several gentle bends, you then traverse a hillside that drops left. In a clearing you meet Charcoal Road, a dirt road that connects Skyline Blvd. with the Table Mountain Trail. Turn left, and after about 100 feet, leave the road to get on an unnamed hiking-only trail.

This single track curves sharply left and climbs into an area of chaparral, including manzanita, toyon, black sage, yerba santa, buckbrush, chamise, and chaparral pea. The trail swings right and follows a rolling ridgetop. The track becomes rocky, and you descend on a gentle grade, enjoying fine views of Stevens Creek canyon, Monte Bello Ridge, and the East Bay hills. Your route alternates between forest and chaparral, and the track varies from a narrow rut to a wide path.

The hiking-only trail shows signs of illegal mountain biking, and this no doubt contributes to the trail's deterioration. During wet weather, even *legal* biking can damage trails.

> **Trees Abounding**
>
> Typical trees in the Santa Cruz Mountains include Douglas-fir, tanbark oak, coast live oak, black oak, canyon oak, California bay, and madrone. California nutmeg, a species uncommon in the Bay Area, is also here.

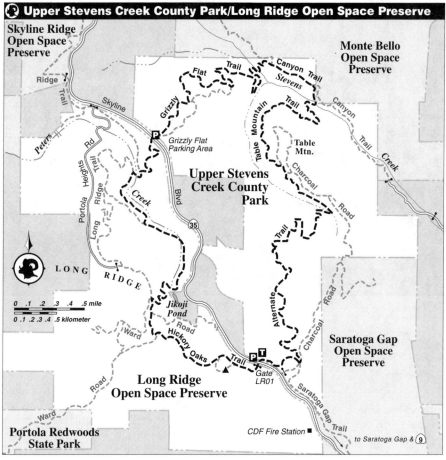

**Upper Stevens Creek County Park/Long Ridge Open Space Preserve**

Skyline Ridge
Open Space
Preserve

Ridge

Monte Bello
Open Space
Preserve

Skyline

Flat

Trail

Canyon Trail

Stevens

Grizzly

Trail

Stevens

Canyon

Trail

Peters

Rd

Grizzly Flat
Parking Area

Table Mountain

Table
Mtn.

Trail

Creek

Portola Heights Trail

Long Ridge Trail

Creek

Blvd

Upper Stevens
Creek County
Park

Charcoal

Road

35

LONG

RIDGE

Trail

Alternate

Charcoal Road

0 .1 .2 .3 .4 .5 mile
0 .1 .2 .3 .4 .5 kilometer

Jikoji
Pond

Road

Ward

Hickory

Oaks

Trail

Gate
LR01

Saratoga Gap
Open Space
Preserve

Long Ridge
Open Space Preserve

Ward

Road

Portola Redwoods
State Park

CDF Fire Station ■

Saratoga Gap Trail

to Saratoga Gap & 9

Peninsula

Using switchbacks, you descend over progressively steeper and more-eroded ground. Plunging into a canyon that holds a seasonal creek, you cross it and then wander through a fern garden on a mostly level grade. At the head of the next canyon, you turn sharply left and cross a hillside—in places, the trail is merely a narrow ledge.

Crossing another seasonal creek—this one meanders through a lovely, fern-filled canyon—you turn left and climb on a moderate and then gentle grade. Soon you come to a grassy clearing dotted with pines, madrones, and cypresses. Climbing steeply along the clearing's left edge, you reach a junction with a dirt road, about 3 miles. Here you join the road by bearing left.

Just ahead, turn left on the unsigned Table Mountain Trail, a single track, and descend moderately and then gently over rough ground. In dense forest, you drop into the canyon holding Stevens Creek, where the plant life is jungle-like, with plenty of ferns and berry vines. Bigleaf maples, sure indicators of ample moisture, tower over the trail.

Eroded switchbacks take you down to a wood bridge over a tributary of Stevens Creek. When you reach Stevens Creek itself, you cross it on rocks or logs. Once across, you have another tributary on your left. Continue on the Table Mountain Trail, a single track, passing an unsigned trail on your right. At the next junction, just ahead,

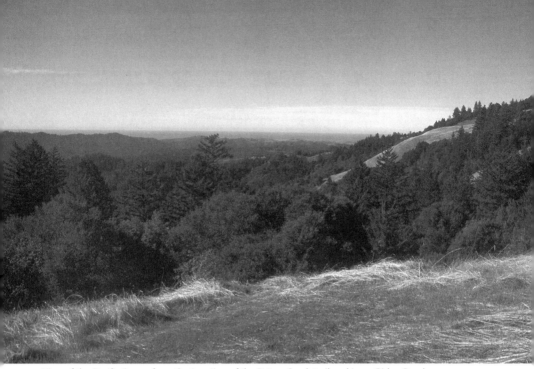
View of the Pacific Ocean from the junction of the Peters Creek trail and Long Ridge Road.

you join the Canyon Trail, a major thoroughfare connecting Page Mill and Stevens Canyon roads.

> **They're Stunners**
> During the rainy season, the seeds of California buckeyes germinate, splitting the pod and producing a long tap root. Often, the root starts out skyward but later bends in search of soil. Buckeye seeds are very poisonous — Native Americans used to place them in streams to stun fish.

Bearing left, you step across the tributary you've been following and then climb on a gentle grade. Gooseberry, mountain mahogany, and hollyleaf cherry grow here, the latter two seeming out of place in this damp, shady environment. The trail runs along the bottom of a narrow canyon whose floor tilts upward at a moderate and then steep angle. After a steady climb, you turn left on the Grizzly Flat Trail.

With another tributary of Stevens Creek on your right, you wind downhill to Stevens Creek, which you cross on rocks or logs. Once across, walk downstream to find the continuation of the Grizzly Flat Trail. A short, moderate climb brings you to a junction at Grizzly Flat, where you stay on the Grizzly Flat Trail by turning right. Grizzly Flat is a ladybug wintering site, and you may see thousands of these colorful creatures attached to leaves and stems of nearby foliage.

The road snakes its way uphill through a mixed-evergreen forest, gaining elevation on a grade that alternates between gentle and moderate. Twice, roads join from the left, but you continue straight. As you near Skyline Blvd., a trail merges sharply from the left. At about 7 miles, you reach a gate and an information board. Just beyond is Skyline Blvd.

Carefully cross Skyline Blvd. and go several hundred feet left to a trailhead for Long Ridge Open Space Preserve.

Follow the Peters Creek Trail, a single track, as it wanders across a hillside that may be colorfully decorated with wildflowers in spring. Soon the trail swings left and descends into a cool, dark forest. At a junction, a trail merges sharply from the right. This is the Ridge Trail, which heads north to Skyline Ridge Open Space Preserve. The Ridge Trail and the Peters Creek Trail (from this point on) are both part of the Bay Area Ridge Trail.

You continue straight and after several hundred feet cross the trail's namesake creek on a bridge. Another couple of hundred feet ahead is the next junction, where the Long Ridge Trail joins from the right. Again you continue straight, passing an amazing fern garden in the creek bed to your left.

Now in the open, you enjoy a level walk past willow thickets that line the creek and the remains of a still-prolific apple orchard that blooms beautifully in spring. Ahead, a dirt road heading sharply right connects to the Long Ridge Trail.

From here, you continue straight on the Peters Creek Trail, now a dirt road, passing several unsigned junctions, left. Soon you cross Peters Creek, which flows under the road through a culvert. Where a gated dirt road angles left to the preserve boundary, you turn right and cross an earthen dam. Built in the 1960s, this 200-foot-long dam turned part of Peters Creek into the cattail-fringed lake on your left. On the far side of the dam, Peters Creek drains water from the lake, and you cross the creek on a wooden bridge.

Now the trail zigzags uphill through forest to a four-way junction atop Long Ridge, at about 9 miles. Here, turn left on Ward Road and climb through a shady grove of Douglas-fir, bay, and coast live oak. At the next junction, leave the road by angling slightly right on a single-track connector to the Hickory Oaks Trail. An expansive view to your right sweeps across a forested sea of parklands and on to the Pacific Ocean. You pass a rest bench, left, and then arrive at the Hickory Oaks Trail, a dirt road.

Turning left, you climb moderately, and in a few spots steeply, over rocky and eroded ground without a whit of shade. A rolling course soon brings you into a forest of bay and madrone. A single-track trail goes right, loops around a hill, and rejoins on the right. Your road descends gently, then comes to a junction where you veer left. (The trail going straight dead-ends.)

Ahead on the left are two information boards and a map holder. Just past them, leave the road and follow a single track that heads left to Skyline Blvd. The main parking area is just across Skyline: cross carefully! The overflow parking area is about 100 yards to your left. To reach it, stay on this side of Skyline and walk facing oncoming traffic. When you are opposite the overflow parking area, cross carefully.

## TRIP2 Long Ridge Open Space Preserve

| | |
|---|---|
| **Distance** | 4.6 miles, Semi-loop |
| **Hiking Time** | 2 to 3 hours |
| **Elevation Gain/Loss** | ±850 feet |
| **Difficulty** | Moderate |
| **Trail Use** | Mountain biking alowed |
| **Best Times** | All year |
| **Agency** | MROSD |
| **Recommended Map** | *South Skyline Region* (MROSD) |

**HIGHLIGHTS** Superb views are the reason to wander uphill from the shady confines of Peters Creek to the dramatically situated Wallace Stegner memorial bench high atop Long Ridge. On a clear day, the scene extends westward over the Pescadero Creek watershed, taking in thousands of acres of protected lands, truly a living monument to the open-space movement. This semi-loop route uses the Ridge, Peters Creek, and Long Ridge trails, along with Long Ridge Road.

**DIRECTIONS** From the intersection of Skyline Blvd. (Highway 35) and Page Mill Road/Alpine Road south of Palo Alto, take Skyline Blvd. southeast 3.1 miles to a roadside parking area on the left. This parking area, sometimes called Grizzly Flat, serves both Long Ridge Open Space Preserve and Upper Stevens Creek County Park.

**FACILITIES/TRAILHEAD** There are no facilities at the trailhead, which is on the southwest side of Skyline Blvd., across from the parking area.

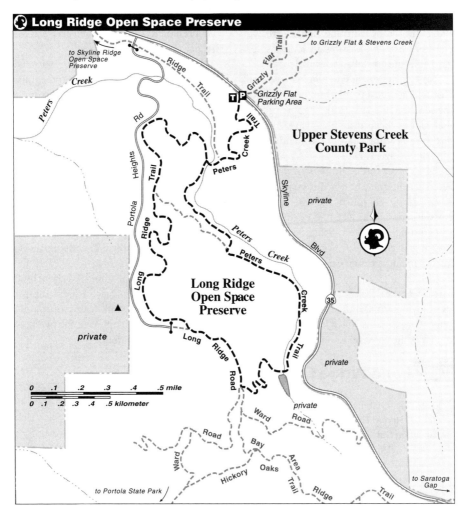

**Long Ridge Open Space Preserve**

F ollow the Peters Creek Trail, a single track, as it wanders across a hillside that may be colorfully decorated with wildflowers in spring. Soon the trail swings left and descends into a cool, dark forest. At a junction, a trail merges sharply from the right. This is the Ridge Trail, which heads north to Skyline Ridge Open Space Preserve. The Ridge Trail and the Peters Creek Trail (from this point on) are both part of the Bay Area Ridge Trail.

You continue straight and after several hundred feet cross the trail's namesake creek on a bridge. This is a lovely area, shaded by stands of bigleaf maple and tanbark oak. Another couple of hundred feet ahead is the next junction, where the Long Ridge Trail joins from the right. Again you continue straight, passing an amazing fern garden in the creek bed to your left.

Now in the open, you enjoy a level walk past willow thickets that line the creek and the remains of a still-prolific apple orchard that blooms beautifully in spring and is often heavily loaded with several varieties of apples in fall. Ahead, a dirt road heading sharply right connects to the Long Ridge Trail. (To shorten this route, turn right, climb gently for 0.4 mile, veer right on the Long Ridge Trail near gate LR12, and follow the description below.)

---

**Long Ridge Flora**

- Coast live oak, canyon oak, tanbark oak, Douglas-fir, California bay, madrone, and bigleaf maple are among the trees found here. Shrubs include toyon, coffeeberry, blue elderberry, hazelnut, buckbrush, and snowberry.
- Search for spring wildflowers such as hound's tongue, milkmaids, shooting stars, mission bells, fairy bells, and a beautiful violet called western heart's ease.

---

From here, you continue straight on the Peters Creek Trail, now a dirt road, passing several unsigned junctions, left. Soon you cross Peters Creek, which flows under the road through a culvert. Where a gated dirt road angles left to the preserve boundary, you turn right and cross an earthen dam. Built in the 1960s, this 200-foot-long dam turned part of Peters Creek into the cattail-fringed lake on your left. Since 1979, the lake has been the property of a Buddhist group, now known as Jikoji, which runs a nearby meditation center. On the far side of

**The Bench**

Wallace Stegner (1909–1993) was one of California's best-loved writers and a tireless advocate for land preservation. In the 1960s, Stegner and others bought about 400 acres of land that later became part of this preserve. The bench was built and dedicated to Stegner's memory by MROSD in 1996 and reads,

> ... to try to save for everyone, for the hostile and indifferent as well as the committed, some of the health that flows down across the green ridges from the Skyline, and some of the beauty and refreshment of spirit that are still available to any resident of the valley who has a moment, and the wit, to lift up his eyes unto the hills.
>
> -Wallace Stegner

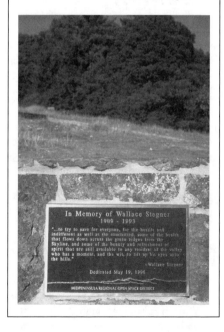

the dam, Peters Creek drains water from the lake, and you cross the creek on a wooden bridge.

Now the trail zigzags uphill through forest to a four-way junction atop Long Ridge, at about 2 miles. Here you turn right on Long Ridge Road and enjoy a fabulous view, which extends westward across the Pescadero Creek drainage to the Pacific Ocean. Soon leaving the ridgetop, you follow a rolling course through mostly open terrain to the Wallace Stegner memorial bench, which is just left of the road. The bench is a great spot to sit and reflect on the value of open space.

Just past the Stegner bench, you veer right on the single-track Long Ridge Trail.

After several hundred feet you enter dense forest and contour across a hillside that drops right. Crossing a saddle, you begin to descend via curves and switchbacks, soon reaching a junction in a clearing. Cross the clearing to find the continuation of the Long Ridge Trail, which eventually descends on a moderate and then steep grade to close the loop at the Peters Creek Trail. Here you turn left and retrace your route to the parking area.

# **TRIP3 South Skyline Region**

| | |
|---|---|
| **Distance** | 6.5 miles, Loop |
| **Hiking Time** | 4 to 5 hours |
| **Elevation Gain/Loss** | ±1500 feet |
| **Difficulty** | Difficult |
| **Trail Use** | Mountain biking allowed[1] |
| **Best Times** | All year |
| **Agency** | MROSD |
| **Recommended Map** | *South Skyline Region* (MROSD) |
| **Notes** | [1]Use alternate trailhead/trails in Skyline Ridge Open Space Preserve. |

**HIGHLIGHTS** This varied and vigorous loop visits four adjoining MROSD preserves — Monte Bello, Coal Creek, Russian Ridge, and Skyline Ridge. Each preserve offers something different: shady oak woodlands, forested canyons, wildflower-strewn slopes, and grassy ridges. The route combines the Skid Road, White Oak, Meadow, Clouds Rest, and Ridge Trails with a short stretch of Alpine Road to explore the heart of the South Skyline Region, where open space acquisitions have made it possible to wander over some of the Bay Area's most beautiful terrain.

**DIRECTIONS** From the intersection of Skyline Blvd. (Highway 35) and Page Mill Road/Alpine Road, take Skyline Blvd. southeast 0.9 mile to an entrance to Skyline Ridge Open Space Preserve on the right. Bear right and go 0.2 mile to a parking area.

**FACILITIES/TRAILHEAD** There is a toilet beside the parking area. The trailhead is about 200 feet east of the parking area, on the north side of the preserve entrance road.

Go about 30 feet from the trailhead to Skyline Blvd., which you carefully cross. Just past gate MB06, you enter Monte Bello Open Space Preserve and turn left on the Skid Road Trail, a rough dirt road that descends gently. Dropping into a dense forest, you soon meet the White Oak Trail. Turn left and descend into a canyon, where a wood bridge helps you across a creek.

After crossing the creek and wandering through a possibly muddy area, the trail makes a rising traverse across a grassy hillside, home to the trail's namesake Oregon, or white, oaks.

Climbing moderately via switchbacks, you gradually win back lost elevation, and this change in perspective provides dramatic views that extend east to Monte Bello Ridge and Black Mountain, and southeast to Mt. Umunhum and Loma Prieta.

Soon you come to a fence and gate, just beyond which is a T-junction. Turn left and

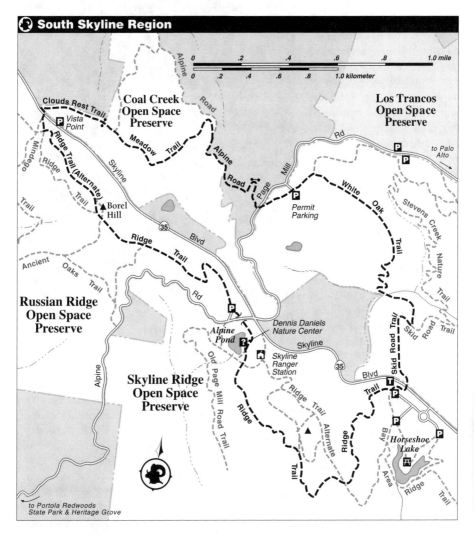

## South Skyline Region

Coal Creek Open Space Preserve

Los Trancos Open Space Preserve

Russian Ridge Open Space Preserve

Skyline Ridge Open Space Preserve

Clouds Rest Trail

Vista Point

Meadow Trail

Alpine Road

Ridge Trail (Alternate)

Borel Hill

Ridge Trail

Ancient Oaks Trail

Page Mill Road

White Oak Trail

Permit Parking

Stevens Creek Nature Trail

Alpine Pond

Dennis Daniels Nature Center

Skyline

Skyline Ranger Station

Ridge Trail Alternate

Skid Road Trail

Horseshoe Lake

to Palo Alto

to Portola Redwoods State Park & Heritage Grove

0  .2  .4  .6  .8  1.0 mile

0  .2  .4  .6  .8  1.0 kilometer

Peninsula

follow the trail, here a dirt road but later a single track, past a paved driveway to a junction and gate MB05. Here, at about 2 miles, you turn right, carefully cross Page Mill Road, and get on Alpine Road. The first 50 feet or so of Alpine Road are paved, but once you pass a driveway, left, and then a gate it changes to dirt and gravel. (This part of Alpine Road is closed to vehicles but gets a lot of bicycle traffic, so stay right.)

At a junction with the Meadow Trail, turn left and enter Coal Creek Open Space Preserve. Climb the shrub-lined trail moderately through meadows to forest, where the grade changes to steep. Where you finally reach level ground the vistas extend from the Peninsula to Mt. Diablo. When you reach the Clouds Rest Trail (may be unsigned), turn left and climb to Skyline Blvd. Now turn left and walk uphill along the road's east shoulder, facing traffic—be very careful of oncoming vehicles!

After about 100 yards, you reach the northwest end of the Caltrans Vista Point parking area. Here, turn right and very carefully cross Skyline Blvd. to reach an entrance to Russian Ridge Open Space Preserve, at gate RR01. Just beyond two information boards is the first of several junctions. Angle left at the first and get on the Ridge Trail, a wide single track. There are two Ridge Trails in this preserve: one is part of the Bay Area Ridge Trail; the other is a 0.5-mile segment of dirt road that traverses Borel Hill, called the Ridge Trail (alternate) in this book.

After about 100 feet, turn left on the Ridge Trail (alternate), an eroded path that snakes its way uphill. At a four-way junction, a trail goes right to a vantage point, but you turn left for the final push to the top of Borel Hill, where a sign shows you are 2572 feet above sea level. When you are ready to leave this dramatic perch, put the elevation sign at your back and follow the

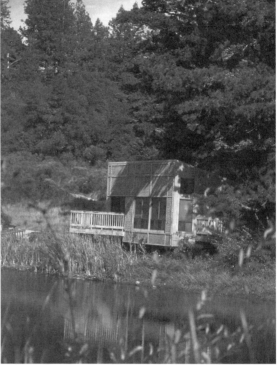

The Daniels Nature Center looks out over Alpine Pond in Skyline Ridge Open Space Preserve.

trail in front of you. It soon joins the Ridge Trail (alternate) at a T-junction. Turn left, and after about 100 feet merge with the Ridge Trail. Soon you pass an unnamed trail, right, not shown on the preserve map.

When you reach a connector, right, to the Ancient Oaks Trail, just past 4 miles, go another 0.5 mile on the Ridge Trail to the Russian Ridge/Skyline Ridge parking area at the corner of Skyline Blvd. and Alpine Road.

A set of steps and also a wheelchair-accessible path lead down from the parking area and join as the Ridge Trail beside an information board. Take the Ridge Trail under Alpine Road through a tunnel and enter Skyline Ridge Open Space Preserve. After passing a gravel road, left, you arrive at Alpine Pond and the nature center. The Pond Loop Trail, a short route around the pond, joins sharply from the right.

Just past the nature center you come to a fork where you bear left. Soon the trail crosses a culvert, angles right, and arrives at a four-way junction with a paved road. You continue straight, passing an unsigned trail and a fenced building, both uphill and left.

## Skyline Flora, Birds

- Early blooming forest wildflowers include trillium, hound's tongue, and slim Solomon. Later in spring, look for western heart's-ease and starflower.
- Oregon oaks are found mostly from farther north in California to Vancouver Island, British Columbia, but a few stands occur in the Bay Area. Identification can be tricky, and it took MROSD personnel several years to decide that trees on a Monte Bello Open Space Preserve hillside were Oregon, and not valley, oaks.
- Savannas, with their combination of wooded groves and open meadows, are great places to look for birds. Some common species found here include spotted towhee, northern flicker, and Steller's jay.

Emerging from the forest, you make a rising traverse across an open hillside. Now the trail makes a couple of bends, crosses a culvert, and curves around a rock outcrop, left. Just beyond a rest bench, left, is a view westward to the Pacific.

From this vantage point you climb steadily on a moderate grade into a zone of chaparral, mostly chamise, toyon, buckbrush, bush monkeyflower, yerba santa, and hollyleaf cherry. California poppies, lupine, checkerbloom, owl's-clover, red maids, bluedicks, and blue-eyed grass may dot the grasslands with color.

After meeting an unsigned trail, left, you round a rock outcrop that looms over a steep slope. Here the trail is buttressed by a concrete footing to hold it in place. There are more fine views from this spot, dubbed "Rattlesnake Point" by some MROSD personnel who encountered the reptiles while building the trail.

A stretch of level trail leads you through extensive groves of manzanita and silk tassel. As the trail curves sharply left, you begin to get sweeping views that extend southeast toward Mt. Umunhum. Monte Bello Ridge, topped by Black Mountain, is northeast. The San Andreas fault and the canyon holding Stevens Creek run parallel to Monte Bello Ridge.

Now you make a gently descending traverse across an open hillside that plunges about 600 feet to Lambert Creek. At a four-way junction with the alternate trail for bicyclists and equestrians, you continue straight and soon regain dense forest. Crossing a culvert, the route bends sharply right and then wanders downhill to the parking area to close the loop.

## TRIP4 Skyline Ridge Open Space Preserve

| | |
|---|---|
| **Distance** | 3.4 miles, Out-and-back |
| **Hiking Time** | 2 to 3 hours |
| **Elevation Gain/Loss** | ±250 feet |
| **Difficulty** | Moderate |
| **Trail Use** | Good for kids |
| **Best Times** | All year |
| **Agency** | MROSD |
| **Recommended Map** | *South Skyline Region* (MROSD) |

Peninsula

**HIGHLIGHTS** This out-and-back jaunt along the Ridge Trail rises from the forested environs of Alpine Pond to a breezy realm of grassland and chaparral where views of Butano Ridge, Portola Redwoods State Park, and the Pacific coast await. The spring wildflowers here are superb, and it is easy to see why this stretch of trail is a Peninsula favorite. The Ridge Trail is part of the Bay Area Ridge Trail, but the segment described here is for hiking only. (Bicyclists and equestrians headed for Horseshoe Lake and beyond must use a trailhead just across Alpine Road and then follow an alternate trail.)

**DIRECTIONS** From the intersection of Skyline Blvd. (Highway 35) and Page Mill Road/Alpine Road south of Palo Alto, take Alpine Road west about 100 yards to a parking area on the right. (This parking area serves both Skyline Ridge Open Space Preserve and Russian Ridge Open Space Preserve. On busy days parking may be unavailable. Additional parking with access to the preserve's trails is available at the parking area for Horseshoe Lake, 0.9 mile southeast on Skyline Blvd.)

**FACILITIES/TRAILHEAD** The David C. Daniels Nature Center, about 0.1 mile south of the parking area on the Ridge Trail, is open to the public on weekends from mid-March through November, and to school groups by arrangement with MROSD. There is a toilet near the trailhead, which is on the south side of the parking area.

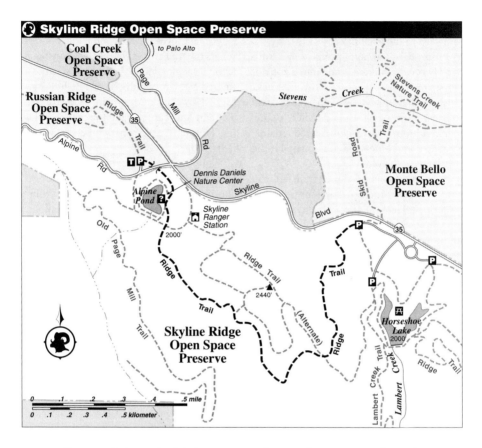

A set of steps and also a wheelchair-accessible path lead down from the parking area and join as the Ridge Trail, beside an information board. Take the Ridge Trail under Alpine Road through a tunnel and soon enter a sheltering forest. After passing a gravel road, left, you arrive at Alpine Pond and the nature center. The Pond Loop Trail, a short route around the pond, joins sharply from the right.

Just past the nature center you come to a fork, where you bear left. Soon the trail crosses a culvert, angles right, and arrives at a four-way junction with a paved road. You continue straight, soon passing an unsigned trail and a fenced building, both uphill and left.

Emerging from the forest, you make a rising traverse across an open hillside. Now the trail makes a couple of bends, crosses a culvert, and curves around a rock outcrop, left. Just beyond a rest bench, left, is a view westward to the Pacific. From this vantage point you climb steadily on a moderate grade into a zone of chaparral, mostly chamise, toyon, buckbrush, bush monkeyflower, yerba santa, and hollyleaf cherry.

> **Alpine Pond**
> This small, serene body of water is an oasis of life, providing habitat for mammals, birds, fish, and amphibians, including red-winged blackbirds, coots, crayfish, bluegills, and western pond turtles.

After meeting an unsigned trail, left, you round a rock outcrop that looms over a steep slope. Here the trail is buttressed by a concrete footing to hold it in place. There

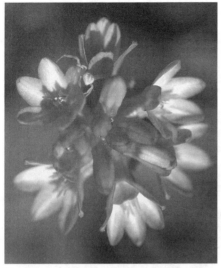

Bluedicks has clusters of small, lavender flowers at the end of a long, slender stem.

topped by Black Mountain, is northeast. The San Andreas fault and the canyon holding Stevens Creek run parallel to Monte Bello Ridge.

The seemingly solid ground on which you stand is part of the Pacific plate, creeping northwest and slowly leaving most of North America behind.

Now you make a gently descending traverse across an open hillside that plunges about 600 feet to Lambert Creek. At a four-way junction with the alternate trail for bicyclists and equestrians, you continue straight and soon regain dense forest. Crossing a culvert, the route bends sharply right and then wanders downhill to a parking area for Horseshoe Lake. From here, retrace your route back to the parking area.

are more fine views from this spot, dubbed "Rattlesnake Point" by some MROSD personnel who encountered the reptiles while building the trail.

A stretch of level trail leads you through extensive groves of manzanita and silk tassel. As the trail curves sharply left, you begin to get sweeping views that extend southeast toward Mt. Umunhum. Monte Bello Ridge,

## TRIP 5 Russian Ridge Open Space Preserve: Ancient Oaks

| | |
|---|---|
| **Distance** | 2 miles, Loop |
| **Hiking Time** | 1 to 2 hours |
| **Elevation Gain/Loss** | ±450 feet |
| **Difficulty** | Moderate |
| **Trail Use** | Mountain biking allowed, Good for kids |
| **Best Times** | All year |
| **Agency** | MROSD |
| **Recommended Map** | *South Skyline Region* (MROSD) |

**HIGHLIGHTS** Justly famous for its wildflowers, this preserve also offers visitors stunning scenic vistas, which take in much of the Bay Area and the often fog-shrouded San Mateo coast. This short loop, using the Ridge, Ancient Oaks, and Mindego trails, merely whets your appetite for further adventures in what many enthusiasts claim is the jewel in MROSD's crown of open space lands. From wind-swept grasslands to shady forest canyons, there is something for everyone on this enchanting route.

**DIRECTIONS** From the intersection of Skyline Blvd. (Highway 35) and Page Mill Road/Alpine Road south of Palo Alto, take Skyline Blvd. northwest 1.1 miles to the Caltrans Vista Point parking area, on your right.

From the intersection of Skyline Blvd. (Highway 35) and Highway 84 in Sky Londa, take Skyline Blvd. southeast 6.2 miles to the Caltrans Vista Point parking area, on your left.

**FACILITIES/TRAILHEAD** There are no facilities at the trailhead, which is on the southwest side of Skyline Blvd., across from the parking area.

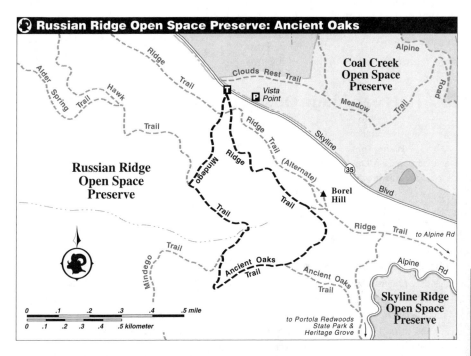

G ate RR01 is where you start this scenic loop. Just beyond two information boards is the first of several junctions. Angle left at the first and get on the Ridge Trail, a wide single track. After about 100 feet, you cross a dirt road heading up Borel Hill, called in this book the Ridge Trail (alternate). Climbing on a moderate grade, the trail winds its way just below the ridgetop, which is left. Soon you reach a junction with a short connector to the Ancient Oaks Trail, right.

Veer right on the connector and after a short stroll reach a T-junction with the Ancient Oaks Trail. Turn right and follow a

**Side Trip**

If you wish to ascend Borel Hill, the highest point in San Mateo County, at the connector with the Ancient Oaks Trail, continue straight on the Ridge Trail for several hundred feet to a junction with the Ridge Trail (alternate). Turn sharply left, go about 100 feet, and then turn right on a single-track trail. A short, moderate climb puts you atop Borel Hill, where 360-degree views await.

ridgetop downhill. The trail curves right and enters a dense forest. Losing elevation

Russian Ridge, west of Skyline Blvd., catches fog blowing in from the Pacific.

on a gentle grade, you soon merge with the Mindego Trail, a dirt road. Go straight and follow the road from forest to open grassland. The road meanders on a mostly level course past a junction with the Alder Spring Trail, left.

Follow the Mindego Trail as it climbs toward a notch in the hills. At a four-way junction with a dirt road, go straight. Just ahead is the junction with the Ridge Trail, right, where you began this loop. From here, retrace your route to the parking area.

---

**Cool and Wet**
- Westerly winds from the Pacific push fog inland to Russian Ridge, where it helps provide water for plants during the Bay Area's dry season. Moisture dripping from trees may cause the ground underfoot to be wet and slippery.
- This preserve hosts shade-loving plants such as trillium, fairy bells, mission bells, and hound's tongue.

---

# TRIP 6 Russian Ridge Open Space Preserve: Borel Hill

|   |   |
|---|---|
| **Distance** | 4.6 miles, Semi-loop |
| **Hiking Time** | 2 to 3 hours |
| **Elevation Gain/Loss** | ±1050 |
| **Difficulty** | Moderate |
| **Trail Use** | Mountain biking allowed |
| **Best Times** | All year |
| **Agency** | MROSD |
| **Recommended Map** | *South Skyline Region* (MROSD) |

**HIGHLIGHTS** This remarkable ramble through what many consider the Peninsula's most scenic preserve uses the Ridge, Ancient Oaks, Mindego, Alder Spring, and Hawk trails. It samples a wide variety of habitats, from the riparian corridor along Mindego Creek to the dazzling wildflower meadows atop Borel Hill, whose displays intensify week by week during spring. Birders will want to have binoculars handy to pick out soaring hawks and falcons. Part of this semi-loop route follows the Bay Area Ridge Trail.

**DIRECTIONS** From the intersection of Skyline Blvd. (Highway 35) and Page Mill Road/Alpine Road south of Palo Alto, take Alpine Road west about 100 yards to a parking area on the right. (This parking area serves both Skyline Ridge Open Space Preserve and Russian Ridge Open Space Preserve. On busy days parking may be unavailable. There is additional parking and access to the preserve's trails at the Caltrans Vista Point parking area, 1.1 miles northwest on Highway 35.)

**FACILITIES/TRAILHEAD** There is a toilet near the trailhead, which is on the west side of the parking area.

Follow the single-track Ridge Trail northwest from the trailhead, then climb via several switchbacks to where the trail becomes a rocky and eroded dirt road. Turn left at a junction with a connector to the Ancient Oaks Trail. Descending on a gentle grade, you wander through a grove of oaks and young Douglas-firs to a junction with the Ancient Oaks Trail. Turning right on a single track, you enjoy a splendid view of the Pacific Ocean as you make a rising traverse across a grassy hillside.

The trail curves left, levels briefly, and then descends to an oak woodland at about 1 mile, where a connector to the Ridge Trail joins on the right. Following a ridgetop

## Russian Ridge Open Space Preserve: Borel Hill

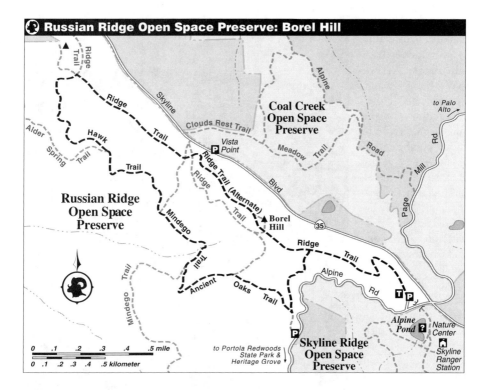

**Leaflets Three**

A thicket of poison oak near the trailhead serves as a reminder that this irritating plant comes in three forms — herb, vine, and shrub. No matter which form it takes, the same rule applies: "Leaflets three, let it be."

downhill, you skirt a steep hillside, left. Soon the trail curves right and enters a dense forest, where many of the oaks and California buckeyes are wrapped with a thick layer of moss. Losing elevation on a gentle grade, you soon reach a junction with the Mindego Trail, a dirt road.

The junction of the Ancient Oaks and Mindego trails, which is near a tributary of Mindego Creek, is a good place to look for California newts during the rainy season.

Go straight on the Mindego Trail, a dirt road that soon bends left and brings you from forest to open grassland. The road wanders over level ground to a junction

with the Alder Spring Trail, also a dirt road. You turn left and enjoy a mostly level walk with views of Mindego Hill and, on a clear day, the Pacific Ocean. Now descending on a moderate grade, the road alternates between wooded and open areas. Listen for the liquid call of the western meadowlark, a grassland bird often found in large flocks.

At a junction, you join the Hawk Trail by continuing straight. The single track makes a rising traverse across a steep, open hillside. The top-of-the-world feeling is enhanced as the trail rises toward a gap in the crest of Russian Ridge. When you meet the Ridge Trail, a dirt road, at about 2.8 miles, turn right and enjoy unrivaled views of the Bay Area. A little more than a mile ahead is Borel Hill, the geographic high point of this route.

In this preserve, the Ridge Trail runs along the spine of Russian Ridge. There is also a 0.5-mile segment of dirt road called the Ridge Trail that climbs up and over

Borel Hill. In this book, designate this as the Ridge Trail (alternate). Where the Mindego and Ridge trails cross, you continue straight and begin a moderate climb. After about 75 feet, a single-track segment of the Ridge Trail veers right, but you stay on the Ridge Trail (alternate), an eroded path that snakes its way uphill.

At a four-way junction, a trail goes right, to a vantage point, but you turn left for the final push to the top of Borel Hill, where a sign shows you are 2572 feet above sea level. When you are ready to leave this dramatic perch, put the elevation sign at your back and follow the trail in front of you. It soon joins the Ridge Trail (alternate) at a T-junction. Turn left, and after about 100 feet merge with the Ridge Trail. Soon you pass an unnamed trail, right, not shown on the preserve map. Close the loop at the next junction, then retrace your route to the parking area.

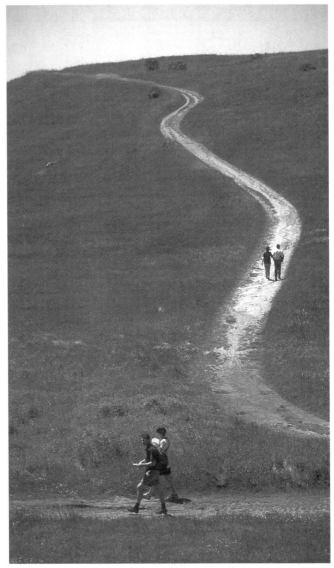

View northwest toward the Ridge and Mindego trails, Russian Ridge OSP.

**Spring Color**
Russian Ridge is famous for its spring-time displays of wildflowers, including California poppy, mule ears, owl's clover, lupine, tidytips, Johnny jump-up, popcorn flower, winecup clarkia, blue-eyed grass, California buttercup, fiddleneck, and checkerbloom.

# TRIP7 Monte Bello Open Space Preserve

| | |
|---:|:---|
| **Distance** | 6 miles, Loop |
| **Hiking Time** | 3 to 4 hours |
| **Elevation Gain/Loss** | ±1400 feet |
| **Difficulty** | Difficult |
| **Trail Use** | Backpacking option |
| **Best Times** | Spring through fall |
| **Agency** | MROSD |
| **Recommended Map** | *Monte Bello Open Space Preserve* (MROSD) |

**HIGHLIGHTS** This challenging but rewarding loop climbs from the riparian corridor along Stevens Creek to the windswept grasslands of Monte Bello Ridge. Using the Stevens Creek Nature Trail, Monte Bello Road, and the Canyon, Skid Road, and Indian Creek trails, the route takes you across the San Andreas fault and then up the ridge that forms the scenic backdrop for Sunnyvale, Cupertino, and Mountain View.

The views from Black Mountain, the summit of Monte Bello Ridge, are superb, and the descent along the Old Ranch and Bella Vista trails offers some of the best hiking on the Peninsula. (During wet weather it may be impossible to cross Stevens Creek, as is required on the first part of this route.)

This preserve is home to the Black Mountain backpack camp, the only site on MROSD lands where visitors can spend the night under the stars. The camp is located atop Monte Bello Ridge near the junction of Monte Bello Road and the Indian Creek Trail. For reservations call the MROSD office: (650) 691-1200.

**DIRECTIONS** From I-280 in Los Altos Hills, take the Page Mill Road/Arastradero Road exit and go south on Page Mill Road 7.2 miles to a parking area on your left.

From the intersection of Skyline Blvd. (Highway 35) and Page Mill Road south of Palo Alto, take Page Mill Road north 1.4 miles to a parking area on your right.

**FACILITIES/TRAILHEAD** There is a toilet near the trailhead, which is on the south corner of the parking area.

Take the Stevens Creek Nature Trail, a single track, to Vista Point, marked by an interpretive sign, where you have a fine view of the canyon holding Stevens Creek, which formed along the San Andreas fault. At a junction, stay on the Stevens Creek Nature Trail by veering sharply right. Now you descend via switchbacks to a forest of California bay, canyon oak, coast live oak, and madrone—a mixed evergreen forest.

As the trail continues to drop into the canyon, you turn right and cross a bridge over a seasonal tributary of Stevens Creek. A sharp left-hand bend brings you to a set of wooden steps leading down to Stevens Creek. After crossing the creek on rocks

> **Frances Brenner**
> The rest bench at the junction honors the late Frances Brenner, a member of the Palo Alto City Council who was active in the conservation movement, especially with regard to protecting watersheds.

(this may be impossible during wet weather) you climb an eroded bank to get back on the trail.

A moderate climb that soon levels brings you to a junction with the Skid Road Trail. Here you bear left on a dirt road, once traversed by teams of oxen dragging huge Douglas-firs and smaller tanbark

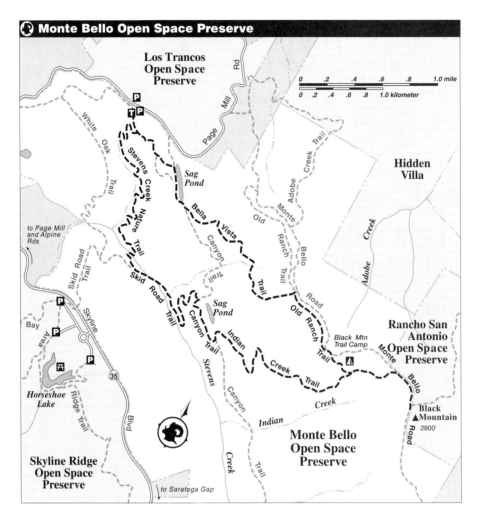

**Monte Bello Open Space Preserve**

oaks felled by loggers. To make the going easier, the road was inlaid with flat-topped logs called "skids," which were then periodically doused with water to reduce friction. In 19th-century Western towns, the neighborhood frequented by loggers, which usually contained saloons, flophouses, and brothels, was often called Skid Road or Skid Row.

Soon you cross Stevens Creek again, this time on a bridge. A moderate climb brings you to a tributary, also bridged, that falls from Monte Bello Ridge. Curving right and climbing steeply, the trail takes you across a precipitous hillside. Now ascending via S-

> **Some Good Newts**
> The creek is a breeding area for the California newt, a member of the salamander family. The California newt is brown with an orange belly and a long, vertically flattened tail. Newts remain mostly hidden in rock crevices and under logs in summer, but during the rainy season they journey to their watery breeding grounds, often in large numbers.

bends, you reach a fence with a gate that prevents access to the Skid Road Trail by bicycles and horses during wet weather.

In a clearing presided over by a large valley oak and several California buckeyes, you find a T-junction with the Canyon Trail, a dirt road. Here you turn right and almost immediately begin a steep climb. Soon, however, the road finds a rolling course through terrain that alternates between wooded and open. At a T-junction at about 2 miles, the Canyon Trail turns right, but you switch to the Indian Creek Trail, also a dirt road, by veering left.

Now you begin a long, steady climb up the side of Monte Bello Ridge. This massive feature, which trends northwest–southeast, parallels the nearby San Andreas fault, which runs through the canyon you recently left. Monte Bello Ridge is topped by Black Mountain, one of many peaks in California with that name. Seen from the cities of Sunnyvale, Cupertino, and Mountain View, Monte Bello Ridge dominates the skyline.

On a mostly moderate grade, you ascend past several gorgeous valley oaks, their twisted and outstretched limbs draped with lace lichen. Gaining elevation, you have ever-improving views of the nearby headwaters of Stevens Creek, and also of distant summits, such as Mt. Umunhum and Loma Prieta. Aiming for a gap on the skyline near the Black Mountain backpack camp, the road soon reaches two closely spaced junctions.

At the first, a single-track trail leads left to Monte Bello Road, bypassing the backpack camp. At the second, a dirt road veers left. To reach the Black Mountain backpack camp and a well-deserved rest spot, turn left on this dirt road. After about 100 feet, you come to a T-junction with a gravel road, where you turn left. The nearby camp has four individual campsites, a group campsite, a chemical toilet, and a phone. (The water available here is non-potable.)

To press on to the summit of Black Mountain, stay on the Indian Creek Trail as it curves right and climbs past the turnoff to the backpack camp. The Indian Creek Trail ends at the next junction, and you join Monte

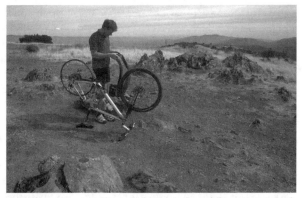

Black Mountain, atop Monte Bello Ridge, draws hikers, runners, and bicyclists.

Bello Road by bearing right. This dirt-and-gravel thoroughfare winds uphill to meet the Black Mountain Trail, left, a dirt road that descends steeply through the upper reaches of Rancho San Antonio Open Space Preserve.

Continuing straight, you soon stand atop Black Mountain, marveling at the 360-degree views from the broad, rocky, and treeless vantage point. On a clear day, you can see most of the San Francisco Bay Area, bounded by Mt. Tamalpais, Mt. Diablo, and Mt. Hamilton. San Jose, Santa Clara, and the southern shoreline of San Francisco Bay lie at your feet. From the preserve's highlands, scan the skies for raptors, especially

---

**A Plethora of Plants**

Four distinct plant communities are represented in this preserve: mixed evergreen forest, Douglas-fir forest, chaparral, and grassland. Factors such as soil type, sunlight, moisture, and wind, along with the effects of logging and fires, determine where different species of plants are found.

during spring and fall migration. After enjoying this splendid summit, retrace your route to the backpack camp turnoff.

At the turnoff, swing right and after about 100 feet meet the gravel road at the T-junction mentioned above. Turn left and walk through the backpack camp, at about 4 miles. Just past the camp, you pass the single-track connector to the Indian Creek Trail, left. At a four-way junction, Monte Bello Road joins sharply from the right, and continues ahead by veering right. Your route, though, is the single-track Old Ranch Trail, which angles left.

The trail contours through grassland and then winds its way gently downhill, offering superb hiking with terrific views. At the next junction, where a short connector goes right about 50 feet to Monte Bello Road, go left on the Bella Vista Trail, a single track. When you reach the Canyon Trail, angle right and follow a level course. To the left of the road is a swampy area, and on the right is sag pond.

Now you pass a rest bench, right, and a junction with a hiking-only trail, left (not

> **Ponder This**
>
> Sag ponds form in fault zones. Here, the Pacific and North American plates slipped past each other and a gap formed, creating a depression. Fed by a spring on Monte Bello Ridge, the pond is gradually becoming overgrown with cat-tails and pond lilies. In the future, it will fill with sediments, becoming first a wet meadow and then a forest, in a process called succession.

shown on the preserve map). Continue straight for about 100 yards and then turn left on the Stevens Creek Nature Trail, a single track closed to bicycles and horses. Now you pass through an old orchard of mostly English walnut trees, soon reaching a junction, left, with the previously mentioned hiking-only trail. Here, bear right and make a rising traverse across an open slope. After closing the loop, simply retrace your route to the parking area.

# TRIP 8 Los Trancos Open Space Preserve

| | |
|---|---|
| **Distance** | 2.3 miles, Loop |
| **Hiking Time** | 1 to 2 hours |
| **Elevation Gain/Loss** | ±500 feet |
| **Difficulty** | Moderate |
| **Trail Use** | Good for kids |
| **Best Times** | All year |
| **Agency** | MROSD |
| **Recommended Map** | *Los Trancos Open Space Preserve* (MROSD) |

**HIGHLIGHTS**  This route combines two scenic loops, the Franciscan Loop Trail and the Lost Creek Loop Trail, to explore a small, wedge-shaped preserve that is rich in geo-logical and botanical interest. The San Andreas fault runs through the preserve. Oaks, bays, bigleaf maples, and Douglas-firs provide a protective canopy for an assortment of native shrubs and wildflowers. Along the way you will descend to the headwaters of Los Trancos Creek, which forms part of the border between San Mateo and Santa Clara counties. (To learn about the area's geology, you can also visit the self-guiding San Andreas Fault Trail, which starts from the west side of the parking area.)

**DIRECTIONS** From I-280 in Los Altos Hills, take the Page Mill Road/Arastradero Road exit and go south on Page Mill Road 7.2 miles to a parking area, on your right. This parking area is just a few hundred feet past the parking area for Monte Bello Open Space Preserve, which is on the left.

From the intersection of Skyline Blvd. (Highway 35) and Page Mill Road south of Palo Alto, take Page Mill Road north 1.4 miles to a parking area on your left. (The parking area for Monte Bello Open Space Preserve is just a few hundred feet past this parking area, on the right.)

**FACILITIES/TRAILHEAD** There is a toilet in the Monte Bello Open Space Preserve parking area, just across Page Mill Road. There are no facilities at the trailhead, which is on the northeast corner of the parking area.

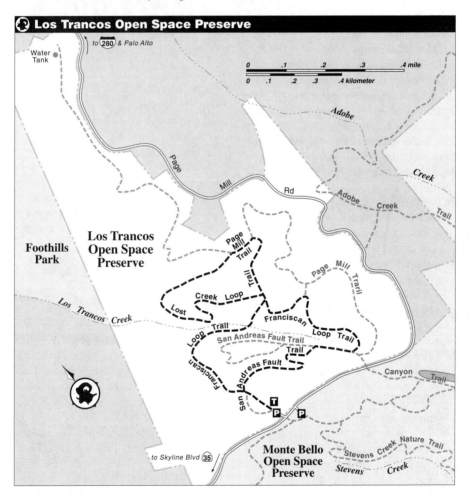

Head north on the Franciscan Loop Trail, and on a clear day you are immediately rewarded with a sweeping view that stretches up the Peninsula to San Francisco and takes in the hulking forms of San Bruno Mountain and Mt. Tamalpais. After about 75 feet the single-track trail forks. The right-hand branch, an unofficial trail, climbs a low rise, offers additional views, and then rejoins the Franciscan Loop Trail. Staying left, you cross a weedy field full of coyote brush, oats, and some thistle.

The depression near the trailhead, marked with white-striped posts to indicate minor fault breaks from the 1906 earthquake, is a sag pond. Sag ponds are found in fault zones and landslide areas where the land has sunk because of earth movement. These ponds often fill with water during winter and become freshwater marshes.

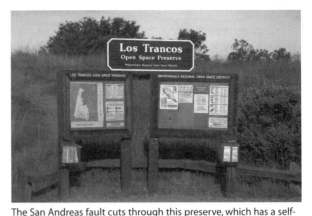

The San Andreas fault cuts through this preserve, which has a self-guiding nature trail.

About 100 yards from the trailhead, the San Andreas Fault Trail merges from the left. At the next junction, where the Franciscan Loop Trail goes both left and straight, you bear left. The unofficial trail mentioned above joins sharply from the right. (The San Andreas Fault Trail, which for part of its length follows the Franciscan Loop Trail, is straight.)

Now you descend through a shady corridor, cross a bridge, and then follow the trail to a T-junction with the Lost Creek Loop Trail. Here, you turn left and after about 75 feet pass the returning end of the Lost Creek Loop Trail on your right. Continuing straight, you follow a gently rolling course and then work your way down a densely wooded ridge via switchbacks to the bank of Los Trancos Creek.

---

**Stepping up to the Creek**

In Spanish, *tranco* means stride or big step, and *tranca* is a bar or barrier. *California Place Names* favors a corruption of the latter to explain this creek's name: Perhaps there were barriers here at one time to prevent cattle from crossing it, or perhaps the creek itself formed a natural barrier.

---

**Los Trancos Flora**

- This preserve is a great place to study native trees, including canyon oak, valley oak, black oak, tanbark oak, madrone, California bay, bigleaf maple, and Douglas-fir.
- Hedge nettle, hound's tongue, milkmaids, Solomon's seal, starflower, bleeding hearts, and trillium are a few of the many forest wildflowers found here.
- A variety of shrubs also thrive in the preserve, including coffeeberry, hazelnut, snowberry, gooseberry, creambush, elk clover, and thimbleberry.

---

Walking downstream, you have the creek on your left. Soon, the trail finds a level course, but the creek cuts its way into an ever-deepening canyon. Now your route curves right and follows a tributary of Los Trancos Creek, which may be dry, upstream. Soon the Page Mill Trail merges from left and joins the Lost Creek Loop Trail for several hundred yards. You continue straight, and at the next junction stay on the Lost Creek Loop Trail by turning sharply right.

Now you ascend via switchbacks into a brighter realm, where a short boardwalk helps you through a marshy area. Reaching a T-junction where the two ends of the Lost Creek Loop Trail join, you turn left and retrace your route for about 75 feet. Here, at a junction with the Franciscan Loop Trail, you continue straight, then curve right and begin to climb. Where a connector to the Page Mill Trail goes left, you stay right.

Passing a very short trail to Page Mill Road, you meet the San Andreas Fault Trail at a T-junction. You turn left and immediately confront a fork. Angling left is a short

trail to the San Andreas Fault Trail's interpretive station 3. During the 1906 earthquake, the ground opened along the San Andreas fault. Later it filled in, forming the flat area, or bench, that is here now.

Bearing right at the fork to stay on the Franciscan Loop Trail, you climb via switchbacks between a line of trees, right, and open meadow, left. At the four-way junction where you began this loop, simply continue straight and retrace your route to the parking area.

## TRIP 9 Windy Hill Open Space Preserve: Hamms Gulch

| | |
|---|---|
| **Distance** | 8 miles, Semi-loop |
| **Hiking Time** | 4 to 5 hours |
| **Elevation Gain/Loss** | ±1650 feet |
| **Difficulty** | Difficult |
| **Best Times** | All year |
| **Agency** | MROSD |
| **Recommended Map** | *Windy Hill Open Space Preserve* (MROSD) |

**HIGHLIGHTS** This adventurous semi-loop uses the Lost, Hamms Gulch, Eagle, and Razorback Ridge trails to explore one of the Peninsula's best-loved preserves. Dropping about 1000 feet in 3 miles, you follow cool and shady Hamms Gulch downhill through a lush forest to the banks of lovely Corte Madera Creek. Aided by many switchbacks, you gradually win back lost elevation. Along the way, look for forest birds flitting through the trees, or study the native plants found along the route. Views from the trail — aided by good visibility and binoculars — sweep northward to San Francisco Bay, three of its bridges, and the cities of Oakland and San Francisco.

**DIRECTIONS** From the intersection of Skyline Blvd. (Highway 35) and Highway 84 in Sky Londa, take Skyline Blvd. southeast 2.3 miles to a parking area on the left.

**FACILITIES/TRAILHEAD** There are picnic tables and a toilet beside the parking area. The trailhead is on the northeast corner of the parking area.

Turn right on the Lost Trail, part of the Bay Area Ridge Trail, and after about 100 feet reach a seasonal gate that prevents access by horses in wet weather. Now the single-track trail climbs on a very gentle grade to a junction with the Hamms Gulch Trail. Turn sharply left and begin descending via switchbacks. Curving right, you pass an unofficial trail leading left to a promontory.

In a dense forest, you continue to descend a ridge by following the twists and turns of its gullies and ravines, some of

**Windy Hill Foliage**
Douglas-firs, California bays, tanbark oaks, California buckeyes, and bigleaf maples tower beside the trail. Native shrubs include toyon, coffeeberry, snowberry, evergreen huckleberry, hazelnut, sticky monkeyflower, thimbleberry, and blue elderberry.

which hold seasonal creeks. Around 2 miles, you reach a rest bench on the left, which

Peninsula

## Windy Hill Open Space Preserve: Hamms Gulch

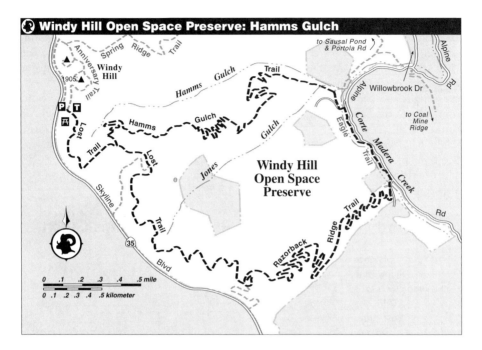

offers a fine view of Windy Hill. This is a great place to take a break. Beyond, the trail continues to lose elevation on a grade that alternates between gentle and moderate, with Hamms Gulch steeply downhill and left. Soon you come to another seasonal equestrian gate.

### Bird Alert

North America's smallest falcon, the American kestrel, is often seen hovering above open fields, searching with its keen eyes for prey such as insects, reptiles, small mammals, and sometimes birds. Also at home here is the northern harrier, told by its long tail, white rump, and low, wobbly flight.

Just beyond the gate, at about 3 miles, a connector to the Spring Ridge Trail goes left. You bear right to stay on the Hamms Gulch Trail, and after several hundred yards reach a bridge over a creek flowing through Jones Gulch. Crossing the bridge, you come to a paved road in about 100 feet. To the

right is the preserve boundary, so turn left and then cross Corte Madera Creek on a stone bridge, which has a paved surface.

Once across the creek, look right to find the start of the Eagle Trail, maintained by the town of Portola Valley and closed to bicycles. This single-track trail parallels the rocky bed of Corte Madera Creek, which is to your right. Before too long, the trail deposits you on Alpine Road. Walk along the road shoulder for about 100 yards, and then regain the trail, which descends to the right.

Soon returning to Alpine Road, follow it for several hundred feet to a paved driveway on the right. After crossing Corte Madera Creek on a bridge, the driveway turns right, but you continue straight and begin to climb a dirt-and-gravel road. After a short, moderate climb, you leave the road on the Razorback Ridge Trail, a single-track marked with a trail post. After about 50 feet, the trail curves right and comes to a seasonal equestrian gate.

The moderate but relentless climb continues, thankfully, via switchbacks in the

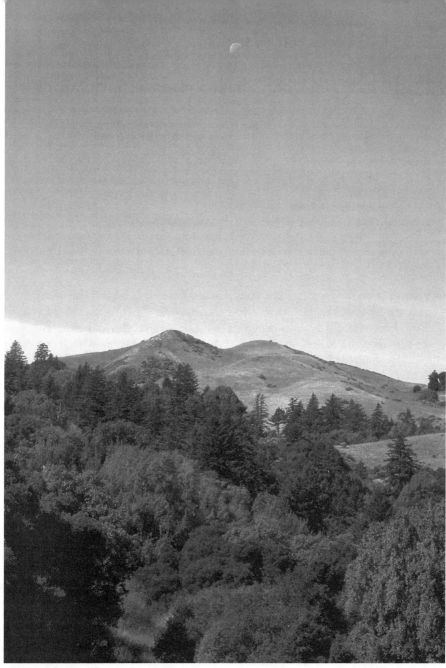

Windy Hill's twin summits are visible from near the junction of the Lost and Hamms Gulch trails.

shade. With the deep canyon holding Damiani Creek to your left, you begin a long, rising traverse to a vantage point with a view of Windy Hill. Now switchbacks take you back and forth across the crest of a ridge, which has an overgrown dirt road running down its spine, fenced to prevent terrain-damaging shortcuts. Someday, traces of the road will disappear completely.

At a junction with the Lost Trail, at about 6 miles, turn right and follow a gently rolling course through a four-way junction to meet the Hamms Gulch Trail, right. From here, retrace your route to the parking area.

# TRIP *10* Windy Hill Open Space Preserve: Spring Ridge

| | |
|---:|:---|
| **Distance** | 7.6 miles, Loop |
| **Hiking Time** | 4 to 5 hours |
| **Elevation Gain/Loss** | ±1400 feet |
| **Difficulty** | Difficult |
| **Trail Use** | Leashed dogs[1] |
| **Best Times** | All year |
| **Agency** | MROSD |
| **Recommended Map** | *Windy Hill Open Space Preserve* (MROSD) |
| **Notes** | [1]Dogs are not allowed on the Betsy Crowder and Anniversary trails, and instead must use the Spring Ridge Trail and the multi-use path that goes west of Windy Hill's summits. |

**HIGHLIGHTS** Using the Betsy Crowder, Spring Ridge, Anniversary, Lost, and Hamms Gulch trails, this leg-stretching loop climbs more than 1000 feet from Portola Valley to the flower-studded slopes of Windy Hill. Windy Hill's twin summits offer unrivaled views of the San Francisco Bay Area and the San Mateo coast. The descent is through densely forested Hamms Gulch. The Anniversary and Lost trails are part of the Bay Area Ridge Trail.

**DIRECTIONS** From I-280 southwest of Palo Alto, take the Alpine Road/Portola Valley exit. Take Alpine Road south 3 miles to a stop sign at the intersection of Alpine and Portola Roads. Turn right and go 0.9 mile to a parking area on the left.

**FACILITIES/TRAILHEAD** There is a toilet near the trailhead, which is on the southwest side of the parking area.

Follow a single-track trail uphill from the parking area to meet an equestrian trail joining sharply from the left. Turn right and go several hundred yards to a T-junction with a dirt road. The Spring Ridge Trail, a multi-use path, is left, but you turn right and almost immediately find the Betsy Crowder Trail on your left. As you start off on this trail, you pass a fence with a seasonal gate that prevents access by horses during wet weather.

The earthen dam that forms Sausal Pond is on your left, partially hidden behind a screen of trees and shrubs. Level at first, the trail now climbs gently to a T-junction with the Spring Ridge Trail, a dirt road. Here, you turn right and begin a curvy ascent through a good birding area—open fields alternating with groves of venerable coast live oaks. Spring Ridge is named for the many springs found nearby, which made the surrounding land valuable to early settlers and ranchers.

> **Notable Trails**
> - The Betsy Crowder Trail honors an MROSD board member who served from 1989 until her death in 2000. She was also active in the MROSD volunteer program, and was one of the authors of *Peninsula Trails*, published by Wilderness Press.
> - The Anniversary Trail, built in 1987, commemorates MROSD's 15th anniversary and also the 10th anniversary of Peninsula Open Space Trust, a local nonprofit land trust that provided major support for the acquisition of this preserve.

Passing a closed trail, left, at about 1 mile, you emerge from a wooded area and have a magnificent view uphill across rolling slopes to the twin summits of Windy Hill. The road, which may be muddy during wet weather, climbs steadily on grades that

## Windy Hill Open Space Preserve: Spring Ridge

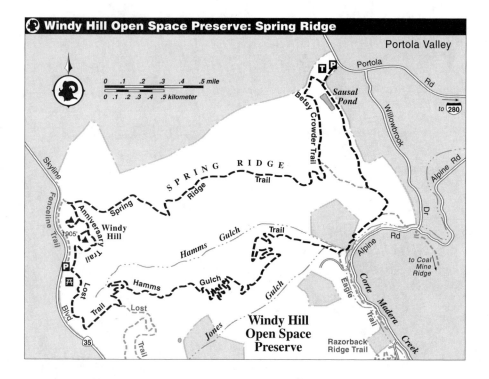

**Windy Hill Foliage, Birds**

- Valley oak, coast live oak, black oak, California buckeye, madrone, Monterey cypress, and eucalyptus are some of the trees growing beside the trail.
- Wildflowers here include California poppies, checkerbloom, lupine, yarrow, bellardia, and fiddleneck.
- You may be lucky enough to spot one or more of this preserve's common raptors — red-tailed hawk, American kestrel, northern harrier, white-tailed kite — patrolling the skies or roosting in a tall Monterey cypress.
- Sausal Pond is home to wood ducks, and large wooden boxes have been placed on nearby trees to provide them with safe nesting sites. Green herons also live here, and sometimes their much larger cousins, great blue herons, drop by for a visit.

run the gamut from gentle to steep. Be sure to stop, turn around, and admire the scenic vista that extends across San Francisco Bay to the East Bay hills.

As you near Skyline Blvd., you may begin to feel the effects of the Peninsula's coastal climate. The wind may increase, and great billows of fog may pour over the ridge. When you reach gate WH01 and an information board, both just east of Skyline Blvd., turn left. Just ahead is a fork, where you bear left on the hiking-only Anniversary Trail.

At around 3 miles you find a rest bench and an unsigned trail, right. To visit the preserve's highest point, turn right and follow the short trail to Windy Hill's north summit. From this impressive vantage point, you have 360-degree views of the San Francisco Bay Area and the San Mateo coast. After enjoying this beautiful spot, return to the Anniversary Trail and bear right.

Now follow the trail as it curves around the base of the north summit. At a saddle where two more rest benches await, you pass a trail to Windy Hill's south summit,

Peninsula

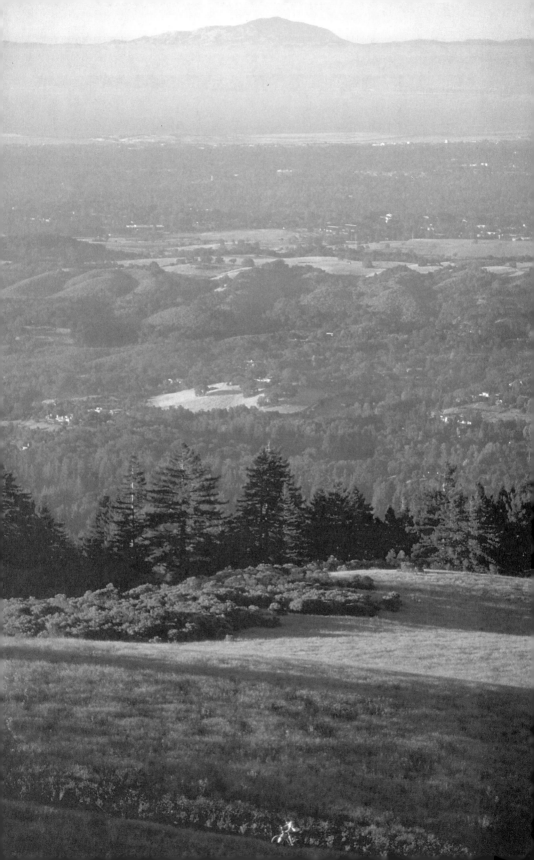

which is about 25 feet lower than its rival. These high vantage points and the hillsides just below them provide great birding opportunities. Spring sightings of lesser goldfinch and lazuli bunting here may encourage you to bring binoculars.

The Anniversary Trail continues from the saddle by clinging to a narrow ledge cut in a hillside. Descending on a gentle grade, the trail makes a sharp bend to the left and brings you to a wood fence with a gap. Just beyond, the multi-use path joins sharply from the right. Now on level ground, you soon reach the end of the Anniversary Trail at its junction with the Lost Trail, which goes left. A parking/picnic area and a restroom are just ahead.

Here, you turn left on the Lost Trail, part of the Bay Area Ridge Trail, and after about 100 feet reach a seasonal gate that prevents access by horses in wet weather. Now the single-track trail climbs on a very gentle grade to a junction with the Hamms Gulch Trail. Turn sharply left and begin descending via switchbacks. Curving right, you pass an unofficial trail leading left to a promontory.

In a dense forest, you continue to descend a ridge by following the twists and turns of its gullies and ravines, some of which hold seasonal creeks. A rest bench, left, offers a great place to relax and enjoy a fine view of Windy Hill. Beyond, the trail continues to lose elevation on a grade that alternates between gentle and moderate, with Hamms Gulch steeply downhill and left. Soon you come to another seasonal equestrian gate. Just beyond the gate, at about 6.3 miles, you bear left on a connector to the Spring Ridge Trail.

Hamms Gulch, which holds a seasonal tributary of Corte Madera Creek, is a lush and lovely area, where Douglas-fir, bay, bigleaf maple, and madrone are joined by snowberry, honeysuckle, berry vines, and ferns. Cross the creek in Hamms Gulch on rocks, then climb gently beside Corte Madera Creek. A dense, riparian corridor borders Corte Madera Creek, but uphill and left is a savanna of mostly valley oaks, giving this part of the route a park-like feel. Many of the oaks are draped with strands of lace lichen, and some hold large clumps of mistletoe.

Continue straight through a four-way junction, now on a dirt road. The next junction, also four-way, is with the Spring Ridge Trail, and again you continue straight. A low-lying, marshy area holding the upper reaches of Sausal Creek is to your left. Sausal Pond, designated a "critical wildlife habitat," is just ahead. Beyond the pond, close the loop and then turn right to the parking area.

## TRIP 11 Wunderlich Park

| | |
|---|---|
| **Distance** | 5.5 miles, Loop |
| **Hiking Time** | 2 to 3 hours |
| **Elevation Gain/Loss** | ±1250 feet |
| **Difficulty** | Moderate |
| **Best Times** | All year |
| **Agency** | SMCP&R |
| **Recommended Map** | *Wunderlich Park* (SMCP&R) |

**HIGHLIGHTS** This loop uses Alambique, Bear Gulch, Meadow, and Redwood trails to explore this compact yet diverse park in the foothills of the Santa Cruz Mountains. The park is a favorite among equestrians, but the trails are closed to horses during wet weather.

View from Windy Hill extends across Portola Valley and San Francisco Bay to Mt. Diablo.

During the first half of the 20th century, the Folger family used this area for recreation, including horseback riding and camping. The park is named for Martin Wunderlich, who bought the land from the Folgers in 1956. In 1974, Wunderlich deeded 942 acres to San Mateo County for park and open space.

**DIRECTIONS** From I-280 in Woodside, take the Woodside Road/Woodside/Highway 84 exit and go southwest 2.8 miles to the park entrance, right. Go about 0.1 mile to a dirt parking area, left.

**FACILITIES/TRAILHEAD** There is a phone beside the park office, just uphill from the parking area. There are water and a toilet near the trailhead, which is on the southwest corner of the parking area.

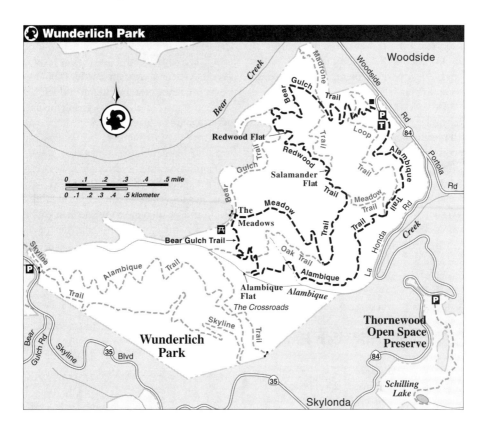

The Alambique Trail, a wide dirt path, follows a level course. The slopes of the Santa Cruz Mountains were once covered with coast redwoods, and this park preserves a remnant of that forest, most of it second-growth. The trail soon begins to climb gently and then moderately into the redwoods, where huge stumps indicate the former stature of the ancient trees. The sparse understory consists mostly of ferns, which thrive in the cool, moist environment.

After passing several unsigned roads, you make a rising traverse across a hillside that drops left and soon reach a junction. Here the Loop Trail goes sharply right, but you bear left to stay on the Alambique Trail, now a dirt road. Where the Meadow Trail heads right, you continue straight, climbing gently beside Alambique Creek. At about 2 miles you reach Alambique Flat, marked by a sign and a grand circle of redwoods. The Alambique Trail continues to the right, and a short trail wanders left toward Alambique Creek.

Follow the Alambique Trail into more open, brighter terrain. Around 2 miles, you reach a junction with the Oak Trail, where you stay on the Alambique Trail by turning left. A short climb via switchbacks brings you to the Bear Gulch Trail, where you turn right. Now you continue to climb on a gentle grade, following a single-track trail out of the forest and into The Meadows. What once may have been a meadow is now overgrown with coyote brush, toyon, coffeeberry, and tangles of berry vines.

This is perfect habitat for the California quail, the state bird. Reluctant to fly, quail often scurry through the underbrush in large coveys. Views from this treeless area extend northeast across San Francisco Bay to the East Bay hills, and southeast along the crest of the Santa Cruz Mountains.

Just after an unofficial trail joins sharply from the left, you come to a four-way junction. Here the Bear Gulch Trail turns left, the Meadow Trail goes right, and an unofficial trail heads straight and uphill. You turn right and follow the Meadow Trail, a dirt road that descends through The Meadows to a T-junction with the Oak Trail. Here you stay on the Meadow Trail by turning left.

Losing elevation on a gentle grade, you soon reach another T-junction, this one with the Redwood Trail. You turn left and almost immediately find yourself back in a dense redwood forest. The Redwood Trail rises on

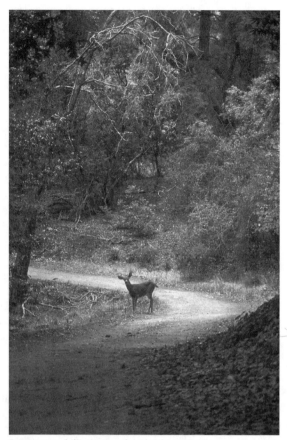

Deer stops while crossing the Alambique Trail.

**Peninsula**

**Creek Lore**

According to historian Frank M. Stanger, Alambique Creek — Spanish for still — was the site of the Peninsula's first bootleg operation and its first sawmill. The mill, a crude, water-driven affair, was built in 1849 for Charles Brown, who owned nearly 3000 acres in the Woodside area, including present-day Wunderlich Park. Steam soon replaced water as a more reliable, year-round source of power and the modern logging era was born. Alambique Creek is also notable, says Stanger, for being the boundary between two large Mexican land grants: Cañada Raymundo to the north and Cañada del Corte de Madera to the south.

> **The Big Trees**
> Redwoods support themselves by inter-locking their roots in a wide but shallow network. Some of the giant redwoods beside the road have partially exposed roots, allowing you to examine their structure. Lacking the deep tap root of other species, redwoods may be knocked down by high winds. Where tanbark oaks and California bays join the redwoods, they grow tall in their search for sunlight.

> **Salamander Studies**
> Amphibians thrive in the cool, moist envi-ronment of a redwood forest. Among the most common are the lungless salaman-ders (family Plethodontidae). As their name implies, these salamanders have no lungs and instead breathe through their skin. Western species live, breed, and lay their eggs on land rather than in water. Most salamanders are sedentary, not straying far from where they were born. Studies show that earth movement along fault lines isolated groups of salamanders and caused them to evolve into separate species.

a gentle grade to a junction with the Madrone Trail, where you stay on the single-track Redwood Trail by angling left. A sign at about 4 miles marks Salamander Flat.

At about 4 miles, you come to Redwood Flat, marked by family circles of redwoods that have sprouted from the stumps of their fallen ancestors. Just beyond Redwood Flat is a T-junction with the Bear Gulch Trail. Here you turn right and follow a single track downhill. At a junction with a short trail to the park boundary, left, you continue straight. Switchbacks take you down to a four-way junction with the Madrone Trail.

Zigzag your way down the Bear Gulch Trail to a seasonal equestrian gate. About 40 feet past the gate is a four-way junction with the Loop Trail, right, and a service road, left. Go straight. After more switch-backs, a bridge helps you across a seasonal creek, and the you follow a dirt road bor-dered by rock walls. To your left is a large brown building, part of a ranch complex formerly owned by San Francisco coffee baron James A. Folger. Ahead are the trail-head and the parking area.

## TRIP 12 Huddart Park

| | |
|---|---|
| **Distance** | 5.2 miles, Loop |
| **Hiking Time** | 2 to 3 hours |
| **Elevation Gain/Loss** | ±1000 feet |
| **Difficulty** | Moderate |
| **Best Times** | All year |
| **Agency** | SMCP&R |
| **Recommended Map** | *Huddart Park* (SMCP&R) |

**HIGHLIGHTS** Visitors encounter three different plant communities — redwood forest, mixed-evergreen forest, and chaparral — on this invigorating loop, which uses the Crystal Springs and Dean trails to explore some of the canyons and hillsides between West Union Creek and Skyline Blvd. (If you have time, also visit the Chickadee Nature Trail, a fully accessible trail that accommodates users of all capabilities; it starts beside the first parking area, the handicapped-only zone, on the right.)

**DIRECTIONS** From I-280 in Woodside, take the Woodside Road/Woodside/Highway 84 exit and go southwest 1.6 miles to Kings Mountain Road. Turn right and go 2.1 miles to the park entrance, right. After 0.2 mile you come to an entrance kiosk and a self-registration station. There are parking areas just ahead on both sides of the road.

**FACILITIES/TRAILHEAD**  The park has group picnic areas, shelters, and youth campgrounds that can be reserved; (650) 363-4021. Phone and water are near the parking areas. Restrooms are about 0.2 mile ahead in the Zwierlein area. The trailhead is several hundred feet north of the parking areas, on the east side of the paved road signed for the Werder, Zwierlein, Madrone, and Miwok areas.

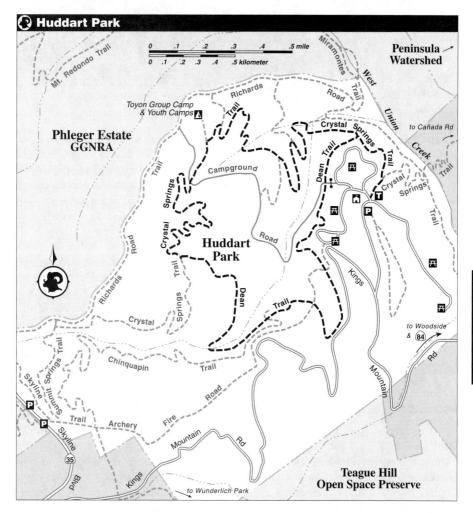

Woodside resident and lumberman James Huddart gave 900 acres for this public park, which the county has operated since 1944. The trailhead here provides access to trails in this park and also to those in the Phleger Estate. You follow a single track that descends to a junction with the

Bay Tree Trail, right. Continuing straight, you pass the Zwierlein picnic area, with restrooms, on your left. Now you reach a junction with the Crystal Springs Trail, a hiking and equestrian route that runs from near the junction of Highway 92 and Cañada Road to just shy of Skyline Blvd. on Kings Mountain.

Bearing left, you follow a rolling course past a junction with the Dean Trail, your return route, left. The cutting of switchbacks has caused severe erosion problems here: please stay on the trail. Now the trail descends on a gentle grade via switchbacks into a canyon holding a seasonal tributary of West Union Creek, shown on the park map as McGarvey Gulch Creek.

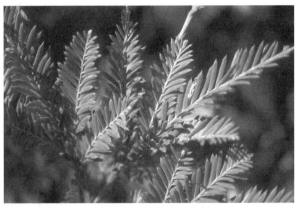

Young coast redwoods produce bright green foliage.

In the canyon bottom, a connector to the Richards Road Trail goes straight, but you turn left and cross a bridge over the creek. Now turning right, you cross a second bridge over another watercourse and then begin to climb on a moderate grade. (A gate here, one of several along the route, prevents access by horses during wet weather.)

---

**Huddart Park Greenery**

- Coast redwoods, Douglas-firs, coast live oaks, madrones, and tanbark oaks are accompanied in this park by hearty shrubs such as manzanita, blue blossom, toyon, and chaparral pea.
- The shady, moist environment is perfect for California bay, coffeeberry, bigleaf maple, hazelnut, ferns, and berry vines.

---

At a junction with the Chaparral Trail, you stay on the Crystal Springs trail by turning sharply left. Passing a junction with the Canyon Trail, left, you enjoy an easy stroll across a hillside that drops right. Switchbacks help you gain elevation, and soon you pass through a grove of manzanitas, many of which are dead. The grade eases and now you follow a level or gently rising course. An inviting rest bench made of rock is on your right.

After a few more switchbacks, you meet a connector to the Richards Road Trail, but

you stay on course by turning left. Ahead is a short trail to the Toyon group camp, but again you veer left to stay on the Crystal Springs Trail. At about 2 miles you cross a dirt-and-gravel road, signed TOYON ROAD but called the Campground Trail on the park map.

The wooded canyons of this park once held magnificent ancient redwoods, and some of the earliest sawmills in the Santa Cruz Mountains operated nearby. Massive stumps near the trail are evidence of this bygone era.

At a junction with a road not shown on the park map, your trail curves right and begins a series of switchbacks to gain elevation. After traversing the wall of a canyon, the trail makes an abrupt left turn and climbs on a moderate grade to a junction with the Dean Trail. You join the single-track Dean Trail by going straight and descending. Before reaching a seasonal creek, you pass McGarvey Flat, a lovely spot with a picnic table and several rest benches hewn from logs.

A level walk soon brings you to a four-way junction (shown incorrectly on the park map), where you bear left to stay on the Dean Trail. McGarvey Gulch Creek, which you crossed near the start of this loop, is downhill and left. Gently descending via S-bends, you soon reach a four-way junction with the Archery Fire Road. Regaining the Dean Trail across the road, you switchback left and again cross the Archery Fire Road, at about 4 miles.

At the edge of a paved road near the Miwok picnic area, your trail turns sharply left and then begins a series of switchbacks, descending past the Madrone picnic area. Now you cross the Campground Trail, a paved road that changes to dirt a few feet to your left. Stay on the Dean Trail, here a wide path, as it makes a curving descent past more picnic areas. At a T-junction with the Crystal Springs Trail, you turn right and retrace your route to the parking area.

## TRIP 13 Phleger Estate

| | |
|---|---|
| **Distance** | 7.9 miles, Loop |
| **Hiking Time** | 3 to 5 hours |
| **Elevation Gain/Loss** | ±1500 feet |
| **Difficulty** | Difficult |
| **Best Times** | All year |
| **Agency** | GGNRA, SMCP&R |
| **Recommended Map** | *Trail Map of the Central Peninsula* (Trail Center) |

**HIGHLIGHTS** This route, using the Crystal Springs, Miramontes, Mount Redondo, Lonely, Summit Springs, Dean, and Richards Road trails, explores the rugged terrain just northwest of Huddart Park, and the contrast between the county park and its GGNRA neighbor couldn't be more extreme. Trading picnic areas and sports fields for a serene forest of coast redwoods, you climb the rugged eastern side of Kings Mountain on the aptly named Lonely Trail, then descend through the heavily wooded county park, a favorite among equestrians.

**DIRECTIONS** From I-280 in Woodside, take the Woodside Road/Woodside/Highway 84 exit and go southwest 1.6 miles to Kings Mountain Road. Turn right and go 2.1 miles to the Huddart Park entrance, right. After 0.2 mile you come to an entrance kiosk and a self-registration station. There are parking areas just ahead on both sides of the road.

**FACILITIES/TRAILHEAD** The county park has group picnic areas, shelters, and youth campgrounds that can be reserved; (650) 363-4021. Phone and water are near the parking areas. Restrooms are about 0.2 mile ahead in the Zwierlein area. The trailhead is several hundred feet north of the parking areas, on the east side of the paved road signed for the Werder, Zwierlein, Madrone, and Miwok areas.

The trailhead here provides access to trails in the Phleger Estate and also to those in Huddart Park. You follow a single track that descends to a junction with the Bay Tree Trail, right. Continuing straight, you pass the Zwierlein picnic area, with restrooms, on your left. Now you reach a junction with the Crystal Springs Trail, a hiking and equestrian route that runs from near the junction of Highway 92 and Cañada Road to just shy of Skyline Blvd. on Kings Mountain.

Bearing left, you follow a rolling course past a junction with the Dean Trail, your return route, left. The cutting of switchbacks has caused severe erosion problems here: please stay on the trail. Now the trail descends on a gentle grade via switchbacks into a canyon holding a seasonal tributary of West Union Creek, shown on the park map as McGarvey Gulch Creek.

In the canyon bottom, where the Crystal Springs trail veers left and crosses the creek,

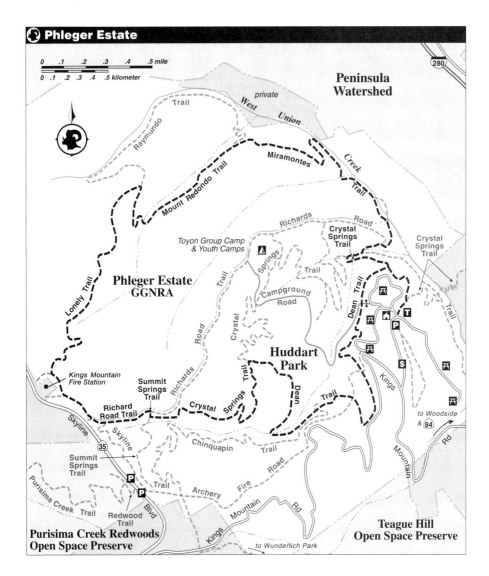

you go straight on a connector to the Richards Road Trail. Soon you merge with the Richards Road Trail and turn sharply left, crossing a culvert that holds the creek. You route, a dirt road, rises steadily to a junction, where you veer right on the Miramontes Trail, a single track. The trail gradually bends left and descends to West Union Creek, which is right, at about 1 mile.

A secluded clearing, marked by a metal sculpture of a Native American on horseback, has a rest bench and a sign with infor-

mation about the 1200-acre Phleger Estate, which you have just entered. Thanks to a combined public and private effort, the estate was purchased in a complex series of transactions, and in 1995 became part of the Golden Gate National Recreation Area. A sign at this clearing reads, "In 1990 the Peninsula Open Space Trust launched a campaign to permanently protect the Phleger Estate and transfer it to the National Park Service. POST's unprecedented efforts culminated on April 29, 1995,

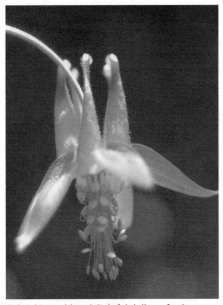

Columbine adds a delightful dollop of color to an otherwise dark redwood forest.

miles, the Raymundo Trail goes straight, but your route, the Lonely Trail, heads left. (For a shorter trip, follow the Raymundo Trail to its junction with the Mount Redondo and Miramontes trails; then retrace your route to the parking area.)

The narrow, single track climbs atop a ridge, then leaves it by curving left. Aptly named, the Lonely Trail wanders through a shadowy sanctuary of redwoods and madrones, far removed from the relatively nearby hustle and bustle of Redwood City, Woodside, and Palo Alto. Now you begin to work your way across a canyon wall that drops steeply left. Near the head of the canyon, your trail wraps left and finds a welcome rest bench set in a clearing. You are now high on the eastern flank of Kings Mountain, a long ridge extending from near Highway 92 southeast to Bear Gulch Road. For part of its length, Skyline Blvd., one of California's premier scenic routes, runs along the summit ridge of Kings Mountain.

when this land was designated as part of one of the greatest national parks in the country, the Golden Gate National Recreation Area."

A thick carpet of redwood needles and twigs, called duff, cushions your steps, and daylight filtering through the forest canopy gives a silvery sheen to the trees' lichen-covered bark. The understory in a redwood forest is sparse—not much else grows in the thick duff. In autumn, the solemn stillness may be interrupted by the nervous chatter of squirrels as they forage for seeds and acorns. Your trail climbs via switchbacks, passing a stand of tall, tropical-looking madrones framed against the sky.

At a junction marked by another beautiful metal sculpture, the Raymundo Trail heads right, but you continue straight, now on the single-track Mount Redondo Trail. With a tributary of West Union Creek to your right, you make a steady, moderate climb that soon eases. Turning right, you cross the tributary and then resume climbing, now aided by switchbacks. At about 3

**Sawmill Country**

About 10 sawmills, among the earliest in the Santa Cruz Mountains, were located on or near West Union Creek and its tributaries. Some of the mill owners are remembered today in the names of local roads, including Whipple Ave. in Redwood City, and Richards Road (now Richards Road Trail), the boundary between the Phleger Estate and Huddart Park.

The trail wanders uphill to avoid a frontal assault on the ramparts of Kings Mountain. But eventually the grade steepens and you switchback left. With the communication towers of the Kings Mountain Fire Station just uphill, you follow a rolling course, passing a trail that joins from the right. Soon you reach the boundary of Huddart Park, marked by the Richards Road Trail, a dirt road that heads right to Skyline Blvd. Go straight on the Richards

Road Trail and descend on a moderate grade past the Skyline Trail, right.

At the next junction, turn right onto Summit Springs Trail. After several hundred feet, you find the Crystal Springs Trail, left, and a rest bench. Here, at about 5 miles, you follow the Crystal Springs Trail past a gate that prevents access by horses during wet weather. The wide path descends gently for about 0.75 mile to the Dean Trail.

You join the single-track Dean Trail by turning sharply right and descending. Before reaching a seasonal creek, you pass McGarvey Flat, a lovely spot with a picnic table and several rest benches hewn from logs.

A level walk soon brings you to a four-way junction (shown incorrectly on the park map), where you bear left to stay on the Dean Trail. McGarvey Gulch Creek is downhill and left. Gently descending via S-bends, you soon reach a four-way junction with the Archery Fire Road. Regaining the Dean Trail across the road, you switchback left and again cross the Archery Fire Road.

At the edge of a paved road near the Miwok picnic area, your trail turns sharply left and then begins a series of switchbacks, descending past the Madrone picnic area. Now you cross the Campground Trail, a paved road that changes to dirt a few feet to your left. Stay on the Dean Trail, here a wide path, as it makes a curving descent past more picnic areas. At a T-junction with the Crystal Springs Trail, you close the loop, turn right, and retrace your route to the parking area.

## TRIP 14 El Corte de Madera Creek Open Space Preserve: Redwood Loop

| | |
|---|---|
| **Distance** | 8.4 miles, Loop |
| **Hiking Time** | 3 to 5 hours |
| **Elevation Gain/Loss** | ±2050 feet |
| **Difficulty** | Difficult |
| **Trail Use** | Mountain biking allowed |
| **Best Times** | All year |
| **Agency** | MROSD |
| **Recommended Map** | *El Corte de Madera Creek Open Space Preserve* (MROSD) |

**HIGHLIGHTS** This strenuous loop uses the Sierra Morena, Methuselah, Giant Salamander, Timberview, and Gordon Mill trails to explore a hidden realm of towering redwoods and massive Douglas-firs. Dropping almost all the way to the preserve's namesake creek, the route then rises to visit one of the few remaining old-growth redwoods on MROSD lands. Not yet complete with this pilgrimage, you drop once more to a lush, creekside canyon before steadily climbing back to Skyline Blvd.

**DIRECTIONS** From the intersection of Skyline Blvd. (Highway 35) and Highway 84 in Sky Londa, take Skyline Blvd. northwest 3.5 miles to roadside parking areas on both sides of the road.

**FACILITIES/TRAILHEAD** There are no facilities at the trailhead, which is at gate CM02 on the southwest side of Skyline Blvd.

Take the Sierra Morena Trail right about 100 feet to a junction with the Methuselah Trail, a dirt road that descends through dense forest. Where the Timberview Trail goes left, you continue straight on the Methuselah Trail as it climbs moderately to a four-way junction. Again you continue straight, now losing elevation over rough

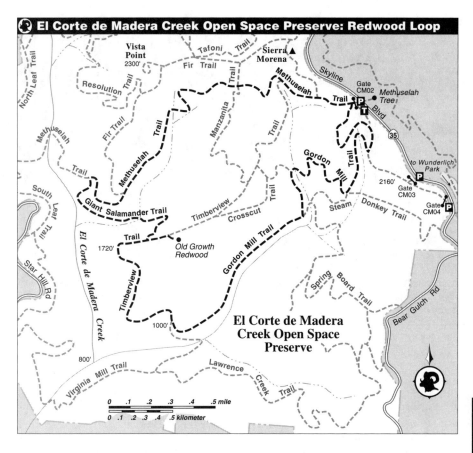

## El Corte de Madera Creek Open Space Preserve: Redwood Loop

El Corte de Madera Creek Open Space Preserve

and eroded ground. The grade here alternates between gentle, moderate, and steep as you follow a tributary of El Corte Madera Creek downhill.

When you reach a clearing, note the towering Douglas-fir nearby and examine it more closely, especially if you have binoculars. This is a granary tree, so called because acorn woodpeckers stash their namesake food supply in holes bored in its trunk. A communal effort, this process involves many birds and hundreds, perhaps thousands, of acorns.

Still descending, you pass the Fir Trail, right, and at the next junction turn left on the Giant Salamander Trail, at about 2.5 miles. Now on a rough, eroded single track, you descend through a jungle-like area of redwoods, huckleberry, ferns, and berry

> **Old Timers**
> The biblical name Methuselah is often used in conjunction with ancient trees, including one about 100 yards from the trailhead on the opposite side of Skyline Blvd. But in the world of coast redwoods, the oldest of which had a life span of more than 2200 years, Methuselah, said to have lived for 969 years, would have been considered a youngster.

vines. El Corte de Madera Creek is to your right but hidden from view. (This stretch of trail may be very muddy during wet weather.)

Coast live oaks, tanbark oaks, Douglas-firs, madrones, and California bays line the first part of the route. A few second-growth

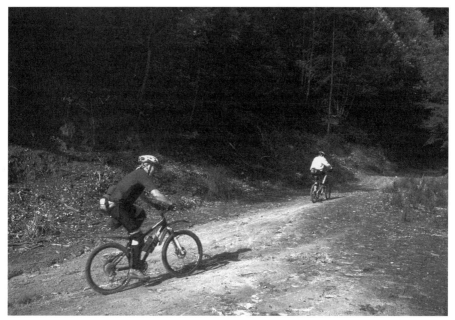

The Methuselah Trail climbs from El Corte de Madera Creek to near Skyline Blvd.

coast redwoods are here too, but most of their ancestors were reduced to stumps during the logging boom of the 19th and 20th centuries.

Curving left and then beginning to climb, you turn away from the creek and follow a tributary upstream on a rolling course. Now you begin a snaking climb on a grade that alternates between moderate and steep. A splendid assortment of ferns, including giant chain fern, adds to the magical quality of the forest here. After crossing a seasonal stream, the trail curves sharply left and reaches a junction with the Timberview Trail, a dirt road.

To visit one of the preserve's remaining old growth redwoods, turn left here and go about 0.1 mile to a clearing, right, marked by a sign that reads TO OLD GROWTH REDWOOD, NOT A THROUGH TRAIL. Turn right into the clearing, and then find a trail on its left-hand edge that leads about 100 feet to a massive coast redwood, approximately 50 feet in circumference at its base. When you have finished paying your respects to this monarch of the forest, return to the junction with the Giant Salamander Trail.

Here you continue straight on the Timberview Trail, descending moderately along a ridgetop. The road leaves the ridge with a sharp left-hand bend, and now you give up all the hard-won elevation gained on the previous trail, plunging on a grade that alternates between gentle, moderate, and steep. The Timberview Trail ends at a junction near another tributary of El Corte de Madera Creek. Here, at about 5 miles, the Lawrence Creek Trail heads right, but you go straight on the Gordon Mill Trail, a dirt road that was the primary haul road when logging was active here, and begin to climb.

Where the Springboard Trail goes right, you continue straight. Just ahead, your route passes a steep and eroded connector to the Timberview Trail, left, and then curves right. Now the road continues gently to gain elevation, passing stands of manzanita and bigleaf maple, two species that usually do not share the same habitat. Manzanitas are usually found on open,

**Feathered Denizens**

- A mature forest is the perfect habitat for band-tailed pigeons, a bird often found in flocks. This species is a larger, more attractively decorated relative of our urban pigeon, or rock dove. When startled, a flock of band-tailed pigeons will often take wing noisily in groups of three or four birds. This, in turn, can easily startle an unsuspecting hiker.

- If you see a bird that looks like a robin, look again. It may be a varied thrush, in the same family as the American robin but sporting a patterned head and wings. The call of the varied thrush — a flute-like note on a single pitch — echoes eerily through the forest.

At about 7 miles, you pass a short connector to the Steam Donkey Trail, right. Soon the road curves sharply right and climbs to a four-way junction. Ahead, the Gordon Mill Trail ends at gate CM03 and Skyline Blvd. The Sierra Morena Trail, a dirt road, angles right to gate CM04. Your route is the single-track branch of the Sierra Morena Trail, which heads left. You cross a grassy area and then return to forest, traveling on a magic carpet of redwood duff, which covers the trail and cushions your steps.

On a rolling course, you reach a junction with a trail veering right and climbing steeply. Ignore this shortcut back to the trailhead (unless you feel in need of further exertion). Your trail curves around a promontory jutting out from the end of a ridge, and here you have another opportunity to admire the preserve's fine trees, in this case massive Douglas-firs. After the shortcut merges sharply from the right, you go another 100 feet or so to the trailhead.

sunny slopes, whereas bigleaf maples prefer moist canyons.

## TRIP 15 El Corte de Madera Creek Open Space Preserve: Tafoni Loop

| | |
|---|---|
| **Distance** | 4.3 miles, Loop |
| **Hiking Time** | 2 to 3 hours |
| **Elevation Gain/Loss** | ±1300 |
| **Difficulty** | Moderate |
| **Trail Use** | Mountain biking allowed[1] |
| **Best Times** | All year |
| **Agency** | MROSD |
| **Recommended Map** | *El Corte de Madera Creek Open Space Preserve* (MROSD) |
| **Notes** | [1]Bicycles are not allowed on the short trail to the sandstone formation. |

**HIGHLIGHTS** An unusual sandstone formation called tafoni is the main attraction of this invigorating loop, which uses the Tafoni, Fir, and El Corte de Madera Creek trails at the north end of the preserve. Along the way, you can visit Vista Point, a scenic overlook with terrific views of the Pacific Ocean and the coastal hills. Towering Douglas-firs and coast redwoods, a sea of chaparral, and a lush riparian corridor near the headwaters of El Corte de Madera Creek are some of the other attractions visitors will enjoy here.

**DIRECTIONS** From the intersection of Skyline Blvd. (Highway 35) and Highway 84 in Sky Londa, take Skyline Blvd. northwest 3.9 miles to the Caltrans parking area at Skeggs Point.

**FACILITIES/TRAILHEAD** There are picnic tables and toilets at Skeggs Point. The trailhead is at gate CM01, on the southwest side of Skyline Blvd., about 100 yards northwest of the parking area.

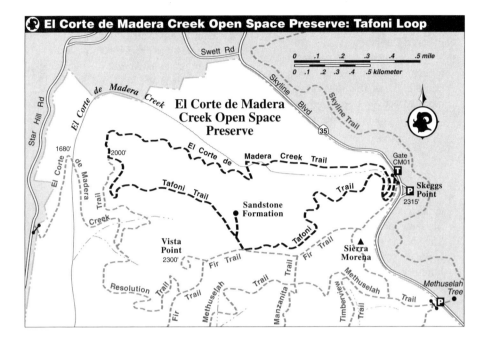

El Corte de Madera Creek Open Space Preserve: Tafoni Loop

Follow the Tafoni Trail, a dirt road that climbs moderately to a junction with the El Corte de Madera Creek Trail, right, which you will use later. The hillside on your right drops steeply into the canyon holding the headwaters of El Corte de Madera Creek. Descending on a moderate grade, the rocky track soon swings sharply left to a T-junction. The left branch is a closed trail, so here you turn right.

Now climbing on a gentle grade, you reach a saddle and a four-way junction in a small clearing. Here the Fir Trail goes left and straight, and the Tafoni Trail goes right.

At about 1.4 miles, turn right (northwest) on the Tafoni Trail, a dirt road, and descend gently to a junction signed SAND-STONE FORMATION. The single-track trail, closed to bicycles and horses, leads to an observation deck with a sign explaining the process that creates tafoni, the eroded sandstone formations you can see from the deck. The formations are fragile: please stay on the trail or the observation deck at all times.

When you have finished enjoying this unusual area, return to the Tafoni Trail and turn right.

In addition to magnificent coast redwoods and Douglas-firs, this preserve is home to coast live oaks, tanbark oaks, California bays, and madrones.

The road makes a long, moderate descent along a ridgetop, then rolls to a fenced restoration area where you turn right to stay on the Tafoni Trail, now a single track. Soon you merge with the El Corte de Madera Creek Trail, which joins sharply from the left. Continuing almost straight, you follow the single-track trail gently uphill through one of the Peninsula's densest forests. You descend and follow the trail as it bends sharply left, then crosses a bridge over El Corte de Madera Creek.

Beyond the bridge is a T-junction, at about 3.5 miles, where you turn right to stay on the El Corte de Madera Creek Trail, now a dirt road. As you climb steadily in a shady,

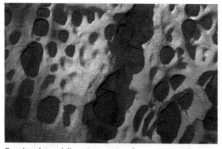

Erosion by acidic rain creates fantastic sandstone formations called tafoni.

**Side Trip**
From the junction of the Tafoni and Fir trails, you can make an easy, 0.6-mile round-trip excursion to Vista Point, where views of the San Mateo coast and the Pacific Ocean await. Take the Fir Trail to a fork, bear right, and at the next fork bear right again.

steep-walled canyon, the creek wanders back and forth under the road through culverts. When you meet the Tafoni Trail, turn left and retrace your route to the parking area. (When walking back to the parking area, carefully cross Skyline Blvd. and use the wide dirt shoulder on the east side of the road.)

## TRIP 16 Purisima Creek Redwoods Open Space Preserve: Purisima Canyon

| | |
|---|---|
| **Distance** | 10.1 miles, Loop |
| **Hiking Time** | 4 to 6 hours |
| **Elevation Gain/Loss** | ±1600 feet |
| **Difficulty** | Very Difficult |
| **Best Times** | All year |
| **Agency** | MROSD |
| **Recommended Map** | *Purisima Creek Redwoods Open Space Preserve* (MROSD) |

**HIGHLIGHTS** One of the premier routes on the Peninsula, this challenging loop uses the North Ridge, Harkins Ridge, Soda Gulch, Purisima Creek, and Whittemore Gulch trails to explore the north half of this expansive preserve. Dropping more than 1500 feet to Purisima Creek, you pass the giant stumps of old-growth redwoods, and can imagine yourself going back in time to an era when the canyons here echoed with the sounds of humans and machinery hard at work harvesting a seemingly endless resource. From the trailhead to Purisima Canyon, this route follows the Bay Area Ridge Trail.

**DIRECTIONS** From the intersection of Skyline Blvd. (Highway 35) and Highway 92, take Skyline Blvd. southeast 4.5 miles to a parking area on the right.

**FACILITIES/TRAILHEAD** There is a phone just northwest of the parking area, in front of the former store. A toilet is beside the trailhead, which is on the southwest corner of the parking area.

Follow a dirt road gently downhill to a junction with the hiking-only North Ridge Trail. Bear right and make a switchbacking descent to a four-way junction where you meet the dirt road you recently abandoned. You go straight, now on the Harkins Ridge Trail. Soon the trail crosses a culvert draining the seasonal creek that flows through Whittemore Gulch. This is one of the many tributaries of Purisima Creek, which eventually deposits its gathered waters into the Pacific south of Half Moon Bay.

After following the trail through several bends, you reach open ground on a scrubby hillside. The Pacific coastline and Half

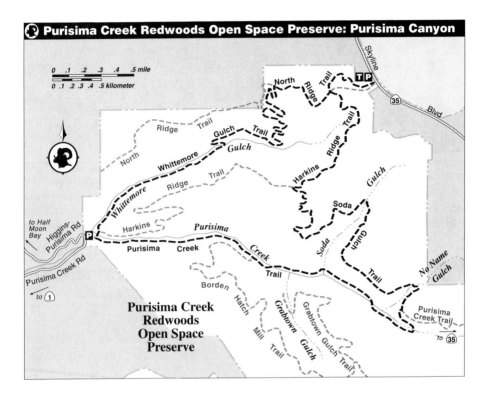

**Purisima Creek Redwoods Open Space Preserve: Purisima Canyon**

Purisima Creek
Redwoods
Open Space
Preserve

Moon Bay, visible on a clear day, are in the distance to your right. At a T-junction with a

**Purisima Plant Life**

- In addition to the preserve's namesake redwoods, the trees here include Douglas-fir, coast live oak, California bay, tanbark oak, madrone, bigleaf maple, willow, and red alder.
- A redwood forest fosters a community of plants that thrive in its moist, shady environment. A thick layer of redwood duff—twigs and needles on the forest floor—inhibits the growth of some species but favors others, including western sword fern, trillium, fairy bells, Pacific star flower, and redwood sorrel.
- California poppy, lupine, goldenrod, aster, blue-eyed grass, paintbrush, Douglas iris, hound's tongue, milk maids, and columbine are among the wildflowers that decorate the preserve.

closed road, left, you turn right and descend to the Soda Gulch Trail. Here, at about 1.4 miles, you turn left and follow the single-track trail, closed to bicycles and horses, across an open slope of coastal scrub.

Now descending via switchbacks, you pass a beautiful stand of coast live oaks, their twisted, gnarled limbs draped with lace lichen. A sudden transition brings you into the realm of the redwoods. A rest bench, left, invites you to spend a few minutes contemplating these towering giants in cool and shady surroundings. Some of the trees are fire-scarred, and some grow in so-called family circles around a fallen ancestor.

As you continue to lose elevation on a gentle grade, you pass a second rest bench and several seasonal creeks. Soda Gulch, another tributary of Purisima Creek, is downhill and right. When you reach Soda Gulch, turn sharply right to cross a bridge, which spans the creek bed. Soon the route emerges briefly onto an open hillside before

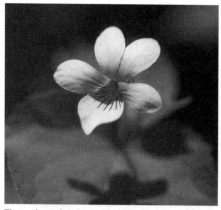

Tiny redwood violets, with yellow flowers, are often found beneath their towering namesake trees

ducking back into the redwoods. You descend to an unnamed tributary of Purisima Creek and cross it on a bridge, then zigzag uphill to meet the Purisima Creek Trail, a dirt road, at about 4 miles.

Join the road by bearing right, then follow it downhill to Purisima Creek, which flows under the road through a culvert. You enjoy a level walk through a riparian corridor lush with red alder, hazelnut, elk clover, and red elderberry. Soon a bridge takes you across Purisima Creek, which is now on your left. The creek from Soda Gulch joins from the right, and you cross it on the next bridge. Look here for tiger lilies in late spring. Wintering ladybugs sometimes gather beside Purisima Creek by the thousands, and you may see them massed on the leaves and branches of trailside plants.

On the left is a remnant of a bridge, which once spanned Purisima Creek and provided a link with the Grabtown Gulch Trail, until it was washed out during a flood. Descend on a moderate grade to the creek and cross it on a bridge, soon passing a junction with the Borden Hatch Mill Trail, left. One of Purisima Canyon's many lumber mills once stood in a nearby clearing. At about 6.3 miles, you pass a toilet, left, and then reach a short connector to the Whittemore Gulch and Harkins Ridge trails. (The Higgins Purisima parking area is about 100 yards ahead.)

Turn right and cross Purisima Creek on a bridge. About 50 feet ahead is a T-junction. Here you turn left on the Whittemore Gulch Trail, a rocky dirt road, and soon pass a fence with a gate that prevents access by bicycles and horses during wet weather. Soon the road curves right, narrows to a single track, and begins to climb. Whittemore Gulch, holding a tributary of Purisima Creek within its steep and narrow walls, is left. (Keep a sharp eye out for descending bicyclists!) It was here in Whittemore Gulch, according to local historian Ken Fisher, that San Mateo's last grizzly bear was killed in 1879, with a piece of poisoned beefsteak.

The grade alternates between moderate and steep as you pass impressive rock cliffs

### That Little B-b-b-bird
Coastal scrub is the perfect habitat for a secretive bird called a wrentit, more often heard than seen. Listen for a stuttering song that sounds like someone trying to start a reluctant car. This small songster is brown with a buffy breast, and has a long tail often held nearly vertical.

on the right. The layers of marine sediments in these cliffs have been tilted almost vertically by geological forces almost too great to imagine. Now on a rolling course, you stroll through stands of redwoods and a forest of red alder. An old-growth redwood grove stands on the opposite side of Whittemore Gulch.

Aided by switchbacks, you continue to gain elevation, passing a short connector to the North Ridge Trail, at about 8.5 miles. After more twists and turns, you come to a T-junction with the North Ridge Trail. Now you bear right on a dirt road and enjoy a mostly level walk through a Douglas-fir forest. At the four-way junction where you started this loop, turn left onto the hiking-only trail and retrace your route to the parking area.

Peninsula

# TRIP 17 Edgewood Park and Preserve

| | |
|---|---|
| **Distance** | 4.5 miles, Loop |
| **Hiking Time** | 2 to 3 hours |
| **Elevation Gain/Loss** | ±850 feet |
| **Difficulty** | Moderate |
| **Best Times** | All year |
| **Agency** | SMCP&R |
| **Recommended Map** | *Edgewood Park and Preserve* (SMCP&R) |

**HIGHLIGHTS** Surprisingly varied for such a small area, the terrain here includes wetland, grassland, oak woodland, and chaparral plant communities; and this route, using the Edgewood, Franciscan, Sylvan, and Serpentine Loop trails, and the Ridgeview Loop, samples them all. It is the grasslands on serpentine soil, however, that produce the park's justly famous display of spring wildflowers. The Natural Resources DataBase, www.nrdb.org, lists more than 470 plant species found in this park and preserve, including a handful of rare, threatened, or endangered ones.

**DIRECTIONS** From I-280 southwest of San Carlos, take the Edgewood Road exit and go northeast 0.9 mile to the park entrance, right. The overflow parking area is immediately on the right, and the main paved parking area is a few hundred feet ahead.

**FACILITIES/TRAILHEAD** There are restrooms, picnic tables, phone, and water uphill from the main parking area. The trailhead is on the this parking area's west side, near its entrance and an information board.

Take the single-track trail that passes to the right of the information board. After 100 feet or so, you come to a T-junction, where you turn right onto the Edgewood Trail, also a single track. As you climb on a gentle grade via switchbacks, look beside the trail for spring wildflowers such as hound's tongue, Ithuriel's spear, soap plant, blue-eyed grass, white globe lilies, yarrow, and bluedicks.

The steady ascent brings you to a four-way junction with a dirt road. You cross it and continue straight on the Edgewood Trail. At the next junction, with a connector to the Sylvan Trail, you also continue straight. Descending gently, the trail reaches a ravine that holds a seasonal creek. Swinging sharply right, you walk through a cool, damp forest.

Along with the rows of houses visible in the distance, traffic noise from I-280 is a reminder that this remarkable preserve has been spared the fate of other formerly open lands.

## Edgewood Flora, Bird Life

- Stands of coast live oak, California bay, toyon, and California buckeye provide shade, but where they are absent, swaths of chaparral and coastal scrub — chamise, buckbrush, chaparral pea, pitcher sage, California sagebrush, bush monkeyflower, golden yarrow, coyote brush, and poison oak — thrive.

- In wooded areas, look for California coast larkspur, a tall member of the genus *Delphinium*, with blue flowers and deeply-cut leaves. Also here is mugwort, a fragrant plant whose crushed leaves are reputed to calm the itching of poison oak.

- This varied habitat attracts birds, including California towhees, spotted towhees, dark-eyed juncos, hummingbirds, chestnut-backed chickadees, bushtits, western scrub-jays, and Steller's jays.

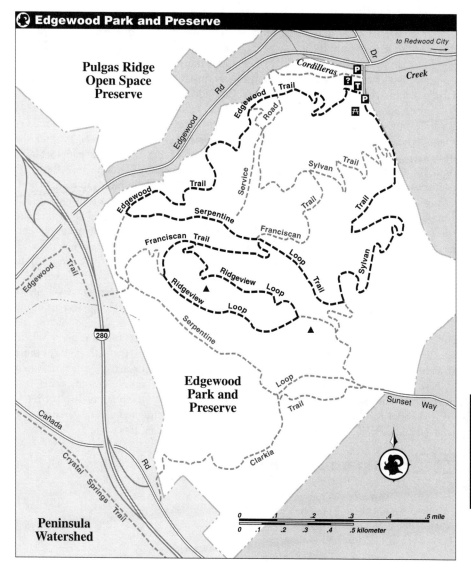

## Edgewood Park and Preserve

Your route makes a sudden transition from forest to grassland. Open grasslands dotted with serpentine rocks wrap around the northwest, west, and southwest sides of the preserve. Purple owl's-clover, mule ears, farewell-to-spring, blow-wives, bellardia, and various lupines are among the flowers attracted to this special combination of sun and soil. Open fields also attract various songbirds, and you may find western bluebirds nearby.

### The Joy of Grass

Grasslands are fragile ecosystems easily damaged by invasive nonnative plants and human intrusion. Efforts are underway to restore the preserve's serpentine grasslands to a more natural state. One of the benefits of this will be improved habitat for the bay checkerspot butterfly, a threatened species.

At a junction with the Serpentine Loop Trail, just past 1 mile, you bear left onto a dirt road. Your view from the gently rising, winding road stretches northeast across San Francisco Bay to the East Bay hills and Mt. Diablo. Behind you rises Kings Mountain, a bastion of open space bisected by Skyline Blvd. Bearing right at a fork with a service road, you descend on a gentle grade to a four-way junction. (To shorten the route, omit the Ridgeview Loop and follow the route description from this junction.)

Turning right at the four-way junction, you follow the Franciscan Trail, a single track that soon switchbacks right, passes a beautifully situated rest bench, and then climbs along the margin between woodland and grassland. At the next junction, a fork, you bear right. The trail loses elevation and then curves left across a sun-baked hillside. The Franciscan Trail veers sharply right to connect with the Serpentine Loop Trail, which is just downhill, but you continue straight on the Ridgeview Loop.

Now climbing on a gentle grade, you soon reach a four-way junction atop a saddle with great views of San Francisco Bay. Here you turn left and continue to climb. As you leave the saddle, look beside the trail for yellow Mariposa lilies. Winding your way uphill, you enter a corridor of chaparral. The trail levels as it nears the wooded ridgetop, then bends sharply right and begins to descend. Close the Ridgeview Loop at the Franciscan Trail, bear right, and then retrace your route to the Serpentine Loop Trail, at about 3 miles.

Now you turn sharply right onto the Serpentine Loop Trail, a wide path that takes you past a hedge of poison oak, coffeeberry, and coyote brush and leads to a T-junction. Leave the Serpentine Loop Trail and turn left on the Sylvan Trail. Wooded areas alternate with open grasslands along your descent, which eventually is aided by switchbacks.

Passing a junction with a closed trail, right, you curve left into a canyon that holds a spring-fed creek. The trail crosses a culvert and then bends right. Along this part of the route, look for creambush, blue witch, yerba santa, virgin's bower, and snowberry. Where a trail joins from the left, you continue straight and soon reach a T-junction with a dirt-and-gravel path. Restrooms, water, and picnic tables are to your left. Turning right, you descend and after several hundred feet reach the parking area.

# TRIP 18 Junipero Serra Park

|  |  |
|---|---|
| **Distance** | 1.7 miles, Loop |
| **Hiking Time** | 1 to 2 hours |
| **Elevation Gain/Loss** | ±300 feet |
| **Difficulty** | Easy |
| **Trail Use** | Good for kids |
| **Best Times** | All year |
| **Agency** | SMCP&R |
| **Recommended Map** | Junipero Serra Park (SMCP&R) |

**HIGHLIGHTS** This delightful stroll on the Quail Loop Trail visits an island of open space within earshot of San Francisco International Airport and the busy I-280 corridor. Spring wildflower displays and hillsides shaded by towering trees are incentives to visit what one park ranger calls "the Golden Gate Park" of the San Bruno area.

**DIRECTIONS** From I-280 northbound in San Bruno, take the San Bruno Ave. exit and turn left on San Bruno Ave. Go under the freeway and turn left to get on I-280 southbound. Immediately exit onto Crystal Springs Road and follow the directions below.

From I-280 southbound in San Bruno, take the Crystal Springs Road exit and stay right. Turn right on Crystal Springs Road and go 0.5 mile to the park entrance, left. There is an entrance kiosk open weekends. Just past the kiosk, turn left and park in the De Anza area, where there is a self-registration station.

**FACILITIES/TRAILHEAD** A small visitor center with natural history exhibits can be reached by turning right just past the entrance kiosk and going about halfway up the road to Iris Point. The park has group picnic areas, shelters, and facilities for youth groups, which can be reserved by calling (650) 363-4021. There are picnic tables, restrooms, and water beside the parking area. The De Anza trailhead is on the northeast corner of the parking area, just across a bridge over El Zanjon Creek. (The Live Oak Nature Trail, a self-guiding route, starts here as well; pick up a brochure at the visitor center.)

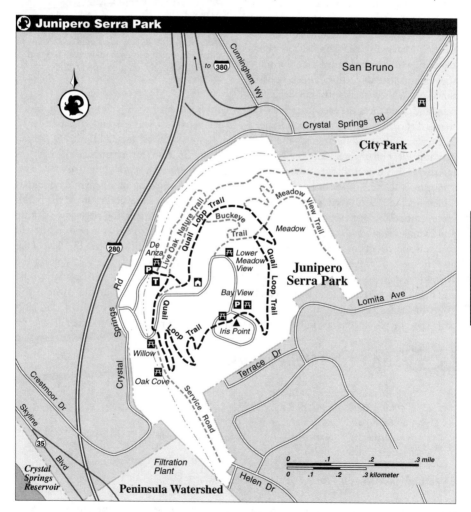

Take the De Anza Trail, a single track that climbs gently through a woodland of coast live oak, California bay, toyon, and Monterey pine. After about 100 feet you come to a four-way junction with the Live Oak Nature Trail, where you continue straight. At a T-junction with the Quail Loop Trail, a dirt-and-gravel path, you turn left and continue climbing on a gentle grade, passing a four-way junction with the Buckeye Trail.

Unfortunately, many of the park's Monterey pines are infected with a fungal disease called pine pitch canker. According to scientists, perhaps 80% of California's Monterey pines will die within the next 30 years.

Passing a trail, left, that goes to San Bruno City Park, you emerge from the woods into a large grassy field with views of San Francisco Bay, San Francisco International Airport, and the San Mateo Bridge. This field is mowed regularly to control invasive nonnative species and to reduce fire danger. Crossing the Meadow View Trail, you soon switchback right and again meet the Meadow View Trail, here a dirt road leading uphill to park headquarters and the parking area for the Lower Meadow View picnic area. Stay on the Quail Loop Trail by turning sharply left.

Enjoy the park's spring wildflowers, which include blue-eyed grass, Ithuriel's spear, checkerbloom, soap plant, yarrow, and Douglas iris.

A surprise awaits, as the trail rises through an unexpected grove of coast redwoods. Beyond the grove, you pass Bay View Shelter and then cross the paved road that circles Iris Point, the park's wooded summit. Just ahead, you cross the paved road again and find the

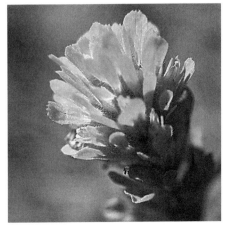

Paintbrush, which comes in many varieties and colors, adds a lively touch to open hillsides.

continuation of the Quail Loop Trail, which veers left. Now you descend via switchbacks across a southwest-facing hillside. El Zanjon Creek (Spanish for channel or slough) is downhill, near the park's boundary.

Shade, welcome on a warm day, signals your approach to several more of the park's picnic areas. Skirting the edge of a parking area, the trail crosses a paved road and comes to a junction. Here the Live Oak Nature Trail goes left, but you stay on the Quail Loop Trail by veering right. Just ahead is the four-way junction where you began this loop. Here you turn left and retrace your route to the parking area.

# TRIP 19 San Pedro Valley Park

| | |
|---|---|
| **Distance** | 2.4 miles, Loop |
| **Hiking Time** | 1 to 2 hours |
| **Elevation Gain/Loss** | ±650 feet |
| **Difficulty** | Moderate |
| **Best Times** | All year |
| **Agency** | SMCP&R |
| **Recommended Map** | *San Pedro Valley Park* (SMCP&R) |

**HIGHLIGHTS**  This surprisingly varied loop, using the Montara Mountain and Brooks Creek trails, climbs through a eucalyptus forest to reach scenic vantage points on a chaparral-cloaked ridge. During the rainy season, a cascading waterfall, visible from the trail, plunges down Montara Mountain.

**DIRECTIONS** From the intersection of Highway 1 and Linda Mar Blvd. in Pacifica, go southeast 1.9 miles on Linda Mar Blvd. to Oddstad Blvd. Turn right and then immediately left into the park. At 0.1 mile you come to an entrance kiosk and a self-registration station. Past the kiosk, turn right and go to a paved parking area, right. (If this area is full, there are others nearby.)

**FACILITIES/TRAILHEAD** The park has two group picnic areas and an overnight area for organized youth groups, available by reservation at (650) 363-4021. There is a visitor center, open weekends and holidays 10 A.M.–4 P.M. Restrooms, picnic tables, phone, and water are beside the parking area. The trailhead is on the west side of the parking area, just right of the restrooms.

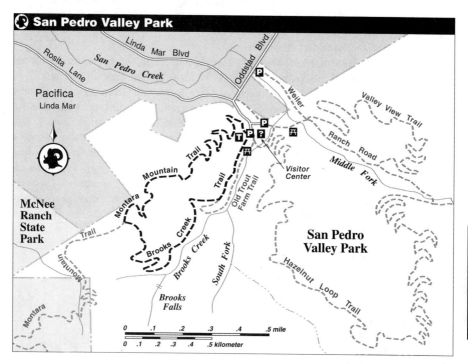

San Pedro Valley Park

Follow a paved path from the trailhead, and after about 25 feet turn left onto a dirt path that skirts the restroom and picnic area. Just ahead is a junction, where you veer right onto the Montara Mountain Trail, a single track. The route climbs gently through a forest of eucalyptus to a paved road, crosses it, and continues steadily to gain elevation, now via switchbacks. Soon you have a view of the Pacific Ocean, framed by the San Pedro Valley.

You climb above the eucalyptus forest for your first good look at Montara Mountain,

actually a long ridge with about half a dozen summits. The trail takes advantage of a ridgetop to gain higher ground, then makes a gently rising traverse across an east-facing hillside that drops left to a ravine. After wandering through a corridor of chaparral and coastal scrub, you come to a junction.

Here the Montara Mountain Trail continues straight, but you turn left on the Brooks Creek Trail, also a single track. The northern wall of Montara Mountain, steep and rugged, rises to your right. The trail traces a curvy course gently downhill, in

---

**San Pedro Foliage**

- Evergreen huckleberry, hazelnut, mountain mahogany, chinquapin, and various species of ceanothus and manzanita thrive on the park's sun-warmed slopes.
- The ravine holding Brooks Creek is lush with thickets of willow, creambush, coffeeberry, yerba santa, and toyon.

---

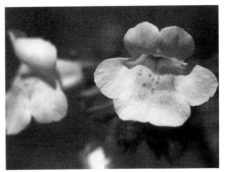

Common monkeyflower, unlike bush monkeyflower, is found in wet areas.

places barely clinging to the precipitous slope. After a switchback left, the route parallels a shady ravine holding a tributary of the South Fork of San Pedro Creek. This tributary is known locally as Brooks Creek.

Several more switchbacks ease the descent, and soon you reach a rest bench. Winter rains create a waterfall that plunges about 175 feet in three tiers down one of Montara Mountain's north-facing ravines, visible from here. Ahead, a bridge takes you across a seasonal creek, and now you reenter the eucalyptus forest that shrouds some of the low-elevation areas of this park.

Where the Old Trout Farm Trail joins from the right, you continue straight on the Brooks Creek Trail, passing another rest bench. After several hundred feet, you pass a closed leg of the Old Trout Farm Trail. Just ahead is the junction with the Montara Mountain Trail, where you began this loop. From here, retrace your route to the parking area.

# TRIP 20 Montara Mountain

|  |  |
|---|---|
| **Distance** | 7.2 miles, Out-and-back |
| **Hiking Time** | 3 to 4 hours |
| **Elevation Gain/Loss** | ±1650 feet |
| **Difficulty** | Difficult |
| **Best Times** | All year |
| **Agency** | CSP, SMCP&R |
| **Recommended Map** | *San Pedro Valley Park* (SMCP&R) |

**HIGHLIGHTS** This route, using the Montara Mountain Trail and North Peak Access Road, starts in a eucalyptus forest in San Pedro Valley Park. Soon you are wandering uphill through chaparral and coastal scrub, until you finally attack the ramparts of Montara Mountain itself. The cleverly constructed trail makes good use of the terrain, so the climbing is not difficult. Views of the Santa Cruz Mountains, the East Bay hills, and some San Francisco landmarks reward your efforts.

**DIRECTIONS** From the intersection of Highway 1 and Linda Mar Blvd. in Pacifica, go southeast 1.9 miles on Linda Mar Blvd. to Oddstad Blvd. Turn right and then immediately left into the park. At 0.1 mile you come to an entrance kiosk and a self-registration station. Past the kiosk, turn right and go to a paved parking area, right. (If this area is full, there are others nearby.)

**FACILITIES/TRAILHEAD** The park has two group picnic areas and an overnight area for organized youth groups, available by reservation at (650) 363-4021. There is a visitor center, open weekends and holidays 10 A.M.–4 P.M. Restrooms, picnic tables, phone, and water are beside the parking area. The trailhead is on the west side of the parking area, just right of the restrooms.

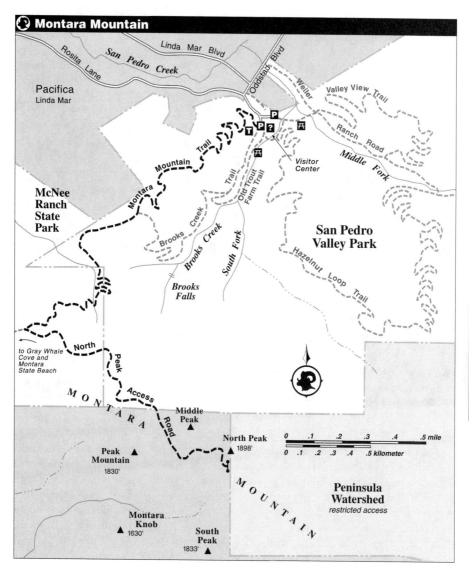

Montara Mountain

Follow a paved path from the trailhead, and after about 25 feet turn left onto a dirt path that skirts the restroom and picnic area. Just ahead is a junction, where you veer right onto the Montara Mountain Trail, a single track. The route climbs gently through a forest of eucalyptus to a paved road, crosses it, and continues steadily to gain elevation, now via switchbacks. Soon you have a view of the Pacific Ocean, framed by the San Pedro Valley.

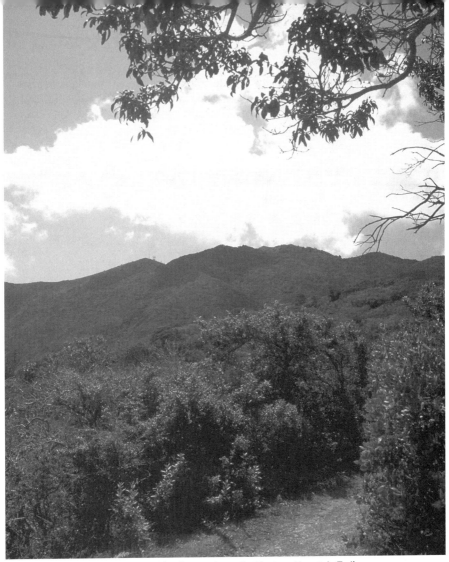

Montara Mountain, actually a long ridge, looms above the Montara Mountain Trail.

You climb above the eucalyptus forest for your first good look at Montara Mountain, actually a long ridge with about half a dozen summits. The trail takes advantage of a ridgetop to gain higher ground, then makes a gently rising traverse across an east-facing hillside that drops left to a ravine. After wandering through a corridor of chaparral and coastal scrub, at about 1.4 miles, you come to a junction with the Brooks Creek Trail.

From here, continue straight on the Montara Mountain Trail. A rest bench, right, invites you to admire a gorgeous panorama of the Pacific Ocean and the coastline sweep-

ing north to Mt. Tamalpais. The route trends southwest, giving you ample opportunities to study Montara Mountain, actually a long ridge crowned by a handful of summits.

Rocky and eroded, the trail runs atop a ridge as it prepares to attack Montara Mountain's formidable ramparts. As you ascend via switchbacks, Mt. Diablo, another Bay Area landmark, appears in the distance, behind Sweeney Ridge. Soon you enter McNee Ranch State Park. To avoid a frontal assault on the mountain's defenses, the trail wanders through ravines and climbs over

**Faulty Mountain?**

Montara Mountain is the northernmost elevation of the Santa Cruz Mountains, a range that straddles the San Andreas fault for most of its length. The fault runs along the Peninsula and enters the Pacific north of Pacifica.

spurs, steadily rising on a grade that alternates between moderate and gentle.

At about 2.5 miles, you reach a junction with the North Peak Access Road (shown on the county park map as Montara Mountain Road); join it by veering left. This road is open to bicycles, so use caution. You are rewarded for your efforts by views of San Bruno Mountain, San Francisco, and the San Mateo coast. The road rises steeply, dips to a saddle, and then climbs gently past a dirt road and an unofficial trail, both right.

Chinquapin, golden yarrow, chaparral currant, and manzanita, including a species found nowhere else, all grow on Montara Mountain.

Sighting southeast, you have an uninterrupted view of the Santa Cruz Mountains down to Mt. Umunhum. To the north, you can pick out features of San Francisco such as the Sunset District, Twin Peaks, and Golden Gate Park. The Berkeley hills, capped by Vollmer Peak and Round Top, are also in view.

Several dirt roads to a communication facility join from the left. You continue straight to a gate at the San Francisco Water Department's Peninsula Watershed boundary, at about 3.6 miles. Montara Mountain's North Peak is just uphill and left, on private property. Mt. Hamilton, with its white observatory domes, graces the distant skyline. From here, retrace your route to the parking area.

## TRIP 21 Sweeney Ridge

| | |
|---|---|
| **Distance** | 4 miles, Out-and-back |
| **Hiking Time** | 2 to 3 hours |
| **Elevation Gain/Loss** | ±850 feet |
| **Difficulty** | Moderate |
| **Trail Use** | Leashed dogs |
| **Best Times** | Spring and fall |
| **Agency** | GGNRA |
| **Recommended Map** | *None* |

**HIGHLIGHTS**  For several centuries, mariners sailed past the fog-shrouded entrance of the San Francisco Bay without suspecting that a great body of water lay just beyond the coastal hills. But in the fall of 1769, Gaspar de Portolá's overland expedition to locate Monterey Bay overshot its mark and found San Francisco Bay instead. From atop Sweeney Ridge, wrote Fr. Juan Crespí, they "beheld the great estuary," one big enough to hold "not only the King's navy but all the navies of Europe." This out-and-back trip uses the Sweeney Ridge Trail, part of the Bay Area Ridge Trail, to visit the San Francisco Bay Discovery Site. Sweeney Ridge, named for a ranch that operated nearby in the late 1800s, rises between Pacifica and San Bruno.

**DIRECTIONS**  From I-280 northbound in South San Francisco, take the Avalon Dr./Westborough Blvd. exit. and go 0.6 mile to Westborough Blvd. Turn left, go under the interstate, and go 1.1 miles to Skyline Blvd. (Highway 35). Turn left, go, 0.7 mile to College Dr., and turn right. At 0.5 mile (Skyline College), turn left and go 0.2 mile to the Student Parking Lot 2 entrance road, left. Go about 100 yards to the parking lot

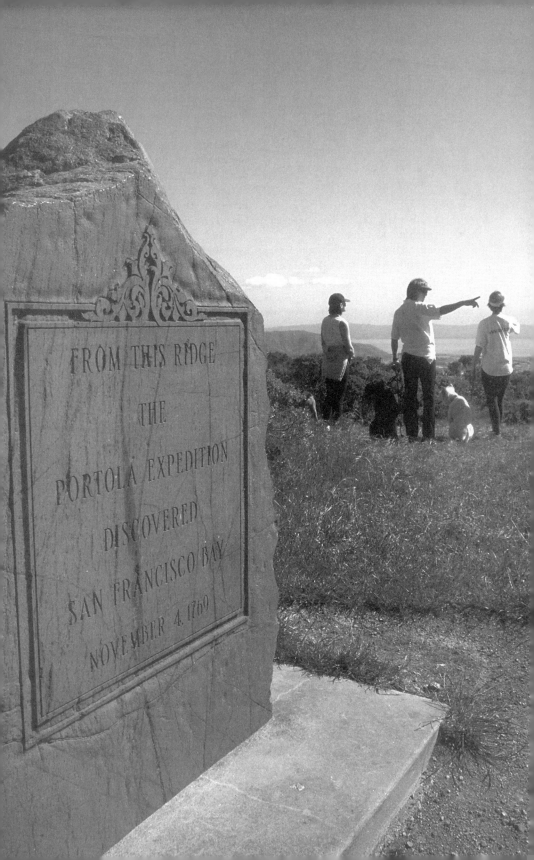

FROM THIS RIDGE
THE
PORTOLA EXPEDITION
DISCOVERED
SAN FRANCISCO BAY
NOVEMBER 4, 1769

entrance. Park in the spaces reserved for GGNRA use, on the left side of the parking lot, near its entrance.

From I-280 southbound, take the Avalon Dr./Westborough Blvd. exit, turn right on Westborough, and then follow the directions above.

**FACILITIES/TRAILHEAD** There are no facilities at the trailhead, which is on the southeast corner of the parking lot.

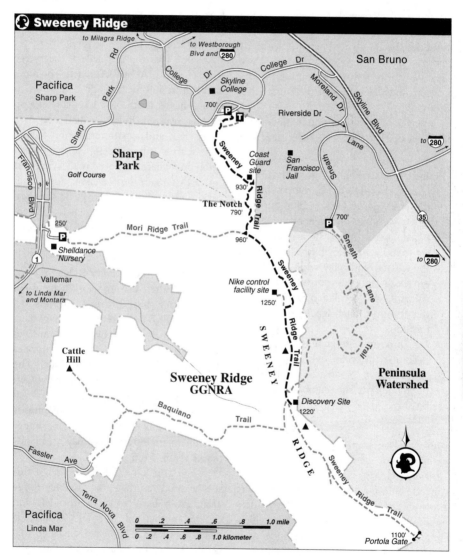

The single-track Sweeney Ridge Trail makes a sharp right turn about 50 feet from the trailhead and then climbs steeply through a grove of Monterey pines. After

From here, members of the Portolá expedition first saw San Francisco Bay.

several hundred yards, you join a dirt-and-gravel road by angling right. The road ascends moderately, providing ever-improving views of Mt. Tamalpais, San Bruno Mountain, San Francisco's Twin Peaks, and the Pacific Ocean.

Above the trees you enter a zone of coastal scrub. Joining the native vegetation in places are stands of cypress and eucalyptus, both species planted here. Curving left and passing several water tanks, you have a view south to Montara Mountain, the northernmost elevation of the Santa Cruz Mountains.

After passing a junction with a road heading sharply left, the grade eases and

---

### Things That Grow and Things That Fly

- Lupine, critical to the development of the endangered Mission blue butterfly's larva, grows on Sweeney Ridge.
- Coastal scrub found here is perfect for many species of birds, including the western scrub-jay, wrentit, northern flicker, and the spotted towhee, a colorful, sparrow-like bird that rustles through fallen leaves searching for food.
- The Discovery Site knoll is beautifully decorated in spring with goldfields, checkerbloom, Douglas iris, California poppy, lupine, sun cups, and paintbrush.

---

you enjoy a scenic panorama of San Francisco and the East Bay hills, the latter crowned by Mt. Diablo. An abandoned concrete building, left, is all that remains of a former Coast Guard site. Just beyond the building you get on a paved path, which curves left and then ends abruptly at a junction with a short dirt road, left. You leave the paved path and descend on trail to a scrub-filled ravine, aided in places by steps.

Now climbing out of the ravine, aided again by steps, you wind uphill to a junction

with a dirt road, at about 1 mile. To the right of this junction, the road is called the Mori Ridge Trail. To the left it is the Sweeney Ridge Trail. Here you angle left and make your way toward several green concrete buildings on a ridge ahead. These are the remnants of a Nike missile command site, used during the Cold War. Today, thankfully, a generation has grown up with a very different association for the Greek goddess of victory.

As you pass the missile site, you merge with a paved road by veering left. The road, a continuation of Sneath Lane in San Bruno, heads south on a level course atop treeless Sweeney Ridge. A dirt road to a water tank and a communication facility joins sharply from the left. Soon you reach a junction where the paved road swings left and a dirt road, the Sweeney Ridge Trail, continues straight. Your goal, the San Francisco Bay Discovery Site, is just ahead. San Andreas Lake, part of the San Francisco Water Department's Peninsula Watershed, is visible from the ridge.

You follow the Sweeney Ridge Trail for several hundred feet to a fork, where you turn left on a short dirt road that rises to a knoll (1220'). There are two stone markers here. As you look out over San Francisco Bay, the marker on the left commemorates the Bay's "discovery" by Europeans. The marker on your right is in memory of Carl Patrick McCarthy, who lobbied for national recognition of the site's historical importance. Atop this marker is a stone cylinder inscribed with the names of Bay Area landmarks visible from here.

When you have finished enjoying this special spot, return to the Sweeney Ridge Trail. From here, you can turn left and explore another mile or so of the trail as it heads southeast to the watershed's Portola Gate. Along the way, you'll pass the Baquiano Trail, which heads west to Pacifica. Or you can simply turn right and retrace your route to the parking area.

# TRIP22 San Bruno Mountain State and County Park

| | |
|---:|:---|
| **Distance** | 3.1 miles, Loop |
| **Hiking Time** | 2 to 3 hours |
| **Elevation Gain/Loss** | ±700 feet |
| **Difficulty** | Moderate |
| **Best Times** | All year |
| **Agency** | CSP, SMCP&R |
| **Recommended Map** | *San Bruno Mountain* (SMCP&R) |

**HIGHLIGHTS** This exploration of San Bruno Mountain, which is actually a long ridge that angles northwest toward Daly City from Brisbane, takes place via the Summit Loop Trail and leads you to an island of open space surrounded by a sea of residential and industrial development. Despite this urban setting, the mountain's rugged canyons and often wind-swept ridges host a remarkable array of rare and/or endangered species. Among these are several species of butterflies and more than a dozen plants, including three manzanitas. When not fogbound, the trails here afford views of San Francisco and beyond, and the spring wildflower displays are sensational.

**DIRECTIONS** From Highway 101 northbound in San Francisco, take the Third St. exit (not well signed). Go 0.5 mile to Paul Ave., turn left, go 0.1 mile to San Bruno Ave., and turn left again. At 0.9 mile San Bruno Ave. joins Bayshore Blvd. Continue straight another 1.5 miles to Guadalupe Canyon Pkwy. and turn right. Go 2.2 miles to the park entrance, right, with an entrance kiosk and a self-registration station. Just past the kiosk, turn right, passing the main parking area, and go 0.2 mile to a second parking area, on the south side of Guadalupe Canyon Pkwy.

From Highway 101 southbound in San Francisco, take the Cow Palace/Third St. exit, staying right toward the Cow Palace. At 0.3 mile you reach Bayshore Blvd. and go straight. Go another 1.8 miles to Guadalupe Canyon Pkwy., turn right, and follow the directions above.

**FACILITIES/TRAILHEAD** There are restrooms, picnic tables, phone, and water at the main parking area. There are no facilities at the trailhead, which is on the south side of the second parking area.

Just south of the trailhead is a junction where you veer right on the single-track Summit Loop Trail. After several hundred feet, a trail splits off to the left and heads back to the native-plant garden. Soon you reach a junction where the Summit Loop Trail divides. Here you stay left and climb through a eucalyptus forest.

Eucalyptus trees are not native to California, and these hardy and adaptable trees present a problem for land managers. Logging here in the 1990s removed some of the mountain's eucalyptus trees, but public pressure stopped this effort. Other nonna-

tives in the park include English ivy, German ivy, and cotoneaster.

Despite the presence of nonnatives, the mountain is deservedly famous for its array of native plants, including colorful spring wildflowers, and for its sprawling hillsides of coastal scrub, sometimes called soft chaparral. Toyon, coffeeberry, snowberry, blue elderberry, ceanothus, bush monkeyflower, lizard tail, and Oregon grape are some of the shrubs here.

You pass the Eucalyptus Loop Trail, left, and as you gain elevation, the views of San Francisco, San Francisco Bay, and the East

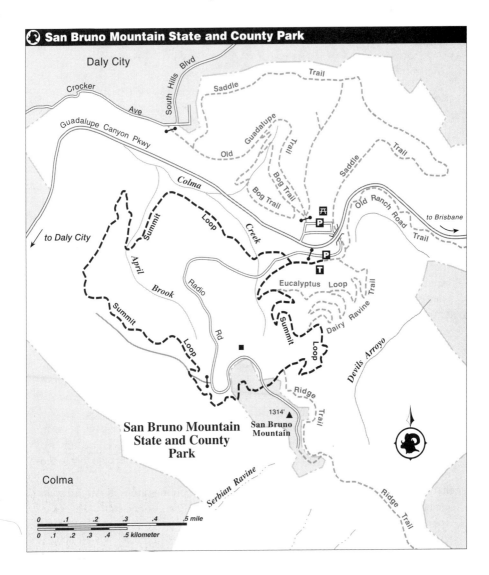

Bay hills become more and more dramatic. Several switchbacks help you climb the ridge that divides Cable and Diary ravines. Where the Dairy Ravine Trail angles left, you follow the Summit Loop Trail as it wraps around a ridge and cuts across a hillside that drops left.

Gaining a ridgetop, you reach a junction. Here the Ridge Trail goes left and dead-ends after another 2.4 miles or so. You continue to the paved road that climbs from the park entrance to just below the moun-

tain's summit. Your route resumes on the other side of the road, just right of a metal gate across a paved driveway. To your right is a concrete-block building. The trail zigzags its way downhill on a gentle grade past communication towers and satellite dishes. A deep canyon is to your left.

Crossing a paved road at about 1.3 miles, you pick up the trail and follow a mostly level course across a hillside of coastal scrub. Notice how the plants grow taller where they are protected from the wind. The extreme

**San Bruno Natives**

- The Mountain is home to more than a dozen rare or endangered plants, including several species of manzanita.
- A native-plant garden near the trailhead, tended by volunteers, grows common coastal plants such as California sagebrush, coast buckwheat, lizard tail, coffeeberry, snowberry, yarrow, and seaside daisy.
- The park also provides habitat for four species of endangered or threatened butterflies — San Bruno elfin, Mission blue, Callippe silverspot, and bay checkerspot.

variability of two common shrubs, coyote brush and coffeeberry, demonstrates this effect. Passing a rest bench, left, the trail rises slightly and then makes a level traverse across the wall of a canyon. This canyon, right, holds April Brook, a tributary of Colma Creek.

Look nearby for broadleaf stonecrop, a succulent with gray-green leaves that clings to rocky outcrops beside the trail. This plant provides food for the larvae of the park's endangered San Bruno elfin butterfly.

You descend along a ridgetop and then follow the trail as it bends sharply right and slices across a hillside. At the bottom of the canyon, the trail crosses April Brook, which flows through a culvert. Now heading downstream, you have the willow-lined brook on your left. Soon your route curves right, climbs on a moderate grade, and then levels. You cross a paved road and then close the loop. Now turn left and retrace your route to the parking area.

Summit Loop Trail on the north side of San Bruno Mountain offers great views of San Francisco.

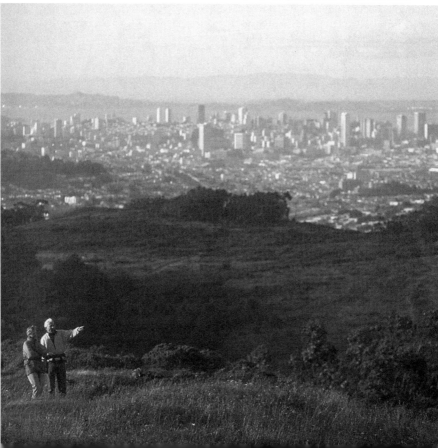

# Appendix 1
# Best Trips

## Geology
Black Diamond Mines Regional Preserve (Chapter 4, Trip 3)
Sibley Volcanic Regional Preserve (Chapter 5, Trip 3)
Almaden Quicksilver County Park (Chapter 7, Trip 9)
Los Trancos Open Space Preserve (Chapter 10, Trip 8)
El Corte de Madera Creek Open Space Preserve: Tafoni Loop (Chapter 10, Trip 15)

## History
Presidio of San Francisco (Chapter 1, Trips 3 & 4)
Angel Island State Park (Chapter 1, Trip 6)
China Camp State Park (Chapter 1, Trip 8)
Olompali State Historic Park (Chapter 1, Trip 15)
Jack London State Historic Park (Chapter 2, Trip 4)
Black Diamond Mines Regional Preserve (Chapter 4, Trip 3)
Almaden Quicksilver County Park (Chapter 7, Trip 9)
Picchetti Ranch Open Space Preserve (Chapter 8, Trip 2)
Fremont Older Open Space Preserve (Chapter 8, Trip 3)
Purisima Creek Redwoods Open Space Preserve (Chapter 9, Trip 6; Chapter 10, Trip 16)
Sweeney Ridge (Chapter 10, Trip 21)

## Peaks
Pine Mountain (Chapter 1, Trip 13)
Mt. Burdell Open Space Preserve (Chapter 1, Trip 14)
Samuel P. Taylor State Park: Barnabe Mountain (Chapter 1, Trip 16)
Pt. Reyes National Seashore: Mt. Wittenberg (Chapter 1, Trip 17)
Sugarloaf Ridge State Park: Bald Mountain (Chapter 2, Trip 2)
Robert Louis Stevenson State Park: Mt. St. Helena (Chapter 3, Trip 1)
Mt. Diablo State Park: Grand Loop (Chapter 4, Trip 7)
Dry Creek Pioneer Regional Park (Chapter 6, Trip 1)
Mission Peak Regional Preserve (Chapter 6, Trip 4)
Russian Ridge Open Space Preserve: Borel Hill (Chapter 10, Trip 6)
Monte Bello Open Space Preserve (Chapter 10, Trip 7)
Windy Hill Open Space Preserve: Spring Ridge (Chapter 10, Trip 10)
Montara Mountain (Chapter 10, Trip 20)
San Bruno Mountain State and County Park (Chapter 10, Trip 22)

## Redwoods
Muir Woods National Monument (Chapter 1, Trips 9 & 10)
Armstrong Redwoods State Reserve/Austin Creek State Recreation Area (Chapter 2, Trip 7)
Redwood Regional Park (Chapter 5, Trip 6)
Butano State Park (Chapter 9, Trip 1)

Portola Redwoods State Park (Chapter 9, Trip 2)
Pescadero Creek Park (Chapter 9, Trip 3)
Sam McDonald Park (Chapter 9, Trip 4)
Memorial Park (Chapter 9, Trip 5)
Purisima Creek Redwoods Open Space Preserve (Chapter 9, Trip 6; Chapter 10, Trip 16)
Wunderlich Park (Chapter 10, Trip 11)
Huddart Park (Chapter 10, Trip 12)
Phleger Estate (Chapter 10, Trip 13)
El Corte de Madera Creek Open Space Preserve (Chapter 10, Trips 14 & 15)

## Waterfalls

Mt. Tamalpais: High Marsh Loop (Chapter 1, Trip 11)
Mt. Diablo State Park: Hidden Falls (Chapter 4, Trip 8)
Uvas Canyon County Park (Chapter 7, Trip 6)

## Wildflowers/Nature Study

Presidio of San Francisco: Ecology Trail (Chapter 1, Trip 3)
Marin Headlands (Chapter 1, Trip 5)
Ring Mountain Open Space Preserve (Chapter 1, Trip 7)
Pine Mountain (Chapter 1, Trip 13)
Mt. Burdell Open Space Preserve (Chapter 1, Trip 14)
Napa River Ecological Reserve (Chapter 3, Trip 3)
Rush Ranch (Chapter 3, Trip 6)
Jepson Prairie Preserve (Chapter 3, Trip 7)
Huckleberry Botanic Regional Preserve (Chapter 5, Trip 4)
Henry W. Coe State Park: Forest Trail (Chapter 7, Trip 4)
Santa Teresa County Park (Chapter 7, Trip 8)
Sierra Azul Open Space Preserve: Woods Trail (Chapter 7, Trip 10)
Fremont Older Open Space Preserve (Chapter 8, Trip 3)
South Skyline Region (Chapter 10, Trip 3)
Skyline Ridge Open Space Preserve (Chapter 10, Trip 4)
Russian Ridge Open Space Preserve (Chapter 10, Trips 5 & 6)
Monte Bello Open Space Preserve (Chapter 10, Trip 7)
Edgewood Park and Preserve (Chapter 10, Trip 17)
San Bruno Mountain State and County Park (Chapter 10, Trip 22)

# Appendix 2
# Recommended Reading

## Bay Area
Heid, Matt, *Camping and Backpacking in the San Francisco Bay Area*. Berkeley: Wilderness Press, 2003.

Lage, Jessica, *Point Reyes*. Berkeley: Wilderness Press, 2004.

Lage, Jessica, *Trail Runner's Guide San Francisco Bay Area*. Berkeley: Wilderness Press, 2003.

Margolin, Malcolm, *The East Bay Out*. Revised ed. Berkeley: Heyday Books, 1988.

Martin, Don, and Kay Martin, *Hiking Marin*. San Anselmo: Martin Press, 1995.

Martin, Don, and Kay Martin, *Mt. Tam*. San Anselmo: Martin Press, 1994.

Martin, Don, and Kay Martin, *Point Reyes National Seashore*. 2nd ed. San Anselmo: Martin Press, 1997.

Rusmore, Jean, *The Bay Area Ridge Trail*. 2nd ed. Berkeley: Wilderness Press, 2002.

Rusmore, Jean, et al, *Peninsula Trails*. 4th ed. Berkeley: Wilderness Press, 2004.

Rusmore, Jean, et al, *South Bay Trails*. 3rd ed. Berkeley: Wilderness Press, 2001.

Spitz, Barry, *Open Spaces*. San Rafael: Marin County Open Space District, 2000.

Spitz, Barry, *Tamalpais Trails*. 4th ed. San Anselmo: Potrero Meadow Publishing Co., 1998.

Stanton, Ken, *Great Day Hikes in & around Napa Valley*. Mendocino: Bored Feet Publications, 1997.

Wayburn, Peggy, *Adventuring in the San Francisco Bay Area*. Revised ed. San Francisco: Sierra Club Books, 1995.

Weintraub, David, *East Bay Trails*. Berkeley: Wilderness Press, 1998.

Weintraub, David, *North Bay Trails*. Berkeley: Wilderness Press, 1999.

Weintraub, David, *Peninsula Tales and Trails*. Los Altos: MROSD, 2004.

Weintraub, David, *Top Trails San Francisco Bay Area*. Berkeley: Wilderness Press, 2004

## History
Lavender, David, *California*. Lincoln: University of Nebraska Press, 1972.

Richards, Rand, *Historic San Francisco*. San Francisco: Heritage House Publishers, 1999.

## Natural History
Alt, David, and Donald W. Hyndman, *Roadside Geology of Northern and Central California*. Missoula: Mountain Press Publishing Company, 2000.

Barbour, Michael, et al, *Coast Redwood*. Los Olivos: Cachuma Press, 2001.

Burt, William H., and Richard P. Grossenheider, *A Field Guide to the Mammals, North America, North of Mexico*. 3rd ed. Boston: Houghton Mifflin Company, 1980.

Clark, Jeanne L., *California Wildlife Viewing Guide*. Helena: Falcon Press, 1992.

Coffeen, Mary, *Central Coast Wildflowers*. San Luis Obispo: EZ Nature Books, 1996.

Faber, Phyllis M., *Common Wetland Plants of Coastal California*. 2nd ed. Mill Valley: Pickleweed Press, 1996.

Faber, Phyllis M., and Robert F. Holland, *Common Riparian Plants of California*. Mill Valley: Pickleweed Press, 1988.

Kozloff, Eugene N., and Linda H. Beidleman, *Plants of the San Francisco Bay Region*. Revised ed. Berkeley: University of California Press, 2003.

Lanner, Ronald M., *Conifers of California*. Los Olivos: Cachuma Press, 1999.

Little, Elbert L., *National Audubon Society Field Guide to North American Trees, Western Region*. New York: Alfred A. Knopf, 1994.

Lyons, Kathleen, and Mary Beth Cooney-Lazaneo, *Plants of the Coast Redwood Region*. Boulder Creek: Looking Press, 1988.

National Geographic Society, *Field Guide to the Birds of North America*. 3rd ed. Washington, D.C.: National Geographic Society, 1999.

Niehaus, Theodore F., and Charles L. Ripper, *A Field Guide to Pacific States Wildflowers*. Boston: Houghton Mifflin Company, 1976.

Pavlik, Bruce M., et al., *Oaks of California*. Los Olivos: Cachuma Press, 1991.

Peterson, Roger T., *A Field Guide to Western Birds*. 3rd ed. Boston: Houghton Mifflin Company, 1990.

Schoenherr, Allan A., *A Natural History of California*. Berkeley: University of California Press, 1992.

Sibley, David Allen, *The Sibley Guide to Birds*. New York: Alfred A. Knopf, Inc., 2000.

Stebbins, Robert C., *A Field Guide to Western Reptiles and Amphibians*. 2nd ed. Boston: Houghton Mifflin Company, 1985.

Stuart, John D., and John O. Sawyer, *Trees and Shrubs of California*. Berkeley: University of California Press, 2001.

## Place Names

Durham, David L., *Place-Names of the San Francisco Bay Area*. Clovis: Word Dancer Press, 2000.

Gudde, Erwin G., *California Place Names*. 4th ed. Berkeley: University of California Press, 1998.

Marinacci, Barbara and Rudy Marinacci, *California's Spanish Place-Names*. 2nd ed. Houston: Gulf Publishing Company, 1997.

# Appendix 3
# Agencies and Information Sources

## Parks and Agencies

California Dept. of Fish & Game (CDF&G)
                Main     (916) 445-0411    www.dfg.ca.gov

California State Parks (CSP)
                Main     (800) 777-0369
     Reservations     (800) 444-7275    http://parks.ca.gov

East Bay Regional Park District (EBRPD)
      Information     (510) 562-7275    www.ebparks.org
  Oakland Reservations     (510) 562-2267
  Hayward Reservations     (510) 538-6470
    Contra Costa County
     Reservations     (925) 676-0192
 Livermore Reservations     (925) 373-0144

Golden Gate National Recreation Area (GGNRA)
                Main     (415) 561-4700    www.nps.gov/goga

Marin County Open Space District (MCOSD)
                Main     (415) 499-6387    www.marinopenspace.org

Marin Municipal Water District (MMWD)
  Sky Oaks Ranger Station     (415) 945-1181    www.marinwater.org
                                              /resourcemanagement.html#recreation

Midpeninsula Regional Open Space District (MROSD)
                Main     (650) 691-1200    www.openspace.org

Palo Alto Dept. of Community Services (PADCS)
                Main     (650) 463-4952    www.city.palo-alto.ca.us/ross

Point Reyes National Seashore
                Main     (415) 464-5100    www.nps.gov/pore

San Mateo County Parks & Recreation (SMCP&R)
      Information     (650) 363-4020    www.eparks.net
     Reservations     (650) 363-4021

Santa Clara County Parks & Recreation (SCCP&R)
      Information     (408) 355-2200    www.parkhere.org
     Reservations     (408) 355-2201    www.gooutsideandplay.org

Skyline Park Citizens Association (SPCA)
                Main     (707) 252-0481    www.skylinepark.org

Walnut Creek Open Space & Trails Division (WCOSTD)
                Main     (925) 943-5860    www.ci.walnut-creek.ca.us/openspace

## Internet Resources

Angel Island State Park
  Ferry from Oakland/Alameda . . . . . . . . . . . . . . . .www.eastbayferry.com
  Ferry from San Francisco . . . . . . . . . . . . . . . . . . . .www.blueandgoldfleet.com
  Ferry from Tiburon . . . . . . . . . . . . . . . . . . . . . . . . .www.angelislandferry.com

Bay Area Hiker  . . . . . . . . . . . . . . . . . . . . . . . . . . . . .www.bahiker.com

Bay Area Open Space Council  . . . . . . . . . . . . . . . . .www.openspacecouncil.org

Bay Area Ridge Trail Council  . . . . . . . . . . . . . . . . . .www.ridgetrail.org

Bay Nature magazine  . . . . . . . . . . . . . . . . . . . . . . . .www.baynature.com

California Native Plant Society  . . . . . . . . . . . . . . . .www.cnps.org

Committee for Green Foothills  . . . . . . . . . . . . . . . .www.greenfoothills.org

Friends of Edgewood Natural Preserve   . . . . . . . . .www.friendsofedgewood.org
                                                  /edgewood.htm

Friends of Recreation & Parks (San Francisco)  . . . .www.frp.org

Golden Gate National Parks Conservancy
  (GGNPC) . . . . . . . . . . . . . . . . . . . . . . . . . . . . . . .www.parksconservancy.org

Greenbelt Alliance . . . . . . . . . . . . . . . . . . . . . . . . . .www.greenbelt.org

Marin Trails . . . . . . . . . . . . . . . . . . . . . . . . . . . . . . .www.marintrails.com

Mount Diablo Interpretive Association  . . . . . . . . . .www.mdia.org

Mt. Tamalpais Interpretive Association  . . . . . . . . . .www.mttam.net

National Audubon Society . . . . . . . . . . . . . . . . . . . .www.audubon.org
  Golden Gate (San Francisco, East Bay) . . . . . . . . .www.goldengateaudubon.org
  Madrone (Sonoma County) . . . . . . . . . . . . . . . . . .www.audubon.sonoma.net
  Marin County . . . . . . . . . . . . . . . . . . . . . . . . . . . .www.marinaudubon.org
  Mt. Diablo area . . . . . . . . . . . . . . . . . . . . . . . . . . .www.diabloaudubon.com
  Napa and Solano counties . . . . . . . . . . . . . . . . . . .www.napasolanoaudubon.org
  Santa Clara Valley . . . . . . . . . . . . . . . . . . . . . . . . .www.scvas.org
  Sequoia (Peninsula) . . . . . . . . . . . . . . . . . . . . . . . .www.sequoia-audubon.org

National Geographic Maps/TOPO!  . . . . . . . . . . . . .http://maps.nationalgeographic
                                                  .com/topo

Natural Resources DataBase  . . . . . . . . . . . . . . . . . .www.nrdb.org

Pease Press . . . . . . . . . . . . . . . . . . . . . . . . . . . . . . . .www.peasepress.com

Peninsula Access for Dogs  . . . . . . . . . . . . . . . . . . . .www.prusik.com/pads

Peninsula Open Space Trust  . . . . . . . . . . . . . . . . . . .www.openspacetrust.org

Point Reyes Bird Observatory  . . . . . . . . . . . . . . . . .www.prbo.org

Responsible Organized Mountain Pedalers  . . . . . . .www.romp.org

Rush Ranch Educational Council  . . . . . . . . . . . . . . .www.rushranch.org

Save Mount Diablo . . . . . . . . . . . . . . . . . . . . . . . . . .www.savemountdiablo.org

Sempervirens Fund . . . . . . . . . . . . . . . . . . . . . . . . . .www.sempervirens.org

Sierra Club
  Loma Prieta (Silicon Valley) . . . . . . . . . . . . . . . . . .www.lomaprieta.sierraclub.org
  Redwood (North Bay) . . . . . . . . . . . . . . . . . . . . . .www.redwood.sierraclub.org
  San Francisco Bay www.sierraclub.org . . . . . . . . . .www.sanfranciscobay.sierraclub.org

Solano Land Trust (SLT) . . . . . . . . . . . . . . . . . . . .www.solanolandtrust.org

Sonoma County Trails Council . . . . . . . . . . . . . . .www.sonomatrails.org/sctc
  Coalition for the Outdoor Recreation Plan . . . . . .www.sonomatrails.org

Strybing Arboretum and Botanical Gardens . . . . . .www.strybing.org

Tamalpais Conservation Club . . . . . . . . . . . . . . . .www.tamalpais.org

Trail Center . . . . . . . . . . . . . . . . . . . . . . . . . . . . . .www.trailcenter.org

University of California Natural Reserve
System (UCNRS) . . . . . . . . . . . . . . . . . . . . . . . . . .http://nrs.ucop.edu/

Weather
  National Weather Service . . . . . . . . . . . . . . . . . . .www.nws.noaa.gov
  Weather.com . . . . . . . . . . . . . . . . . . . . . . . . . . . .www.weather.com

Whole Access (to increase recreational
opportunities for people with disabilities) . . . . . . . .www.wholeaccess.org

Wilderness Press . . . . . . . . . . . . . . . . . . . . . . . . . .www.wildernesspress.com

## Maps

It would be nice if high-quality maps existed for each park covered by this guide, but that is not the case. The maps used to navigate the trails varied from topographic ones that were professionally drawn to sketch maps lacking contour lines and other features. In a few cases, no maps were available. When you visit a park that has a staffed entrance kiosk or visitor center, check there for a map. Sometimes maps and trail guides will be found in dispensers near the trailhead. Not surprisingly, bigger, more well-known parks have the best maps. Check the website of the agency administering the park or open space you plan to visit to see if downloadable maps are available.

As an alternative, you can print your own customized maps using TOPO!, a computer program from National Geographic Maps, *http://maps.nationalgeographic.com/topo*. TOPO! uses USGS maps on CD-ROM combined with software that allows you to draw routes, insert text, meas-ure distance, plot elevation gain and loss, and locate landmarks. There is an interface that allows a GPS unit to transfer data to and from your computer. This allows you to load waypoints from a map into your GPS, so you can find them in the field, and also to take waypoints stored in your GPS during a hike and plot them on a map.

Getting to the trailhead requires some navigation too. The California State Automobile Association (CSAA) gives its members free road maps. Most useful for the routes in this book are *San Francisco Bay* and *Monterey Bay*, in the California Regional Series. The Thomas Guide's *Metropolitan Bay Area Street Guide and Directory* is helpful for driving around the Bay Area.

### NORTH BAY

The best map for Mt. Tamalpais, the Marin Headlands, and Muir Woods is the Olmsted *Trails of Mt. Tamalpais the Marin Headlands*, available at REI stores. *Pt. Reyes National Seashore and Surrounding Area,* a recreation map, is available from Wilderness

Press. A Point Reyes National Seashore trail map is available at the visitor center. Maps for California state parks are problematic—sometimes they are available only at entrance kiosks or visitor centers, and these may be closed during the week. Marin County Open Space District has maps available by mail and from its website. Lands of the Marin Municipal Water District are covered by Olmsted's *Mt. Tamalpais* map. The *Skyline Wilderness Park* map is available at the entrance kiosk and from the Skyline Park Citizens Association website. *Trails of Northeast Marin County,* from Pease Press, shows China Camp and Mt. Burdell Open Space Preserve.

### EAST BAY

A trail map of Mt. Diablo State Park is available at the park's visitor centers and from the Mt. Diablo Interpretive Association. The East Bay Regional Park District has maps available at its trailheads, by mail, and from its website. There are two Olmsted maps for the East Bay, northern and central sections, available at REI stores.

### SOUTH BAY

Henry W. Coe State Park has a map available for sale at the visitor center. Santa Clara County Parks has maps at its trailheads and downloadable maps on its website; these are also available by mail. Midpeninsula Regional Open Space District maps are available at its trailheads, by mail, and from its website.

### PENINSULA

Maps for the Presidio of San Francisco are available at the Presidio's visitor centers and from the Golden Gate National Recreation Area's website. Trail maps for the central and southern Peninsula, produced by the Trail Center, are available from Wilderness Press and REI. Pease Press publishes *Trails of the Coastside and Northern Peninsula,* showing San Bruno and Montara mountains. Midpeninsula Regional Open Space District maps are available at its trailheads, by mail, and from its website. San Mateo County Parks has maps available at trailheads, by mail, and on its website.

# Index

# About the Author

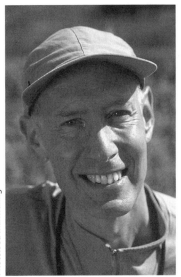

David Weintraub is a writer, editor, and photographer based in South Carolina and Cape Cod. A former long-time San Francisco resident, he has authored a number of books for Wilderness Press, including *East Bay Trails, North Bay Trails, Monterey Bay Trails, Adventure Kayaking: Cape Cod and Martha's Vineyard*, and *Top Trails San Francisco Bay Area*, a guide to the best hiking routes in the North Bay, East Bay, South Bay, and Peninsula.